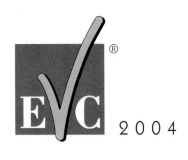

2004

HYBRID VASCULAR PROCEDURES

Blackwell Publishing, Inc., 350 Main Street, Malden, Massachusetts 02148-5018, USA
Blackwell Publishing Ltd, 9600 Garsington Road, Oxford OX4 2DQ, UK
Blackwell Publishing Asia Pty Ltd, 550 Swanston Street, Carlton, Victoria 3053, Australia

04 05 06 07 5 4 3 2 1

ISBN: 1-4051-2489-X

Library of Congress Cataloging-in-Publication Data

EVC 2004 (2004 : Amsterdam, Netherlands)
    EVC 2004 : hybrid vascular procedures / edited by Alain Branchereau & Michael Jacobs.
        p. ; cm. -- (European vascular course ; EVC 2004)
Includes bibliographical references and index.
    ISBN 1-4051-2489-X (hardcover : alk. paper)
1. Blood-vessels--Surgery--Congresses. 2. Laparoscopy--Congresses. 3. Robotics in medicine--Congresses. 4. Virtual reality in medicine--Congresses.

    [DNLM: 1. Vascular Surgical Procedures--Congresses. 2. Laparoscopy--Congresses. 3. Robotics--Congresses. 4. Video-Assisted Surgery--Congresses. WG 170 E918 2004]
I. Title: Hybrid vascular procedures. II. Branchereau, Alain, MD . III. Jacobs, Michael, MD.
IV. Title. V. Series.

    RD598.5.E93 2004
    617.4'13--dc22
                                        2004002000

A catalogue record for this title is available from the British Library

Acquisitions: Jacques Strauss
Production: Joanna Bellhouse
Typesetter: Odim, in France

For further information on Blackwell Publishing, visit our websites:
www.blackwellfutura.com
www.blackwellpublishing.com

Notice: The indications and dosages of all drugs in this book have been recommended in the medical literature and conform to the practices of the general community. The medications described do not necessarily have specific approval by the Food and Drug Administration for use in the diseases and dosages for which they are recommended. The package insert for each drug should be consulted for use and dosage as approved by the FDA. Because standards for usage change, it is advisable to keep abreast of revised recommendations, particularly those concerning new drugs.

HYBRID VASCULAR PROCEDURES

Edited by

ALAIN BRANCHEREAU, MD

University Hospital, Marseille, France

&

MICHAEL JACOBS, MD

University Hospital, Maastricht, The Netherlands

LIST OF CONTRIBUTORS

Karim AISSI
Service de Chirurgie Vasculaire
Centre Hospitalier Universitaire Nord
Chemin des Bourrelly
13915 Marseille Cedex 20, France

Yves ALIMI
Service de Chirurgie Vasculaire
Centre Hospitalier Universitaire Nord
Chemin des Bourrelly
13915 Marseille Cedex 20, France

Eric ALLAIRE
Département de Chirurgie Vasculaire et Imagerie
Hôpital Henri Mondor, Université Paris XII
94000 Creteil, France

Jens-Rainer ALLENBERG
Bereich für Gefässchirurgie
Chirurgische Universitätsklinik Heidelberg
Im Neuenheimer Feld 110
D-69120 Heidelberg, Germany

Bruno AUBLET-CUVELLIER
Hôpital Gabriel Montpied
Centre Hospitalier Universitaire
63003 Clermont-Ferrand Cedex 1, France

Amine BAHNINI
Groupe Hospitalier Pitié-Salpêtrière
47-83, boulevard de l'Hôpital
75651 Paris Cedex 13, France

Xavier BARRAL
Service de Chirurgie Cardiovasculaire
Centre Hospitalier Universitaire Nord
Avenue Albert Raimond
42055 Saint-Etienne Cedex 2, France

Pierre BARTHÉLEMY,
Service de Chirurgie Vasculaire
Centre Hospitalier Universitaire Nord
Chemin des Bourrelly
13915 Marseille Cedex 20, France

Jean-Pierre BECQUEMIN
Département de Chirurgie Vasculaire et Imagerie
Hôpital Henri Mondor, Université Paris XII
94000 Creteil, France

Rachel BELL
Department of General and Vascular Surgery
Guy's & St. Thomas' Hospital
Lambeth Palace Road
London SE1 7EH, United Kingdom

Albert-Claude BENHAMOU
Groupe Hospitalier Pitié-Salpêtrière
47-83, boulevard de l'Hôpital
75651 Paris Cedex 13, France

Luca BERTOGLIO
Chirurgia Vascolare
IRCCS H. San Raffaele, Via Olgettina, 60
20132 Milano, Italy

Sylvain BEURTHERET
Faculté de Médecine de Marseille
Université de la Méditerranée, Assistance Publique
Hôpitaux de Marseille, Hôpital de la Timone
Service de Chirurgie Vasculaire
264, rue Saint-Pierre
13385 Marseille Cedex 05, France

Jan BLANKENSTEIJN
410 Department of Surgery
Radboud University Nijmegen Medical Center
PO Box 9101
6500 HB Nijmegen, The Netherlands

Mourad BOUFI
Service de Chirurgie Vasculaire
Centre Hospitalier Universitaire Nord
Chemin des Bourrelly
13915 Marseille Cedex 20, France

Didier BOURRA
Service de Chirurgie Cardiovasculaire
Centre Hospitalier Universitaire Nord
Avenue Albert Raimond
42055 Saint-Etienne Cedex 2, France

Alain BRANCHEREAU
Faculté de Médecine de Marseille
Université de la Méditerranée, Assistance Publique
Hôpitaux de Marseille, Hôpital de la Timone
Service de Chirurgie Vasculaire
264, rue Saint-Pierre
13385 Marseille Cedex 05, France

Ivo BROEDERS
Department of Surgery
University Medical Center Utrecht, Postbus 85500
3508 GA Utrecht, The Netherlands

Giovanni de CARIDI,
Service de Chirurgie Vasculaire
Centre Hospitalier Universitaire Nord
Chemin des Bourrelly
13915 Marseille Cedex 20, France

Gustavo CASERTA
Instituto Cardiovascular, Hospital Clínic
Universidad de Barcelona, Villarroel 170
08036 Barcelona, Spain

Manuel CASTELLÁ
Instituto Cardiovascular, Hospital Clínic
Universidad de Barcelona, Villarroel 170
08036 Barcelona, Spain

Jean-Michel CHEVALIER
Service de Chirurgie Vasculaire
Hôpital Edouard Herriot, Place d'Arsonval
69008 Lyon, France

Laurent CHICHE
Groupe Hospitalier Pitié-Salpêtrière
47-83, boulevard de l'Hôpital
75651 Paris Cedex 13, France

Roberto CHIESA
Chirurgia Vascolare
IRCCS H. San Raffaele, Via Olgettina, 60
20132 Milano, Italy

Efrem CIVILINI
Chirurgia Vascolare
IRCCS H. San Raffaele, Via Olgettina, 60
20132 Milano, Italy

Albert CLARÁ
Sevei de Cirurgia Vascular
Hospital del Mar, Paseo Maritimo 25-29
08003 Barcelona, Spain

Martin CLARK
Department of Radiology
St Mary's Hospital, Praed Street
London W2 1NY, United Kingdom

Philippe CLUZEL
Groupe Hospitalier Pitié-Salpêtrière
47-83, boulevard de l'Hôpital
75651 Paris Cedex 13, France

Mark COWLING
Department of Radiology
St Mary's Hospital, Praed Street
London W2 1NY, United Kingdom

Miguel CUESTA
Department of Surgery
Vrije Universiteit Medical Center, PO Box 7057
1007 MB Amsterdam, The Netherlands

Pascal DESGRANGES
Département de Chirurgie Vasculaire et Imagerie
Hôpital Henri Mondor, Université Paris XII
94000 Creteil, France

Laurence DESTRIEUX-GARNIER
Département de Chirurgie Vasculaire et Imagerie
Hôpital Henri Mondor, Université Paris XII
94000 Creteil, France

Hans-Henning ECKSTEIN
Bereich für Gefässchirurgie
Klinikum rechts der Isar, Ismaninger Straße 22
D-81675 München, Germany

John EDOGA
95 Madison Avenue, Suite 103
07960 Morristown, New Jersey, USA

Jean-Pierre FAVRE
Service de Chirurgie Cardiovasculaire
Centre Hospitalier Universitaire Nord
Avenue Albert Raimond
42055 Saint-Etienne Cedex 2, France

Patrick FEUGIER
Service de Chirurgie Vasculaire
Hôpital Edouard Herriot, Place d'Arsonval
69008 Lyon, France

Natalia de la FUENTE
Sevei de Cirurgia Vascular
Hospital del Mar, Paseo Maritimo 25-29
08003 Barcelona, Spain

Cesar GARCÍA-MADRID
Instituto Cardiovascular, Hospital Clínic
Universidad de Barcelona, Villarroel 170
08036 Barcelona, Spain

Carlos GRACIA
Department of Surgery
UCLA Center for the Health Sciences
Los Angeles, California, USA

Rolf GÜNTHER
Bereich für Röntgendiagnosis
Universitätsklinik, Pauwelsstrasse 30
D - 52057 Aachen, Germany

Patrick HAAGE
Bereich für Röntgendiagnosis
Universitätsklinik, Pauwelsstrasse 30
D - 52057 Aachen, Germany

Michiel de HAAN,
Department of Radiology
University Hospital Maastricht, PO Box 5800
6202 AZ Maastricht, The Netherlands

Werner HACKE
Bereich für Neurologie
Ruprecht Karls University Heidelberg
Neurologische Universitätsklinik
Im Neuenheimer Feld 400
D-69120 Heidelberg, Germany

Olivier HARTUNG
Service de Chirurgie Vasculaire
Centre Hospitalier Universitaire Nord
Chemin des Bourrelly
13915 Marseille Cedex 20, France

Mathieu HERMIER
Hôpital Gabriel Montpied
Centre Hospitalier Universitaire
63003 Clermont-Ferrand Cedex 1, France

Gwan HO
Department of Vascular Surgery
Amphia Hospital Breda, Langedijk 75
4819 EV Breda, The Netherlands

Chantal van der HORST
Amsterdam Medical Center
Center Plastic Surgery G4/224
PO Box 22700
1007 MB Amsterdam, The Netherlands

Krassi IVANCEV
Department of Radiology, Endovascular Center
Malmö University Hospital
S-205 02 Malmö, Sweden

Michael JACOBS
Department of Surgery
University Hospital Maastricht, PO Box 5800
6202 AZ Maastricht, The Netherlands

Miguel JOSA
Instituto Cardiovascular, Hospital Clínic
Universidad de Barcelona, Villarroel 170
08036 Barcelona, Spain

Milla KALLIO
Department of Vascular Surgery
Helsinki University Central Hospital
P O Box 340
00029 HUS, Finland

Edouard KIEFFER
Groupe Hospitalier Pitié-Salpêtrière
47-83, boulevard de l'Hôpital
75651 Paris Cedex 13, France

Hischam KOBEITER
Département de Chirurgie Vasculaire et Imagerie
Hôpital Henri Mondor, Université Paris XII
94000 Creteil, France

Ralf KOLVENBACH
Bereich für Gefässchirurgie und Phlebologie
Augusta Hospital, Amalien Strasse 9
40472 Düsseldorf, Germany

Fabien KOSKAS
Groupe Hospitalier Pitié-Salpêtrière
47-83, boulevard de l'Hôpital
75651 Paris Cedex 13, France

Koen van LANDUYT
Department of Reconstructive Surgery
University Hospital, De Pintelaan 185
9000 Gent, Belgium

Bengt LINDBLAD
Department of Vascular Diseases
Malmö University Hospital
S-205 02 Malmö, Sweden

Denis LYONNET
Service de Radiologie Vasculaire et Urologique
Hôpital Edouard Herriot, Place d'Arsonval
69008 Lyon, France

Serguei MALIKOV
Faculté de Médecine de Marseille
Université de la Méditerranée, Assistance Publique
Hôpitaux de Marseille, Hôpital de la Timone
Service de Chirurgie Vasculaire
264, rue Saint-Pierre
13385 Marseille Cedex 05, France

Martin MALINA
Department of Vascular Diseases
Malmö University Hospital
S-205 02 Malmö, Sweden

Mariangela de MASI,
Service de Chirurgie Cardiovasculaire
Centre Hospitalier Universitaire Nord
Avenue Albert Raimond
42055 Saint-Etienne Cedex 2, France

Germano MELISSANO
Chirurgia Vascolare
IRCCS H. San Raffaele, Via Olgettina, 60
20132 Milano, Italy

Volker MICKLEY
Bereich für Gefässchirurgie
Stadtklinik Baden-Baden, Balger Strasse 50
D-76532 Baden-Baden, Germany

Frans MOLL
Department of Vascular Surgery
University Medical Centre Utrecht
Heidelberglaan 100
3584 CX Utrecht, The Netherlands

Issifou MOUMOUNI
Hôpital Gabriel Montpied
Centre Hospitalier Universitaire
63003 Clermont-Ferrand Cedex 1, France

Jaume MULET
Instituto Cardiovascular, Hospital Clínic
Universidad de Barcelona, Villarroel 170
08036 Barcelona, Spain

Andres OTERO
Service de Chirurgie Vasculaire
Centre Hospitalier Universitaire Nord
Chemin des Bourrelly
13915 Marseille Cedex 20, France

Mathieu POIRIER
Hôpital Gabriel Montpied
Centre Hospitalier Universitaire
63003 Clermont-Ferrand Cedex 1, France

Samy POUGET
Hôpital Gabriel Montpied
Centre Hospitalier Universitaire
63003 Clermont-Ferrand Cedex 1, France

Jan RAUWERDA
Department of Surgery
Vrije Universiteit Medical Center, PO Box 7057
1007 MB Amsterdam, The Netherlands

Vicente RIAMBAU
Instituto Cardiovascular, Hospital Clínic
Universidad de Barcelona, Villarroel 170
08036 Barcelona, Spain

Peter ROBLESS
Regional Vascular Unit
St Mary's Hospital, Praed Street
London W2 1NY, United Kingdom

Begoña ROMÁN
Faculdad de Filisofía
Universitat Ramon Llull, C/Claravall 1-3
08022 Barcelona, Spain

Eugenio ROSSET
Hôpital Gabriel Montpied
Centre Hospitalier Universitaire
63003 Clermont-Ferrand Cedex 1, France

Olivier ROUVIÈRE
Service de Radiologie Vasculaire et Urologique
Hôpital Edouard Herriot, Place d'Arsonval
69008 Lyon, France

Jelle RUURDA
Department of Surgery
University Medical Center Utrecht, Postbus 85500
3508 GA Utrecht, The Netherlands

Thomas SCHMITZ-RODE
Bereich für Röntgendiagnosis
Universitätsklinik, Pauwelsstrasse 30
D - 52057 Aachen, Germany

Hardy SCHUMACHER
Bereich für Gefässchirurgie
Chirurgische Universitätsklinik Heidelberg
Im Neuenheimer Feld 110
D-69120 Heidelberg, Germany

Geert Willem SCHURINK
Department of Surgery
University Hospital Maastricht, PO Box 5800
6202 AZ Maastricht, The Netherlands

Karl SCHÜRMANN
Bereich für Röntgendiagnosis
Universitätsklinik, Pauwelsstrasse 30
D - 52057 Aachen, Germany

Francesco SETACCI
Chirurgia Vascolare
IRCCS H. San Raffaele, Via Olgettina, 60
20132 Milano, Italy

Luuk SMEETS
Department of Vascular Surgery
University Medical Centre Utrecht
Heidelberglaan 100
3584 CX Utrecht, The Netherlands

Björn SONESSON
Department of Vascular Diseases
Malmö University Hospital
S-205 02 Malmö, Sweden

Peter TAYLOR
Department of General and Vascular Surgery
Guy's & St. Thomas' Hospital
Lambeth Palace Road
London SE1 7EH, United Kingdom

Yamume TSHOMBA
Chirurgia Vascolare
IRCCS H. San Raffaele, Via Olgettina, 60
20132 Milano, Italy

Erkki TUKIAINEN
Department of Plastic Surgery
Helsinki University Central Hospital
P O Box 266
00029 HUS, Finland

Carlos URIARTE
Instituto Cardiovascular, Hospital Clínic
Universidad de Barcelona, Villarroel 170
08036 Barcelona, Spain

Nicolas VALÉRIO
Faculté de Médecine de Marseille
Université de la Méditerranée, Assistance Publique
Hôpitaux de Marseille, Hôpital de la Timone
Service de Chirurgie Vasculaire
264, rue Saint-Pierre
13385 Marseille Cedex 05, France

Frank VERMASSEN
Department of Vascular Surgery
University Hospital, De Pintelaan 185
9000 Gent, Belgium

Francesc VIDAL-BARRAQUER
Sevei de Cirurgia Vascular
Hospital del Mar, Paseo Maritimo 25-29
08003 Barcelona, Spain

Marco VOLA
Service de Chirurgie Cardiovasculaire
Centre Hospitalier Universitaire Nord
Avenue Albert Raimond
42055 Saint-Etienne Cedex 2, France

Joachim WILDBERGER
Bereich für Röntgendiagnosis
Universitätsklinik, Pauwelsstrasse 30
D - 52057 Aachen, Germany

Willem WISSELINK
Department of Surgery
Vrije Universiteit Medical Center, PO Box 7057
1007 MB Amsterdam, The Netherlands

John WOLFE
Regional Vascular Unit
St Mary's Hospital, Praed Street
London W2 1NY, United Kingdom

X

PREFACE

The management of vascular diseases has rapidly evolved into a hybrid speciality combining both open and endovascular techniques as well as laparoscopic and robotic procedures. This year's European Vascular Course is the first event ever to highlight the concept of hybrid procedures.

This book Hybrid Vascular Procedures has embraced the importance of these new technologies and their integrated application since it will determine the future of vascular surgery.

The first chapter describes the operating room of the future as the new arena in which vascular specialists will work with these advanced and innovative technologies. The next chapter philosophically looks beyond evidence-based surgery and considers hybrid vascular procedures as paradigmatic examples of how the art of practice may flourish in dialogue with science.

Following, combined treatment of supra-aortic trunks and cerebral arteries by means of surgery, angioplasty and thrombolysis are discussed. In the chapters addressing the thoracic aorta, type B dissection and repair of arch, descending and thoraco-abdominal aneurysms are treated by ingenious combinations of surgical and endovascular techniques. Management of abdominal aortic pathology is currently aiming for the least invasive and most optimal technique associated with adequate long-term outcome. Seven chapters describe the available technology, including laparoscopic, robotic-assisted and endovascular modalities as well as their integrated application with open surgery. In arterial disease of the lower limbs, hybrid procedures combine standard bypass surgery with percutaneous recanalization, remote endarterectomy, free vascular flap and assisted thrombectomies. Finally, venous thrombectomy and iliocaval stenting, embolization and surgery for vascular malformations and hybrid solutions in access surgery are discussed.

We would like to thank the authors who are the pioneers in this first book on hybrid vascular procedures. Major effort and editorial assistance was provided by Bertrand Ede and Dirk Ubbink. Blackwell Publishing/Futura and especially Joanna Levine, Gina Almond and Jacques Strauss significantly contributed with editorial support. Marie-France Damia and the ODIM-team have succeeded again in printing the high quality English and French version of the book. We are greatly indebted to our secretaries Annie Barral and Claire Meertens who invested tremendous energy in the preparation of this book. Jean-Pierre Jacomy is, as a medical artist, responsible for the drawings. Iris Papawasiliou is highly appreciated for the organization of the European Vascular Course.

This textbook would not have been possible without the substantial support of the biomedical industry. We are very greatful to our major sponsors for their contribution and confidence in this project.

Maastricht - Marseille, 2004

Michael Jacobs   -   Alain Branchereau

CONTENTS

XIV

1

THE OPERATING ROOM OF THE FUTURE

IVO BROEDERS, MICHAEL JACOBS

The evolution in computer science has generated challenging options for vascular surgeons in an era that focuses strongly on minimally invasive interventions. Vascular surgery is shifting from direct access to image-guided treatment, while craftsmanship is slowly being replaced by advanced technology.

Computer-aided surgery has enabled surgeons to prepare their interventions precisely, and to perform them as planned. Various imaging techniques are being combined to optimize less invasive visualization of the arterial segment of interest. Although feasibility has been demonstrated for computer-aided surgery, clinical application is limited because of the complexity of advanced technology.

Surgeons should be able to concentrate on surgical performance in a plug and play *environment without the annoyance of equipment failure, or difficult and time-consuming instrument handling. The current operating theaters are not equipped to deal with upcoming surgical technology and require extensive adaptation to meet the standards of top-level care.*

In this chapter the authors describe the operating room (OR) of the future that will allow surgeons to work with advanced surgical technology in an efficient and safe manner, with a focus on pre-operative planning, data handling, and the surgeons' working environment.

Pre-operative planning

Image processing of volumetric computed tomography (CT) and magnetic resonance angiography (MRA) datasets have provided the tools to optimize preparation of endovascular procedures. Especially in case of aneurysms, surgeons can exactly define the extent of the disease and the necessity of surgical intervention. In case surgery is warranted, dedicated programs can be applied to select the optimal endograft and to prepare the surgical intervention. One can draw lines through the center of the vessels and explore reconstructions exactly perpendicular to this so-called central lumen line in order to define the exact arterial diameter at any level. Measuring the length of the line reveals the optimal length of the endograft. This allows selection of the optimal size and type of the prosthesis for the individual patient. Three-dimensional (3-D) reconstructions will help the operating team to understand the anatomy of the arterial segment of interest. With this information one can select the optimal access site and anticipate on challenges in endovascular interventions due to complex anatomy.

While these computer programs have already proven to be most supportive, unavailability, user unfriendliness, and the time consuming process of image processing hinder applicability. It takes an experienced image processor with a vascular background about 20 minutes to measure the arterial segment of choice and select the optimal endograft, while 5 more minutes are required to guide the semi-automated process of 3-D reconstruction. The workstations used for image processing are usually located at the department of radiology and, for logistic or political reasons, are not always available. Additionally, it takes time and effort to learn how to handle these programs.

The basic requirement for optimal pre-operative planning is therefore an adequate hospital information system including a digital patient file and an integrated public-access computer system (PACS) of a digital radiology database. The future surgeon can prepare his or her procedures from behind their desk or at home, with all essential patient information available in digital format, and with the programs installed to process CT and MRA datasets. With information available at any time from any computer in the hospital, the threshold to use dedicated software for surgical planning will decline. The motivation to learn how to handle these programs will increase and growing feedback on program optimization will lead to better, faster, and easier planning applications.

The next step is using these applications for emergency surgery. The number of reports on endovascular treatment of ruptured aneurysms is growing and results are at least promising. In an optimal scenario, the surgeon will gather all information required to make a basic choice between an open or an endovascular approach, and to select the most suitable, off the shelf, endograft in case of endovascular treatment. Even in stable patients, the time required for this process should be minimized. Large medical centers that deal frequently with these patients should ideally have a multislice CT scan available at the emergency center. A CT investigation with today's equipment will cause a delay of about 5 minutes. Meanwhile, the surgeon can go to the operating theater and use the OR workstation to analyze and process the images with his or her PACS access. The endograft is selected on the spot while the patient is transported to the OR and prepared for surgery.

The elements for this approach are available, but implementation depends on optimization of the hospital digital network and the willingness to invest both personally and financially in a minimally invasive approach to live threatening disease.

Surgery in the era of information technology

High-tech surgery holds promising options for improvement of care but it also increases the complexity of the preparation and the actual performance of surgical interventions. Surgeons will use a number of digital sources to gather information and prepare the procedure. During surgery, they will have to control delicate equipment from within the sterile field, and they will thrive to store essential visual information. Dealing with digital information is therefore a key issue for the operating theater of the future. One of the biggest challenges is to develop a central computing system that controls all incoming and outgoing digital information. This OR "nerve center" should be accessible for all members of the OR team, and all disciplines should be able to gather and store the information that is essential for part of the procedure (Fig. 1).

When following a patient from first visit to recovery room, the process could ideally go as follows. At the time of the first visit, the surgeon will import the essential data in the digital patient file. If surgery is planned, all essential materials required for the procedure, such as stents, endografts, or specific introducers or guidewires, will be listed on the operation preparation file. In case pre-operative image processing of CT/MRA scans of angiography is performed, the plan will be linked to the patient file. The surgeon can also give directions for logistic issues such as the positioning of equipment relative to the OR table.

At the time of surgery, OR nurses will prepare the digital environment of the operating theater by entering the patient number in the central computer, using a OR workstation positioned in one of the OR walls. They can prepare the procedure based on the information from the operation preparation file. All material used will be stored and linked to the individual procedure with two purposes. First, the OR material stock will be under direct control to allow for a small stock, which nevertheless guarantees availability of all items at any time. Secondly, all costs incurred for the individual patient can be accounted to visualize true expenses of treatment for the hospital and the insurance company. This also includes an exact overview of time spent in the OR with differentiation for preparation, surgery, and convalescence.

The anesthesiologist will use the same system for a variety of purposes. First, the essential patient information such as the pre-operative anesthesiology file, X-rays, and pulmonary or cardiac tests will be readily available from the anesthesiology workstation. This should address the annoyance of missing paperwork or X-ray maps including essential information. The anesthesiology team can prepare the OR set-up according to the surgeon's proposal in the operation preparation file. During surgery, all essential information of vital functions and anesthesia details will be stored and linked to the digital patient file, allowing standardized and thorough documentation. Using picture-in-picture applications, the anesthesiologist can follow the progress of the procedure with images from the OR light camera or projections from the endoscopic view or the fluoroscopy images. This will lead to better communication between surgeon and anesthesiologist, earlier anticipation of complications, and an earlier start of the awakening process.

The surgeon will use the OR workstation to get a final update and check the pre-operative plan. During surgery, he or she will use the central computing system for three purposes. First, all existing information can be used by scrolling through smart selection menus with a sterile mouse, a touch screen with sterile cover, or by voice control. Essential information regarding the procedure itself, such as video sequences of fluoroscopy or endoscopy, or digitally recorded verbal commands, will be stored in a temporary database. The surgeon can also use the central computing system to communicate from the sterile field with the outside world. Pagers can be answered using headsets, and colleagues inside and outside the hospital can be contacted for support. Using the intranet and Internet, anyone with permission can follow the images acquired during surgery to support verbal communication. The same digital network will provide a solid base for teleconferencing and live case transmission.

Finally, the central computing system will allow the surgeon to control basic and dedicated equipment from within the sterile field. This includes OR lights, table position, all equipment used for endoscopic surgery, but also all image acquisition devices and complex systems such as fluoroscopy units, ultrasonography, and navigation tools.

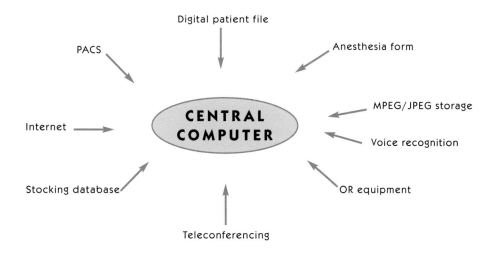

FIG. 1 Dealing with a large number of digital formats is a major challenge for "operating room of the future" programs.

Immediately after the procedure the surgeon will use the OR workstation to select images or verbal comments and link these files to the digital patient file. The procedure report is finalized by using a standardized digital selection sheet or by verbal recording and automated transition in written language.

At the moment of transport to the recovery room, all essential information on the procedure is available to any person with access permission from any computer linked to the intranet or Internet.

THE OPERATING COMPLEX OF THE FUTURE: DEDICATED TECHNOLOGY IN A DEDICATED WORKPLACE

Although the majority of routine procedures are still performed with instruments that strongly resemble those of the early years of surgery, complex technological devices are increasingly integrated in more complex interventions. Surgery follows developments in consumer society and industry with prudence, but appealing new techniques are adapted to improve surgical outcome. Clear examples are lasers, navigation technology, and robot-assisted surgery systems. These demanding devices have been introduced in clinical practice within a logistic environment that is based on a "one theater fits all" concept. Equipment is usually stored away and brought to the theater when needed. This leads to time loss, damage, and inefficient use resulting from logistic inadequacy.

The operating complex of the future will comprise a number of workplaces that are fully dedicated to specific type of surgical technology. These theaters are no longer surgeon dedicated, but are used by a multidisciplinary group of specialists who share the investment in technology that can be applied for a variety of disorders.

Today's examples are theaters with ceiling-mounted fluoroscopy equipment or theaters dedicated to endoscopic surgery. Theaters focusing on laser surgery, navigation technology, and medical robotics will follow in the upcoming years.

The advantages of technology-dedicated theaters are threefold. Most importantly, the room can be adapted to the technology of choice to guarantee optimal logistics, resulting in efficient and safe use. The equipment can be positioned in a fixed set-up, and all supportive equipment that is not directly required in the OR itself will be stored in an outside control room. This will result in a spacious and clean OR with no cables crossing the floor and without unnecessary obstacles blocking the way of the

team and the sterile tables. Wireless anesthesia will also assist in this purpose.

A set-up with a flexible OR table and a ceiling-mounted anesthesia tower will allow optimal positioning of the patient relative to the equipment of choice without compromising the workspace of the anesthesiologist and the OR team. The central computing system can be adapted to the theme of the individual operating theater to optimize equipment control from within the sterile field. Using these basic concepts, one can develop an intervention theater designed for endovascular surgery that combines a logical approach to both surgery and fluoroscopy, with a relatively small and light ceiling-mounted C-arm under the full control of the team at the table.

A logical consequence of technology-dedicated theaters is differentiation of OR staff. Computer-aided surgery is reaching a level of complexity that demands special skills for the surgeon, but also from supportive OR personnel.

OR nurses will start focusing on a limited field of the surgical spectrum, but their education and capacities will increase to the level appropriate for a more demanding surgical environment. Finally, concentrating high care in an OR complex with dedicated theaters will result in more and more efficient workflow and a reduction in total investment in OR equipment.

Technology in the operating room of the future: what can we expect?

Minimally invasive surgery is the key research and development topic in most surgical fields for the upcoming decade. Within this perspective, surgical technology programs will focus on enhancement of visualization and precision while reducing surgical trauma. Next to computer-steered fluoroscopy suites, we can expect integration of 3-D ultrasound and navigation technology to visualize vascular pathology. The basic concept is the goal to use pre-operative 3-D CT and MRI images as a guide for endovascular interventions.

In order to use pre-operative images as a virtual reality roadmap during the actual surgical intervention, one must integrate a navigation system in the OR set-up. A C-arm or ultrasonography probe coupled to the navigation system may serve to link the pre-operative roadmap to the actual procedure. This technology is readily available, but the challenge is to deal with deformation of the arteries during manipulation with guidewires or introducers. For this purpose, 3-D ultrasound will be used to analyze the actual situation and to adapt the high-resolution pre-operative roadmap to the changes in vascular anatomy at the time of surgery. The ultimate goal is to use a high-resolution 3-D imaging device interactively during surgical intervention. MRI would be the ideal technology because of its absence of ionizing radiation, but progress has been slow due to unfavorable patient access during surgery and insufficient speed of image processing, which hinders true interactive surgery. Futuristic concepts for MRI intervention suites explore the options to incorporate the hardware in the OR walls with a concentration of the magnetic field at the OR table to allow optimal access for the surgical team (Fig. 2). With numerous issues to attend to the field of image-guided surgery, and an increasing number of reports on long-term failure of en-

dovascular aneurysm repair, the direct approach to arteries by use of endoscopic techniques is gaining more interest. Robotic surgery systems may prove to play an important role in this field, especially when it comes to endoscopic suturing or delicate handling of automated anastomosis devices. The currently available robotic systems will be vastly improved and miniaturized, with inclusion of force feedback and semi-automated task performance (Fig. 3).

Exciting new technology is within reach, so one should thrive to develop the operating theater of the future that not only demonstrates feasibility of new techniques, but also supports the future surgeon in providing top-level care in a safe, reproducible, and efficient manner.

Surgical robotics

The OR of the future will increasingly be guided by surgical robots performing complex endoscopic

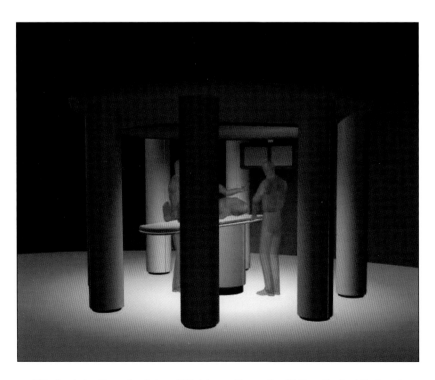

FIG. 2 Animation of a future MRI intervention suite *(Philips Medical Systems)*.

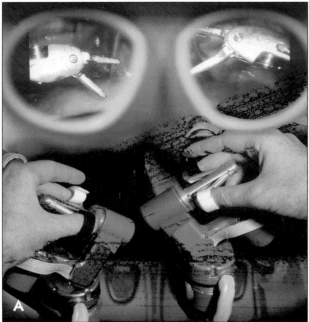

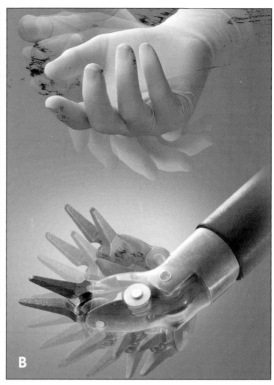

FIG. 3 A - Robotic instruments as seen through the eyes of the console, directed by the hands of the surgeon. B - Freedom of movements: human hand and direct translation to robotic instrument.

procedures by means of telemanipulation systems. The drawbacks of laparoscopic and thoracoscopic techniques include the inverted response at the tip of the instrument, the discrepancy between the small movement outside and major movement inside the patient, limited degrees of freedom, and indirect 2-D vision. The goals of robotic surgery are to apply the advantages of minimally invasive surgery and add direct 3-D vision, to correct the inverted response of instruments, to provide a high level of precision, to neutralize vibrations ("virtual stillness"), and to increase the degrees of freedom. Connection of the robotic arms and camera to the surgical console via digital highways offers the already existing option of telesurgery. With the surgeon in any geographical location and assistance from centers of expertise, education and training can be performed via connected systems. The previously described pre-operative CT and MRI computer data transition into a virtual reality setting will allow for image-guided robotic interventions. Connecting this virtual reality dataset to on-line, intra-operative assessment will navigate the robot to perform procedures with high precision.

Transition from the current OR to the OR of the future

During the last decades, the uniform format of construction of the OR department consisted of identical operating rooms with multifunctional OR tables. Standard equipment such as anesthesia instruments is an integral part of the room, whereas additional equipment like microscopes, heart-lung machine, fluoroscopy, endoscopy tower, laser, etc. is stored elsewhere. The continuous emerging technologies have created chaos with cables, tools, towers, and storage- and space-consuming machines. Obviously, these traditional rooms had the main advantage that they were usable for many surgical specialties.

The OR of the future will combine uniformity and selective furnishing based on the type of specialty and type of intervention. The "umbrella" construction principle will contain all elements of side equipment like the robot, imaging, and data acquisition instruments. Specific elements, such as the surgical robot, are connected as a module to the central "cockpit".

The pilot of this cockpit is the surgeon, controlling the working environment and surgical field. The surgeon regulates all side equipment and is connected on-line with the surgical planning laboratory (pre-operative data) and continuously connected with on-line acquisition systems. Control of the surgical environment can be either through manual control (joysticks, touchscreens, remote), voice control, or eyeball position tracking.

Operating room of the future: contemplation

The OR of the future should be considered as a concept. Many technical and innovative techniques will determine the architecture of the OR of the future, which is therefore not limited to one standard format. In any case, the goals of the OR of the future should be to allow efficient and functional surgery and to offer advanced and safe treatment with a better result for the patient. Many side studies must be performed as well, including cost-benefit analyses and assessment of quality of life.

2

BEYOND EVIDENCE-BASED SURGERY: THE CASE FOR HYBRID AND UNUSUAL VASCULAR PROCEDURES

ALBERT CLARÁ, BEGOÑA ROMÁN
NATALIA DE LA FUENTE, FRANCESC VIDAL-BARRAQUER

Hybrid vascular procedures (HVPs) are combinations of different technologies by which experienced and skilled vascular surgeons try to provide suited-to-case therapeutic solutions for complex vascular problems. HVPs emerge as a response to the potential complexity of individual cases and are paradigmatic examples of how medicine is primarily perceived by the particular (the patient) and secondly interested in the general (the knowledge). This simple but significant issue allows for the differentiation of medicine, and thus surgery, from pure and applied sciences. The frequent oblivion of this primary scope may make surgeons feel uncomfortable when facing the possibility of performing one of these infrequently generalizable procedures, like HVPs used to be, within the present climate of scientific evidence myth. Obviously, the low frequency, special idiosyncrasy, and variability of many HVPs make them unlikely aims of the critical look of evidence-based medicine (EBM). However, this fact, rather than a limitation, is a good example of the uniqueness of our profession, which is destined to join, without pre-established hierarchies, hard evidence, practical wisdom, skillfulness, system and professional features, and patient values and preferences, to provide an adequate therapy for particular patients. Underlying many HVPs, there is a sincere epistemological effort for combining rational-based evidence with the reasonable-based practical wisdom. This approach, at the very end, is the basis by which reflective surgeons *have long been able to decide every day with every patient in the everlasting conditions of uncertainty.*

Are hybrid vascular procedures problematic or is the problem just in our minds?

We live in an era where evidence-based hard data and their interpretation are not only considered a valid basis for therapeutic decisions, but claim to be the most valid or even the almost unique basis on which individual patients should be treated. Any physician's attempt to make different therapeutic decisions for individual patients on the basis of physiological, pathological, or anatomical characteristics, or taking in consideration the concurrence of other diseases or treatments, is frequently discouraged and may even become prohibited in some institutions or other "guideline"-based clinical settings [1].

In this context, it may be not surprising that the majority of HVPs, as many other suited-to-case treatments, are considered exceptional, non-generalizable, non-validated, unproven, and perhaps avoidable procedures within the adversarial climate created by EBM. HVPs represent a "callous" for the current conception of medicine as an applied science: they can be neither easily absorbed because of their usual infrequent practice, special idiosyncrasy, and variability, nor avoided because they emerge directly from the core of surgical practice. HVPs are paradigmatic examples of how medicine is primarily perceived by the particular (the patient) and secondly interested in the general (the knowledge). This simple but significant issue differentiates medicine, and thus surgery, from pure and applied sciences and has enormous consequences in the epistemology and ethics of our profession.

The "fundamental misconception": medicine as an applied science

Since the 19th century, a growing number of physicians have been persistently engaged to gain the admission of our ancient profession in to the realm of scientific disciplines. In our post-modern western society, science has become the myth that represents one of the single existing truths, and medicine could not stay out of its shadow. The consequences of this approach have been spectacular: technical advances farther than anyone could anti-

cipate, an improvement in patient's quality of life, and a sharp increase in life expectancy. In this sense, this conception of medicine as on its way to becoming a science has been useful and therefore considered to be worthy. However, the recognition of medicine as an applied science has also brought conceptual and practical problems, some of which have emerged over the last decades, and others that may arise in the near future.

Though there is not a generally accepted analysis of what makes a discipline or an enterprise a science, pure science, as it is usually understood, tries to acquire knowledge and understanding of the world by establishing general theories and laws based on observations (induction) and/or mathematical deduction. Its scope is the truth. Particular cases are only important for the internal development or the confirmation of theories. Applied science, on the other hand, aims to obtain knowledge about things of importance to the interests of humans. Here the scope appears to be the usefulness. The question of truth or falsity of theories is not of such vital importance. Once more, particular cases are only important for the verification of the usefulness of the technological development, technology being the application of applied science.

As opposite to sciences (concerned with the general), medicine, as it has been anciently understood, is concerned with the particular case. Clinical practice brings the generalized body of knowledge (pure and applied science) together with other epistemic issues frequently enrolled in the art of practice, to bear benefit for an individual. Medicine may be partially indistinguishable from science in its research activities and contributions to knowledge, but the use of "scientific methods" themself does not make an activity a science. Medicine is beyond its cognitive content. While the aim of scientists is the epistemic one of theoretical or applied knowledge, the aim of physicians is to promote the health of their patients. Therefore, the patient becomes the primary concern of the physician and any search for the truth, the usefulness, or the efficaciousness constitutes an honorable scope for future patients but a systematically secondary consideration. Medicine as an activity is an inappropriate subject for reduction as opposite to biology or any other science [2]. Medicine approaches science not because its scope has to become a scientific discipline but for its practical purposes insofar as sciences currently provide the basis for a successful practical action in achieving its unique aim: the welfare of particular patients.

Consequences of the "fundamental misconception"

THE DISEASE AS A POTENTIALLY KNOWLEDGEABLE AND THUS CONTROLLABLE ENTITY

The consideration of medicine as an applied science has brought the legitimate but probable positivist utopia by which diseases will become completely understood, and thus controlled, by scientific methods. This conviction is based upon the assumption that diseases can be reduced to somewhat complex equations, and is rooted in the 19th century medicine. In this sense, Rudolf Virchow, the famous German physician and scientist, stated: *"If biology were completed, if we would comprehend exactly the laws of life and the conditions of its manifestation, if we would know with certainty all the consequences of each and every change in these conditions, then we would have obtained a rational therapy and the unity of medical science would be established"* [3].

The confidence in the possibility of a new rational therapy to be grounded in some scientific theory (cellular pathology, microbiology, genetics, and so forth) has long been (and is) believed to significantly diminish, or even abolish, the disliked uncertainty of clinical practice, and has had many implications for medical research and education [4]. Unfortunately, this hoped "rational therapy" has yet to emerge out of the enormous accumulation of newly gained scientific knowledge.

In addition, the same concept of disease is problematic:
1 - diseases, like any concept, do not exist entirely "out there" but rather, to some degree, are mental constructs for putting in order our knowledge;
2 - diseases are not always all-or-none propositions;
3 - and sometimes it may be difficult to distinguish between the disease and non-disease status [5,6].

All these difficulties result from the fact that what does essentially exist in the real world are ill people and to date neither pure nor applied sciences have been able to capture their uniqueness. The achievement of such goal would simply imply the resolution of the everlasting problem of human nature.

EFFICACY OR PATIENT'S DIGNITY: WHAT DOES FAVOR EVIDENCE-BASED MEDICINE?

Medical epistemology seeks to ascertain how we can justify our knowledge, belief, or understanding of the disease process. Its practical goal is to reveal the mechanisms whereby doctors arrive at diagnoses and management plans. Prior to a decade ago, medical epistemology used to be grounded in basic research, patient-centered clinical research, and clinical expert opinion. Since knowledge can never be disinterested or even infallible, the opinion of clinical experts allowed to counterbalance in some way the weight of evidence-based data. Clinical experts provided not only the limits of the application of scientific data in the real world, i.e., outside research studies, but also evidence for all those uncertain issues which appear in the healing of particular individuals, some of them potentially knowledgeable by scientific methods while some other not. Both a clinical expert opinion and a patient-centered clinical research mainly based in non-true-experimental designs allowed the possibility of preserving the primary concern of medicine with the particular patient as a keystone of the epistemological research. Currently, however, this concern with the particular could be on the way of becoming broken with the raising of EBM movement.

EBM has been classically defined as: *"... the conscientious, explicit and judicious use of current best evidence in making decisions about the care of individual patients"* [7]. This definition appears to be ambitious but misfortunate for what has been called to be a new paradigm in medical practice. The best physicians have long sought the best empirical evidence available on which to base their decisions. What essentially separates EBM from other approaches is the priority it gives to certain forms of evidence, in particular to randomized controlled trials (RCTs) [8]. Connected to this idea is the "democratizing" feature of EBM by which medical epistemological authority is being wrested from clinical expert opinion. However, the hierarchization of evidence, as seen by EBM, is problematic.

Clinical expert opinion seems to be valuable not only when scientific evidence is lacking, but even when hard data seems to be available. Hard data can be frequently reconverted to softer data by appealing to the indefiniteness of many observable empirical events, that is non-classifiably in exact classes [6], publication bias, flawed study design, interests of third parties, recruitment problems, shift of patients among the arms of treatment, design of the statistical analysis, and so forth. At the very end, there is always some "interpretation" of hard data by expert physicians in the issue of EBM (epidemiologists, statisticians, some journal editors, among others), raising a new form of what they used to criticize as opinion-based medicine. To surpass the gap between interpreted hard data and real practice, the opinion of clinical experts still appears to be very important. Hard data does not use to challenge what a comprehensive personal clinical experience uses to reveal. But if it does, it should not be directly considered for clinical practice without some "approval" of clinical experts uninvolved in the study. Clinical experts may share some hidden interests, but so do investigators and evidence experts. Knowledge can never be disinterested and only through an explicit recognition of fallibility and a dialogic process (in equipoise) among all involved parties a reasonable consequence for medical practice is to emerge.

While the role of clinical experts in the hierarchy of evidence may be suitable for revision, there is an additional concern with the distinctive features of EBM that may be more difficult to resolve: RCTs challenge the core of the patient-physician relationship. Any patient seeking help wishes to obtain from his trusted physician what, to his wisdom (scientific evidence, practical wisdom, and so forth) is to be the best therapeutic option for him. Uncertainty is (and will be) always present in medical decisions but this has never been a reason for making clinical decisions by tossing a coin. Physicians with experience have very reasonable grounds to state which of the therapeutic options may be the best in general and the best for a particular patient. In addition, the patient has his own values and may prefer one of the therapeutic options, not necessarily the most effective, or may simply wish to trust his physician's choice. All these features of the patient-physician relationship are challenged by RCTs, which shift the interest of the physician from the particular to the general and whose recruitment success seems to be directly related to a particular way of disclosing uncertainty in which the patient perceives that his physician has no idea at all of what to do. Experimental designs may have the potential of revealing harder data but attempt to the core of the patient-physician relationship. Accepting RCT as the most desirable source of evidence makes the whole community of physicians, though not directly involved in research, accomplices of this ethically undesirable research method.

FURTHER LIMITATIONS OF EVIDENCE-BASED PRACTICE IN SURGERY

The previous reflection should suffice to reconsider some of the grounds by which evidence search is perceived today. In surgery evidence-based practice may be still more problematic. Surgery differs from medicine by the fact that its procedures are not easy like giving a pill, though some have not yet realized this. The methodology of any surgical procedure cannot be ever completely translated to words so there is always a potential gap in the reproducibility of a study. Some of the observed differing results among surgical series may thus result from unnoticed variations in how surgery was performed. Every surgical procedure is composed by a pleiad of hand movements, logic steps, and so forth, that may vary from one surgeon to another. Some of them may be irrelevant to the patient's outcome but some others surely not. Surgeons may have a reasonable idea of what works in their own technique but any attempt to reduce the procedure to an explicit process with known steps and variables is condemned to failure. It was the scientist and philosopher Michael Polanyi, whose greatest work *Personal knowledge* was published nearly 50 years ago, who said something seemingly relevant to this issue. Moving from his knowledge of a problem to knowledge of a skill [9], Polanyi would probably have asserted that every vascular surgeon may know perfectly well how to use needleholders, clamps, and so forth, but is unable to articulate the particulars of what he knows explicitly. And if he attempts to concentrate on the particulars of his movements and perceptions, he would become incapable of accomplishing them at all in a similar way, as the pianist who concentrates on the individual finger movement ceases to play. This part of knowledge is left unsaid, even in principle.

To this conceptual limitation of scientific research in surgery, some other methodological problems may account for the scarce number of RCTs published by operative specialties (3.4% of publications in the leading surgical journals, from which 55.9% compared medical therapies within surgical patients) [10]. This number is too small to be significantly grounded in an adverse predisposition of surgeons to EBM, as it has been suggested, because of commercial competition and personal prestige, lack of funding and experience in data collection, and lack of education in clinical epidemiology [11]. More evident methodological obstacles for performing RCTs in surgery may include:
1 - the learning curve if randomization is held between a familiar and an unfamiliar operation,
2 - variations on a same operation reflecting surgeon's preferences or the constant evolution of surgical procedures,
3 - difficulties in enforcing quality control monitoring of surgical procedures,

4 - patient and surgeon preferences,
5 - blinding,
6 - and placebo.

To conclude, regardless of any need to reconsider the epistemological grounds of current medical research, the rules of evidence for surgery could not even necessarily be the same ones.

A PERSPECTIVE OF HUMBLENESS FOR MEDICAL SCIENTIFISM: IS CHAOS AT THE END?

In the previous sections an epistemology of medicine that preserves some equipoise between scientific evidence and practical wisdom has been defended. Of course, there are many physicians, probably not so many surgeons, persistently engaged in Virchow's rational therapy who would not accept this position. Their enthusiasm, however, could be on the way to becoming deceived if scientific medicine simply follows the steps of other scientific disciplines. While philosophers of science are still wondering what this thing called science is, the complexity rises as new discoveries and theories about the world become available. It might seem that nature is resistant to human efforts to unmask its intimacy. Something similar could happen with "medical science".

The Newtonian mechanistic scientific world view still dominates our ideas on health and disease. This model presupposes predictable outcomes and summation of parts to equal the whole (mathematical linearity). Interaction terms, approximations, and statistical manipulations are used to adjust for discrepancies while limitations reflect inadequacies, omissions, bias, or randomness [12]. However, in vascular as in many other diseases, genes seem to interact dynamically with the environment. The interactions are probably multilevel, complex, numerous, and feed back into each other. Despite some predictability, such complexity seems to be not adequately expressed by linear models and perhaps could be better described by the mathematics of nonlinear dynamics or chaos theory, which would suggest both caution and optimism for intervention and change [13]. Chaotic systems are not totally random. The outcomes they produce are variable and complex but may stay within bounded parameters. We may know, for example, some predictive variables associated with lower limb bypass patency. However, our predictive abilities break down when we attempt more precise predictions about individual patients. Chaos theory could give us a powerful tool for understanding why precise predictions of which patient will have his bypass occluded are so

difficult. If such complexity ultimately governs our intimate nature, and thus illness, both caution and humbleness would appear to be important virtues even for those enthusiasts of Virchows's belief.

Progress and knowledge are completely legitimate scopes and of course are very welcome, but physicians on the way to becoming scientists should
1 - attenuate their fanaticism and pay more attention to the foreseeable limitations of their approach;
2 - base their scientific research on observational and non-true-experimental designs to keep the trust that should ground every patient-physician relationship;
3 - and investigate the art of practice of medicine, frequently ignored over the last decades, if they intend to practice the medical profession in its genuine uniqueness.

Grounding the epistemology of medicine from the primary concern with the particular patient

The majority of limitations of the scientifism approach to medicine can be easily recognized:
1 - its primary interest in the general without which no particular's need could be satisfied;
2 - and its belief that medical epistemic issues beyond the analysis of scientific methods will be reduced or even abolished.

However, as it has been shown before, medicine has long been primarily concerned with the particular, even before science existed, and continues to be an uncertain business and peculiarly practical. Without the simple scene of an ill person seeking help and the physician trying to help, any epistemic search in medicine could be equalized to the study of the diseases, for example, of the amoeba. Therefore, any search to ascertain how we can justify our knowledge, belief or understanding of the disease process
1 - is a very important but secondary consideration;
2 - and should be grounded directly from the real clinical practice.

This position has two consequences:
1 - patient-centered clinical research should be based mainly on observational and non-true-experimental designs rather than on true experimental ones (RCTs);

2 - and there is a pleiad of issues concerning this primary concern with the particular (physician attitudes and practical wisdom; patient attitudes, preferences and values) which have been forgotten for decades and should be approached with appropriate study designs, for example by qualitative methods.

In the present section, a concise overview on the convenience of all these designs for medicine and surgery in general, and for the case of innovative and unusual procedures in particular, will be provided in the belief that the reader will easily find a more comprehensive review of these methodologies in other bibliographic sources.

OBSERVATIONAL DESIGNS

In observational studies (OS), the investigator simply observes the natural course of events and records the results without trying to influence them. Properly conducted, OS are important in modifying clinical practice by informing clinicians about unanticipated or unrecognized dangers of medical or surgical therapies. There is evidence that OS can be designed with rigorous methods that mimic those of RCTs. The "restricted cohort" design [14], for example, identifies a "zero time" for determining a patient's eligibility and baseline features, uses inclusion and exclusion criteria, adjusts for differences in baseline susceptibility to the outcome, and uses statistical methods similar to those of RCTs. Concato et al. [15] have recently shown that, contrary to prevailing beliefs, the "average results" from well-designed OS did not significantly overestimate the magnitude of the associations between exposure to treatment and outcome as compared with the results of RCTs on the same topic.

Observational studies provide very useful information and are frequently the first methodological design for evaluating surgical innovations. Some therapeutic interventions may have such a large effect that observational data alone may be sufficient evidence of effectiveness. In addition, OS can be reinforced by systems of quality control, using instruments such as *cusum* or *variable life-adjusted display* (VLAD) plots, to evaluate the learning process of a new procedure.

The cusum method [16] provides both numerical and graphical representation of a learning process. In cusum charts, successive cases are recorded on the horizontal axis. The line moves up for successes and down for failures according to a set target value for the level of performance. More failures than

expected result in an increase in the cusum. If improvement in performance occurs, the cusum will reverse that appearance.

As a refinement of the cusum method, VLAD plots [17] provide information about both success and failure in the learning process, taking into account the expected risk associated with each particular case. For each case there is a previous risk score that determines the magnitude by which the graph ascends or descends. If the patient was at high risk of failure, the surgeon's success rates are not unduly penalized, but success figures are penalized when a procedure in a low-risk patient fails. VLAD can show also the difference between the expected and actual cumulative failure curve.

QUASI-EXPERIMENTAL DESIGNS

The recent emphasis on RCT may have led to a depreciation and misunderstanding of the role of non-true-experimental designs in patient-centered analytic research. It has been widely said that non-true-experimental designs do have the potential for bias and that it may never really be known whether any observed change could have occurred without the intervention. Contrary to this position, it has been suggested that this attitude is not well founded in epistemological grounds and that randomization is not a panacea and is by no means sufficient for causal inferences [18]. While RCTs may have the potential to provide harder data, information from non-true-experimental designs may be particularly useful when a moderate to large effect size is observed between the exposure to treatment and outcome. An estimate higher than 2 for the relative risk or the odds ratio between two rates is generally deemed to be "clinically important". It is at this estimate level that the effect size could be unlikely explained on the basis of bias or chance alone, provided that adequate matching of patients and control for confounding factors is done. RCT may have the potential to perceive lower effect sizes although this advantage could be questioned by appealing to whether this effect size is indeed important enough to break the trust in the patient-physician relationship.

The analytic designs that use non-randomized control groups for comparison between treatments suitable for surgical research may include after-only studies with non-randomized control group, time series studies using different samples (historical controls), and controlled before and after studies. With after-only studies, the effect of the new procedure is assessed by measuring it only after the group has been exposed to it, and it is compared with an appropriate control group. Matching of participants of both groups and covariance adjustment may help to remove the potential bias. With time series studies, a group of participants who are given a new procedure are compared with a group of participants who had previously been given an alternative procedure. Analysis of a time series involves checking for changes in either the level or slope of the series after the introduction of the innovation. Time series data can provide useful and inexpensive monitoring of an innovation and can even furnish evidence of causal effects. Finally, with controlled before and after studies patients with similar characteristics to the study population and with no access to the innovative procedure in their referral institutions, because of surgeon preferences or absence of consensus or technology for implanting it, act as the comparison group to patients treated in the institution with the innovative treatment. Data are collected in both populations contemporaneously using similar methods before and after the intervention is introduced in the study population. Matching of participants according to patient characteristics, indication for surgery, and so forth, together with covariance adjustments, are needed to control potential biases.

In summary, because there is no agreed upon analytical solution to the problem of baseline selection differences, probably the best that innovative surgeons can currently do is to use several methods of analysis. If the results from the various methods are congruent, evaluators may state conclusions about the effectiveness of the surgical innovation with appropriate caution. The global accuracy of this approach, if properly designed, may not be very different to that obtained from RCT, though it may require more time and effort to obtain grounded epistemological evidence. This cost appears to be very low if the prize is to maintain the integrity of the context in which care is provided.

THE VERY LAST RESORT: RANDOMIZED CONTROLLED TRIALS

To consider RCTs as a poorly desirable method for clinical research does not mean, however, that they cannot be ever done. Dualist positions force the dialogue further than reasonable. There may exist very occasional issues in which uncertainty or equipoise raise deep concerns within the whole community of clinical experts, not just within some

colleagues or third parties, and where no other research design seems possible for clarifying the problem, for example when the difference between two treatments appears to be small and one of the treatments is medical and the other one surgical. The need to resolve the value of these potentially modest shifts in efficacy and/or safety of new treatments should be necessarily shared by National Health Providers and by some sort of adequately represented "jury" of ill people. The ethical cost of an RCT is too high to be decided by just part of the interested parties. The design and interpretation of these RCTs should be done by experts uninvolved in its steering committee and, of course, no remuneration should be offered to recruiter-physicians. Finally, ethics committees should be specialized in the involved issue and specifically named for each RCT. In this way, RCTs would become an issue of society interest and would be reserved for very ad hoc epistemological concerns, while the main body of clinical research could be left to well collected observational studies and non-true-experimental designs.

INVESTIGATING THE ART OF PRACTICE

Beyond the enormous accumulation of newly gained scientific knowledge, clinical medicine, and especially surgery, continue to be an uncertain business and peculiarly practical, and it will be so in the foreseeable future. Though poorly defined, the art of practice includes all such skills and mental abilities partly acquired from experience by which physicians take into account scientific evidence (basic and patient-centered), practical knowledge yet to be scientifically proven, practical knowledge probably non-scientifically testable, patient and professional values, and system features for making particular decisions in conditions of uncertainty. Even as science progresses and our evidence-based knowledge increases, our epistemological uncertainty does not seem to decrease (perhaps it even increases). It is widely known that each answer promotes always some new questions, as seen for example with the Malthusian growth of uncertainty when multiple technologies are combined into clinical strategies. Take two technologies and they can be used in two different sequences; take five technologies and the number of possible sequences are 120. The gray areas of knowledge and the need to decide every day with every patient warrant the role of practical wisdom in the epistemology of medicine. It has been suggested that evidence and experience are not essentially different categories of knowledge, the first being a systematic approach of the second [19]. However, as it has been seen, clinical experience provides physicians the epistemic opportunity to expand their knowledge beyond what is at that moment scientifically proven or what may remain non-reducible to scientific methods. Basic sciences and clinical studies provide a framework of knowledge that does not exhaust the knowledgeable of illness. A great effort will be needed in the future to counterbalance a century of scholarly disinterest in the field of medical practice [4].

Hybrid vascular procedures are not only a good opportunity to confirm how medicine is primarily concerned with the particular but also a paradigmatic example of how the art of practice may still flourish in dialogue with scientific evidence. New technologies progressively increase the chances for suited-to-case surgical treatments and their combination will make it more difficult to achieve generalizable hard data. This unavoidable particularization of surgical practice not only demands an active attitude of the whole community of surgeons to squeeze the possibilities of observational and quasi-experimental designs by means of registries of innovative procedures and so forth, but also to explore the gray epistemic areas of practice without complexes. Ultimately, there is probably some need for changing the rational intolerant attitude to uncertainty rooted in the enlightenment for another one more everlasting and grounded on a balance between rationality and reasonableness.

FACING UNCERTAINTY THROUGH QUALITATIVE STUDIES: THE DELPHI PROCESS

The process of developing a consensus in areas of medicine where hard evidence is scarce (i.e., innovation) or contradictory or in issues difficult to approach by scientific methods, can be problematic. The traditional method for dealing with complicated problems has been to use committee meetings or steering groups to reach a consensus and then formulate guidelines. There are clearly drawbacks with this approach. Committees may be influenced by the nature of interpersonal interactions within the group. Dominant personalities, who do not equal more expertise, may impose their views on other members, while those in positions of responsibility may find it difficult to shift their position. Consensus methods may help to avoid these difficulties and attempt to assess the extent of agreement and to resolve disagreement between

experts. The three best-known consensus methods are the Delphi process, the nominal group technique, and the consensus development conference.

The Delphi process [20] is a consensus method that allows synthesis of existing evidence with expert opinion without a physical concurrence of involved experts. The Delphi process is characterized by anonymity, iteration, controlled feedback, and statistical aggregation of group response. Anonymity is achieved through the expert's private answer of a structured questionnaire. Iteration occurs through the submission of the questionnaire over a series of rounds, usually three, allowing members to change their opinions. Controlled feedback occurs between rounds. The results of each round are analyzed by a central researcher and the responses for each given statement are fed back to all experts of the Delphi group. This allows members of the group to reassess their views in light of the group's responses. Finally, the statistical aggregation of group response is obtained at the end of the procedure. This is an expression of the degree of consensus of the group on the particular issue. The Delphi process should not be seen as a quick fix to complicated issues and it is not always an easy process. It requires enthusiasm from both the respondents and organizers, but the results can be satisfying and informative for both.

Grounding ethics from the primary concern with the particular patient Ethics of innovation

At the beginning of the chapter, it was asserted that medicine is a distinctive discipline whose primary concern is the particular patient and that this has important consequences in the issues of epistemology and ethics. In the previous sections, it has been shown how an epistemology of medicine grounded from the concern with the particular case can be threatened by a conception of medicine being on the way of becoming a scientific discipline. Although the present chapter has been primarily focused on epistemological issues, it would be inadequate to conclude this discussion without at least some general considerations about ethics of innovation. Epistemology and ethics are related but distinct studies. While epistemology seeks to ascertain how we can justify our knowledge, belief, or understanding, ethics tells us how to conduct ourselves, that is how to decide rightly in the collection, dissemination, and use of both certain and uncertain knowledge.

THREATS TO GROUNDING ETHICS FROM THE PRIMARY CONCERN WITH THE PARTICULAR PATIENT

Grounding ethics from the primary concern with the particular patient may have the potential threat of an overemphasis in the general, in this case the society. This is not a common problem among physicians but it may be the case for the growing number of experts in the issues of meso- and macro-resource allocation that frequently incommode rather than promote the quality of healing activities of physicians "in the trench". Fortunately, there seems to still be a great number of physicians who believe that:

1 - their responsibilities toward patients (fiduciary duty) are, to begin, "ahead" of any other consideration;

2 - any restriction in care delivery to their patients on the basis of reasonable resource allocation should be stated beforehand, through a dialogic process among interested parties and not at the bedside;

3 - and it is possible to adhere sincerely to the principle of justice by simply choosing tests and interventions known to be beneficial, by choosing the test or intervention with the least cost among equally beneficial options, and by resolving occasional conflictive claims for scarce resources on the basis of need and benefit (micro-allocation).

At least as important as this overemphasis for the general, the potential interests of other particulars, in this case the physicians, may also threaten the primary concern with the particular patient in clinical decisions. This problem can be especially relevant in the issues of innovation. Currently, there is a declining interest in the excellence of the patient-physician relationship in hospital settings. Patients are sometimes seen as objects of interest for research purposes. Reference and university hospitals and scientific associations seem to promote a model of physician more characterized by his scientific curriculum and innovative potential than by the satisfaction, or even sometimes the outcome of his patients. As a result, a growing number of hospital physicians may become progressively more sensitive to their academic flourishing than to the excellence of their healing activities. This problem can be illus-

trated by the explicit example of the hospital physician who must refer an ill close relative to another hospital colleague. Frequently, the chosen physician is not precisely characterized by his scientific curriculum or his dedication to publishing articles or attending meetings, but for his skillfulness, clinical expertise, reasonable decision-making, empathy with patients, and especially for his dedication to clinical practice. If these latter features are not met, it is not possible to guarantee the primary concern with the particular patient, and any attempt for research, innovation, etc. should be seriously reconsidered.

THE ETHICS OF INNOVATION

Innovation is highly valued in progressive societies. In surgery, a certain level of innovation is expected in the daily practice when the surgeon encounters unanticipated findings. However, surgeons are generally conservative guardians of routines and techniques that have been validated by years of experience engendering a profound trust in their relationship with the patient. This trust creates a dangerous situation for the patient and the surgeon when innovative treatments are introduced. Throughout many decades, many surgical innovations have been achieved by means of what has been called informal research [21]. Informal research consists of interventional studies with several common characteristics:

1 - they consist of a series of patients;

2 - outcome measures are common clinical parameters, the type usually obtained during routine clinical follow;

3 - formal written protocols do not exist;

4 - and because these activities are viewed as clinical care, they are invisible to institutional review boards.

Currently there is an increased concern in ethical and legal issues and, opposite to what might occur in the origins of vascular surgery, present innovations intend to improve the therapeutic efficacy and/or safety for conditions for which often a satisfactory treatment already exists. So, while innovation may consist of technical improvements or variations in existing techniques, some modifications of the "informal research" method could suffice for updating this design to the current ethical and legal requirements; but if an innovation represents a significant departure from previous practice, it should be regarded as a new approach to the problem. In such circumstances, the assessment of the procedure should follow a rigorous audit.

Farther than animal and mechanical testing, if appropriate, the introduction of every new surgical procedure in clinical practice should be controlled from the first suitable case and evaluated by some sort of register, as does for example *the Australian Safety and Efficacy Register of New Interventional Procedures-Surgical* (ASERNIP-S) established by the Royal Australian College of Surgeons in 1998, before final recommendations about safety and efficacy can be set. The ASERNIP-S provides a rigorous methodology for assessing new procedures by a prior evaluation of the technique, and the training and experience of the involved institutions, the monitoring of the learning curve and the informed consent, and the register and evaluation of consecutive cases.

Registers like ASERNIP-S provide an adequate ethical framework for surgical innovative techniques, but may fail to be useful for unusual procedures such as many HVP can be. In such circumstances, and provided that no international register yet exists, far from using rules and regulations, the most reliable protection for patients seems to be the presence of an informed, conscientious, compassionate, and responsible surgeon. As a general rule, the surgeon must always be on guard against fashion and avoid the willingness of patients to try something new in a desperate situation. By means of a proper auto-critical thinking, every innovative surgeon should be able to decide whether to go on or forego the new technique by asking himself:

1 - whether there is really a need for such procedure in such patient, which implies bibliographic search, own attitudes discernment and safety and efficacy expectation;
2 - whether he is the adequate person for doing it;
3 - whether his department has the adequate stability, cohesion, and clinical and research trajectory;
4 - whether his institution is going to provide sufficient technical, logistic, and ethical support for undertaking such a step;
5 - whether some sort of specialized peer review of the idea has been foreseen;

6 - and whether an adequate informed consent is going to be provided to suitable patients, which implies that the patient (and family) need to be a) advised that the technique is new and/or experimental, and b) provided with information about alternative available treatments and previous experience with the proposed treatment. Under these circumstances, innovation can be ethically grounded in the primary concern with the particular patient.

Conclusion

1 - HVPs are paradigmatic examples of the distinctive nature of medicine as an activity whose primary concern is the particular patient rather than as a science whose primary interest is the knowledge.
2 - The search for scientific knowledge in medicine (basic and patient-centered) is a legitimate and honorable scope. However, this objective should be respectful to the primary commitment of physicians, thus avoiding true-experimental studies that may challenge the trust in the patient-physician relationship.
3 - The practical wisdom of clinical experts is an additional prominent source of knowledge whose oblivion impoverishes any epistemic search in medicine and handicaps the learning of the practical management of clinical uncertainty.
4 - Hybrid and unusual vascular procedures can be paradigmatic examples of how the art of practice may flourish in dialogue with science.
5 - Innovation should be respectful to the primary commitment of medicine. Currently there are adequate methods for controlling and auditing innovative processes, although they may fail to be useful for many hybrid and unusual vascular procedures because of their rarity, special idiosyncrasy, and variability.

Ultimately, far from using rules and regulations, the most reliable protection for patients may well be the presence of an informed, conscientious, compassionate, and responsible surgeon.

REFERENCES

1 Resnick LM. Why we can't translate clinical trials into clinical practice in hypertension. *Am J Hypertens* 2003; 16: 421-425.

2 Munson R. Why medicine cannot be a science. *J Med Philos* 1981; 6: 183-208.

3 Virchow R. Die Einheitsbestrebungen in der wissenschaftlichen Medizin. Berlin, Reimer, 1849.

4 Wiesing U, Welie JV. Why medicine should consider a theory of practice? Introduction to the issue. *Theor Med Bioeth* 1998; 19: 199-202.

5 Norman GR. The epistemology of clinical reasoning: perspectives from philosophy, psychology and neuroscience. *Acad Med* 2000; 75: S127-S135.

6 Widder J. The fallibility of medical judgment as a consequence of the inexactness of observations. *Med Health Care Philos* 1998; 1: 119-124.

7 Sackett DL, Rosenberg WM, Gray JA, et al. Evidence based medicine: what it is and what it isn't. *BMJ* 1996; 312: 71-72.

8 Sehon SR, Stanley DE. A philosophical analysis of the evidence-based medicine debate. *BMC Health Serv Res* 2003; 3: 14.

9 Saunders J. Validating the facts of experience in medicine. In: Evans M, Finlay I (eds). *Medical Humanities*. London, BMJ Books 2001: pp 223-235.

10 Wente MN, Seiler CM, Uhl W, Buchler MW. Perspectives of evidence-based surgery. *Dig Surg* 2003; 20: 263-269.

11 McCulloch P, Taylor I, Sasako M, et al. Randomised trials in surgery: problems and possible solutions. *BMJ* 2002; 324: 1448-1451.

12 Philippe P, Mansi O. Nonlinearity in the epidemiology of complex health and disease processes. *Theor Med Bioeth* 1998; 10: 591-607.

13 Rambihar VS, Baum M. A new mathematical (chaos and complexity) theory of medicine, health and disease: refiguring medical thought. In: Rambihar VS (ed). *A New Chaos Based Medicine Beyond 2000: the response to evidence*. Toronto, Vashna Publications 2000.

14 Horwitz RI, Viscoli CM, Clemens JD, Sadock RT. Developing improved observational methods for evaluating therapeutic effectiveness. *Am J Med* 1990; 89: 630-638.

15 Concato J, Shah N, Horwitz RI. Randomized, controlled trials, observational studies and the hierarchy research designs. *N Engl J Med* 2000; 342: 1887-1892.

16 Van Rij AM, McDonald JR, Pettigrew RA, et al. Cusum as an aid to early assessment of the surgical trainee. *Br J Surg* 1995; 82: 1500-1503.

17 Lovegrove J, Valencia O, Treasure T, et al. Monitoring the results of cardiac surgery by variable life-adjusting display. *Lancet* 1997; 350: 1128-1130.

18 Abel U, Koch A. The role of randomization in clinical studies: myths and beliefs. *J Clin Epidemiol* 1999; 52: 487-497.

19 Parker M. Whither our art? Clinical wisdom and evidence-based medicine. *Med Health Care Philos* 2002; 5: 273-280.

20 Jones J, Hunter D. Consensus methods for medical and health services research. *BMJ* 1995; 311: 376-380.

21 Margo CE. When is surgery research? Towards an operational definition of human research. *J Med Ethics* 2001; 27: 40-43.

3

CAROTID ENDARTERECTOMY COMBINED WITH INTRA-ARTERIAL THROMBOLYSIS OR STENTING

JENS-RAINER ALLENBERG, HARDY SCHUMACHER
HANS-HENNING ECKSTEIN, WERNER HACKE

The efficacy of elective carotid endarterectomy (CEA) in symptomatic high-grade extra-cranial carotid stenosis is well proven as secondary prevention of ischemic stroke. The benefit of CEA in patients with additional intracranial atherosclerotic disease is uncertain. Within the patient population of the North American Symptomatic Carotid Endarterectomy Trial (NASCET), intracranial atherosclerotic disease was observed in one third of the patients, although the NASCET protocol excluded severe intracranial atherosclerotic disease. The data analysis of this subpopulation showed that intracranial atherosclerotic disease is an independent risk factor for subsequent stroke. There are nearly no data on patients operated for carotid stenoses with associated cranial stenosis. Similarly, there are no data showing whether simultaneous thrombolysis, intra-operative transluminal angioplasty, or stenting in combination with CEA is of advantage or improves clinical outcome. Emergency CEA for acute or progressive stroke is still a matter of debate [1-4]. As a result of disappointing experience in the 1960s, including the Joint Study of Extracranial Arterial Occlusion, with unacceptable high surgical mortality and cerebral hemorrhage rates between 29% and 50%, carotid desobliteration for acute stroke was considered to be contra-indicated [5-8]. Inadequate patient selection with poor pre-operative identification of the degree of cerebral injury in the era before computed tomography (CT) and magnetic resonance imaging, combined with insufficient control of postoperative hypertension, may have been significant contributors to the high incidence of peri-operative hemorrhagic complications. Recently, the potential benefit of emergency CEA was shown in patients with fluctuating neurological deficit or progressive stroke, showing satisfactory clinical outcome (no or mild neurological deficit) in up to 84% and an overall mortality rate of 6% to 20% [9-15]. The main prognostic predictors for good clinical outcome in these patients were timing of surgery, absence of cerebral coma, quality of collateral blood flow, and co-existence of simultaneous arterio-arterial embolization in the middle cerebral artery (MCA).

Thrombolysis and CEA

Several studies have shown that thrombolytic agents given either intravenously or intra-arterially can be successful in recanalizing an acute occlusion of the MCA [16-30]. As thrombolytic therapy cannot be effective in the treatment of an embolizing carotid focus, a combined approach consisting of thrombolysis and extracranial CEA, either as a staged or simultaneous procedure, might be a promising therapeutic option in the management of an acute carotid-related ischemic stroke [31]. Additionally, intra-operative thrombolysis might be indicated in elective CEA complicated by intra-operative intracranial embolism [32,33]. Table I summarizes the indications and types of combined procedures at the internal carotid artery (ICA).

In this chapter we address our initial experiences with staged procedures (thrombolysis prior to CEA) and simultaneous procedures including patients with a carotid-related stroke (emergency CEA and throm-

bolysis simultaneously) and patients with elective CEAs complicated by intra-operative and postoperative intracranial embolic vessel occlusion (surgical re-exploration and intra-operative thrombolysis, and stent application).

Personal experience

PATIENTS

Between January 1994 and January 2003, a total of 845 carotid reconstructions were performed. In 20 patients (2.4%), a combined therapeutic approach consisting of intracerebral thrombolysis and CEA was performed. In one case, distal stenting after elective CEA was done during the same procedure.

In 8 patients thrombolysis for acute ischemic stroke was performed first. CEA was carried out after clinical improvement at the earliest interval (4 to 21 days). In 8 patients intracerebral thrombolysis was performed intra-operatively during emer-

Table I	INDICATIONS AND TYPES OF COMBINED PROCEDURES AT THE INTERNAL CAROTID ARTERY

Indications

    Symptomatic intracranial internal carotid tandem stenoses

    Intimal flap with distal occlusion after proximal eversion endarterectomy

    Petrous carotid artery dissection after balloon angioplasty or endoluminal shunt insertion

    Correction of endovascular or open procedural complications

    Non-atherosclerotic lesions of the ICA including fibromuscular dysplasia

Type of procedures (simultaneous or staged)

    Proximal endarterectomy and distal angioplasty

    Proximal endarterectomy and selective thrombolysis

    Proximal endarterectomy and distal stenting

    Systemic thrombolysis and secondary endarterectomy

gency CEA for acute carotid-related stroke (n = 6) and in 2 patients with CEA and immediate complications at completion angiography. Four patients underwent re-exploration and thrombolysis after elective CEA with complicated outcome after surgery. In one patient revision after completion angiography was necessary and resulted in primary stenting of a distal dissection caused by insertion of the shunt.

DIAGNOSIS

To exclude both intracerebral hemorrhage and early signs of already established major ischemic infarction, all patients were analyzed by cerebral CT scans. These early signs include hypodensity of the MCA territory, obscuration of the lentiform nucleus, focal brain swelling, loss of insular ribbon, or the so-called hyperdense internal carotid sign, which indicates occlusion of the ICA and/or the MCA [12].

In all staged procedures (n = 8) carotid angiography was performed prior to the procedure. In all other patients, emergency surgery was done without pre-operative angiography. Diagnosis of carotid occlusion was obtained by doppler or duplex studies and by neurological examination. Intracerebral embolization was revealed by intra-operative on-table angiography (digital subtraction arteriography), and was performed in all patients by puncture of the common carotid artery after completion of the reconstruction. After aspiration of blood to ensure proper endoluminal placement of the needle, 5 to 10 mL contrast medium was injected into the common carotid artery while antegrade flow was maintained. Imaging of the carotid bifurcation and the intracranial vessels including the intracranial ICA, the intracranial carotid bifurcation, the MCA, and the anterior cerebral artery were performed in two different projections.

In staged procedures, patency of the MCA after thrombolysis was assessed by transcranial doppler and confirmed by intra-operative angiography during early CEA. In 13 simultaneous procedures, postoperative patency of the reconstructed ICA and the MCA was confirmed by duplex scans, transcranial doppler, and/or angiography/CT angiography three to five days after the procedure.

SELECTION

Selection criteria for initial thrombolysis in acute ischemic stroke were adopted from the ECASS study and included a time window of less than six hours between onset of stroke and thrombolysis, exclusion of cerebral bleeding, and/or early signs of an established ischemic infarction greater than one third of the territory of the MCA and evidence of an intracerebral embolism and/or thrombus [12].

Similarly, emergency surgery for stroke was indicated in patients with evidence of carotid occlusion or high-grade stenosis, absence of cerebral coma, and exclusion of intracerebral hemorrhage and/or established ischemic infarction on the pre-operative CT scan of the brain. Intra-operative thrombolysis was performed after on-table angiography and visualization of middle or anterior cerebral artery embolization. A delay of more than six hours since onset of symptoms did not exclude patients from surgery as long as no signs of infarction were detectable on the CT scan.

Patients with a postoperative stroke within the first hours after elective CEA were re-explored under emergency conditions to exclude a technical failure of the carotid reconstruction unless other reasons for the postoperative deficit existed (malignant hypertension, cholinergic syndrome). In order to avoid delay, cerebral CT was not repeated and angiography was performed intra-operatively.

THROMBOLYTIC AGENTS

Recombinant tissue plasminogen activator (rt-PA) was administered as intravenous lysis therapy with doses depending on the body weight (80 to 100 mg intravenously). Intra-operative thrombolysis was performed using urokinase, which was administered via the ICA (locally) or selectively via a microcatheter (Tracker®-18, 2.5 F, *Target Therapeutics Inc., Fremont, CA, USA*). As no accepted dose regimen for intra-operative use of thrombolytic agents exists, 500 000 to 750 000 IU urokinase were given in the majority of patients. Individually, a lower dose of 150 000 IU urokinase was used in a 81-year-old woman. Higher doses (1 million IU urokinase) were used in two patients in whom the MCA was catheterized selectively but no recanalization was achieved.

OPERATIVE DETAILS

In all operative procedures a bolus of 5000 IU heparin was given intravenously prior to cross-clamping of the ICA. In all emergency procedures, continuous heparinization was maintained by infusion of 1.000 to 1.500 IU intravenously per hour in order to double activated partial thromboplastin time.

Neuromonitoring was performed routinely during elective CEA by recording somato-sensory-evoked potentials (SSEP). Loss of SSEP in elective CEA always guided toward shunt insertion and on-table angiography of the major extracranial and intracranial vessels.

Results

STAGED PROCEDURES: THROMBOLYSIS FOR ACUTE/PROGRESSIVE STROKE AND EARLY CEA AFTER NEUROLOGICAL IMPROVEMENT

Eight patients were admitted to the Department of Neurology with symptoms of an acute hemiplegia or acute or progressive hemiparesis. On the base of a modified Rankin scale, the neurological deficit was defined before the intervention. In one case Rankin 2 was found, in three cases Rankin 3, in three Rankin 4, and in one Rankin 5. The initial cerebral CT excluded hemorrhagic infarction and/ or early signs of a major ischemic infarction in all cases. Within an interval of 2.5 to 5 hours, angiography was performed to confirm occlusion of the ICA (n = 2/8) and occlusion of the intracranial carotid bifurcation or MCA (n = 6/8) as suspected by doppler or duplex scanning. In three cases 80 mg rt-PA was administered intravenously, in four 100 mg rt-PA and in one patient 1 million IU urokinase. In the Department of Vascular and Endovascular Surgery, CEA was performed at the earliest day after neurological improvement. The time interval differed between 4 and 21 days and the procedure was uneventful in all patients. The postoperative CT showed a wide range, varying from absence of lesion (n = 2) to minimal lesion (n = 2) and infarction (n = 4). The recanalization was patent in all cases except one, in whom the MCA was opened by thrombolysis but the ICA could not be re-opened by surgery. In that case a simple CEA of the external carotid artery was performed. The neurological deficit was improved in the early postoperative phase in three of eight patients, and in six of eight patients after six months (Table II).

COMBINED EMERGENCY CEA AND INTRA-OPERATIVE THROMBOLYSIS FOR CAROTID-RELATED STROKES

Six patients were primarily submitted to the surgical department and treated simultaneously by CEA and intra-operative thrombolysis. Three patients suffered from an acute hemiplegia with Rankin 5, and three others showed a progressive stroke (one Rankin 4, two Rankin 5). CEA was done in all cases

and urokinase was administered in a dosage of 150 000 IU up to 1 million IU locally or selectively by intracranial catheterization. Two patients died postoperatively. One patient who was treated 3 hours after the onset of symptoms (Rankin 5) by CEA selectively received 500 000 IU urokinase and died from intracerebral hemorrhage in the early postoperative period. The other patient suffered from a massive infarction (8 centimeter diameter) and died.

Patients no. 9 and no. 10 (Table II) clearly illustrate the practical performance of combined emergency CEA and thrombolysis.

Case patient no. 9 is a 66-year-old man with a symptomatic stenosis greater than 90% of the left ICA (hemispheric transient ischemic attacks) who suffered from a severe left hemispheric stroke with complete hemiplegia of the right side, global aphasia, and progressing lack of consciousness. Acute carotid occlusion was diagnosed and emergency operation by thrombectomy and CEA was performed after exclusion of intracerebral hemorrhage and/or major ischemic infarction by means of CT scanning. Intra-operative needle angiography following eversion endarterectomy revealed subtotal occlusion of the MCA. Via the reconstructed ICA, intra-operative lysis therapy was performed with 500 000 IU urokinase. Three hours after the procedure, the patient's hemiplegia and aphasia gradually diminished, and after 24 hours the patient recovered nearly completely. A selective carotid angiogram three days later depicted a normal intracerebral vascular architecture without residual thrombo-embolisms. At discharge from hospital the patient was free of complaints. A CT scan of the brain showed neither intracerebral hemorrhage nor ischemic infarction. A last neurological examination only indicated a minimal weakness of a facial branch and signs of dysdiadochokinasis of the right arm. Some weeks later, no neurological deficit could be detected (Rankin 0, published as case report in 1995 [31]).

Case patient no. 10 was a 70-year-old man who was waiting for elective CEA because of a symptomatic high-grade stenosis of the ICA. He suffered from a progressive neurological deficit with severe hemiparesis, and acute carotid occlusion was suspected by doppler assessment. After exclusion of cerebral bleeding by CT, re-establishment of carotid flow was achieved three hours after onset of stroke by emergency desobliteration. During surgery it appeared that the ICA was occluded. Completion angiography showed embolic occlusion of the MCA mainstem

Table II PERSONAL EXPERIENCE

N°	Age/Gender	Site of occlusion	Symptoms (mod. Rankin-scale*)	Therapy	Interval** (hours)	Recanalization (angio, CTA, duplex)	Postoperative CT	Outcome (mod. Rankin-scale*) Early	≥6 months
1	41/m	Right carotid-T ECA stenosis 90%	Acute hemiplegia (Rankin 5)	1 - 100 mg rt-PA i.v. 2 - CEA day 6 (uneventful)	4	Yes	After thrombolysis: minimal ischemic lesion	0	0
2	79/m	MCA occlusion ICA stenosis 90%	Acute hemiparesis (Rankin 3)	1 - 100 mg rt-PA i.v. 2 - CEA day 5 (uneventful)	3	Yes	After thrombolysis: diameter 2 cm ischemic infarction	3	3
3	58/m	Left ICA MCA occlusion	Acute hemiparesis (Rankin 4)	1 - 80 mg rt-PA i.v. 2 - CEA of ECA day 14 °	2.5	ICA reoccluded MCA yes	After thrombolysis: diameter 3 cm ischemic infarction	3	3
4	67/m	Right ICA ICA stenosis 80%	Acute hemiplegia (Rankin 2)	1 - 80 mg rt-PA i.v. 2 - CEA day 6 (uneventful)	4.5	Yes	No lesions	2	1
5	75/f	Left MCA ICA stenosis 70%	Acute hemiparesis (Rankin 4)	1 - 1 Mill. UI UK sel 2 - CEA day 21 (uneventful)	3	Yes	After thrombolysis: diameter 5 cm ischemic infarction	2	1
6	68/f	Left MCA ICA stenosis 80%	Acute hemiplegia (Rankin 3)	1 - 100 mg rt-PA i.v. 2 - CEA day 7 (uneventful)	5	Yes	After thrombolysis: minimal ischemic lesion	3	2
7	70/m	Right MCA ICA stenosis 99%	Progressive hemiparesis (Rankin 4)	1 - 80 mg rt-PA i.v. 2 - CEA day 4 (uneventful)	3	Yes	After thrombolysis: diameter 4 cm ischemic infarction	4	2
8	54/m	Left ICA	Acute hemiplegia (Rankin 3)	1 - 100 mg rt-PA i.v. 2 - CEA day 12 (uneventful)	4	Yes	No lesions	3	3

STAGED PROCEDURES

Table II   PERSONAL EXPERIENCE

N°	Age/Gender	Site of occlusion	Symptoms (mod. Rankin-scale*)	Therapy	Interval** (hours)	Recanalization (angio, CTA, duplex)	Postoperative CT	Outcome (mod. Rankin-scale*) Early	≥6 months
9	66/m	Left ICA MCA	Acute hemiplegia (Rankin 5)	CEA **and** 500.000 UI UK loc	3	Yes	No lesion	0	0
10	70/m	Right MCA ICA stenosis 90%	Progressive hemiparesis (Rankin 5)	CEA **and** 750.000 UI UK loc	3	Yes	Ischemic infarction diameter 4 cm□	2	1
11	81/f	Left ICA MCA	Progressive hemiparesis (Rankin 4)	CEA **and** 150.000 UI UK loc	5	Not done	Not done	3	3
12	55/m	Left ICA MCA	Progressive hemiparesis (Rankin 5)	CEA **and** 600.000 UI UK sel	12	Yes	Ischemic infarction diameter 4 cm	4	2
13	60/f	Left carotid-T ICA stenosis > 90 %	Acute hemiplegia (Rankin 5)	CEA **and** 1 Mill. UI UK sel/loc	3	ICA/ACA yes MCA no	Ischemic infarction diameter 8 cm	6	-
14	69/m	Intra-operative MCA	Acute hemiplegia (Rankin 5)	CEA **and** 500.000 UI UK sel	3	Yes	Intracerebral hemorrhage	5	6
15	74/m	Intra-operative right ACA	Completion angio intra-operatively	CEA **and** 500.000 UI UK loc	< 1	Yes	No lesion	0	0
16	60/m	Intra-operative right MCA	Completion angio intra-operatively	CEA **and** 500.000 UI UK loc	< 1	Not done	No lesion	0	0

SIMULTANEOUS PROCEDURES

Table II   PERSONAL EXPERIENCE

POSTOPERATIVE COMPLICATIONS

N°	Age/Gender	Site of occlusion	Symptoms (mod. Rankin-scale*)	Therapy	Interval** (hours)	Recanalization (angio, CTA, duplex)	Postoperative CT	Outcome (mod. Rankin-scale*) Early	Outcome (mod. Rankin-scale*) ≥6 months
17	72/m	Intra-operative MCA	Hemiplegia immediately after elective CEA (Rankin 5)	Revision **and** 500.000 UI UK sel	3	Not done	Ischemic infarction diameter 8 cm	6	–
18	53/m	Postoperative right ICA MCA	Hemiplegia after aorto-carotid bypass (Rankin 5)	Revision **and** 1 Mill. UI UK sel	12●	Yes	Ischemic infarction diameter 8 cm	5	5
19	64/f	Postoperative right ICA MCA	Hemiparesis 2 h after elective CEA (Rankin 4)	Revision **and** 500.000 UI UK loc	80 min.	Yes	Ischemic infarction diameter 3 cm	2	1
20	55/m	Postoperative right ICA MCA distal branch	Hemiplegia 3 h after elective CEA (Rankin 5)	Revision **and** 500.000 UI UK loc	50 min.	Yes	Ischemic infarction diameter 2 cm	2	3
21	67/m	Intra-operative petrous left ICA (dissection)	Completion angio intra-operatively	Revision **and** primary stenting (4 x 40 mm coronar stent)	40 min.	Yes	No lesion	0	0

ACA: anterior cerebral artery
ECA: external carotid artery
i.v.: intravenously
loc: locally via internal carotid artery (ICA)
MCA: middle cerebral artery (M1/M2 segment)
sel: selectively by microcatheter
UK: urokinase (IU)

* Modified Rankin scale:
0 – no deficit
1 – minimal deficit
2 – mild, non-disabling deficit
3 – moderate deficit, but little support in daily activities
4 – disabling, not walking alone
5 – severe deficit, confined to bed
6 – peri-operative death

** Interval: interval between onset of symptoms and thrombolysis.
○ Patient 3: internal carotid artery re-occluded after several days without a new neurological deficit.
● Patient was ventilated mechanically for 8 hours and neurological deficit was unknown.
○ No SSEP loss during clamping of the common carotid artery.
□ Partial hemorrhagic transformation of the ischemic infarction.

3
27

which guided us to apply 750 000 IU urokinase locally in the ICA. After the intervention, the patient recovered step by step, and only showed a minor neurological deficit at discharge (Rankin 2). Six months later no functional deficit existed (Rankin 1). The postoperative CT scan of the brain revealed a secondary hemorrhagically transformed ischemic infarction but no parenchymatous cerebral bleeding. Patency of the ICA and the MCA was evidenced by CT angiography four days postoperatively.

ELECTIVE CEA COMPLICATED BY PERI-OPERATIVE INTRACRANIAL EMBOLISM AND OCCLUSION

Of 845 elective patients for CEA, outcome after surgery was complicated in 4 cases. The neurological deficit was detected immediately or some hours after surgery and was classified as Rankin 4 and 5. In three other cases, arterial occlusion was found during completion angiography and the reconstruction was done immediately within a time frame of a few minutes up to 40 minutes. While the outcome of the latter three patients was excellent, the neurological deficit in the four patients with a complicated course was poor. One patient died from a cerebral infarction with a diameter of 8 centimeters, one patient suffered from an infarction with Rankin 5, one with Rankin 3, and one with Rankin 2. In the late follow-up the remaining patients stayed at the same level or were slightly better.

INTRA-OPERATIVE STENTING OF THE PETROUS ICA AFTER COMPLICATED EXTRACRANIAL ENDARTERECTOMY WITH DISTAL CAROTID DISSECTION AFTER ENDOLUMINAL SHUNTING (Figure)

Patient no. 21 (Table II) was a 67-year-old male complaining of recurrent amaurosis fugax attacks due to a symptomatic high-grade (superior to 90%) ICA stenosis on the left and an asymptomatic 60% contralateral ICA stenosis; elective conventional CEA and carotid reconstruction using a 6 millimeter interposition dacron graft was performed. Completion angiography depicted a distal occlusion of the petrous ICA after secondary endoluminal shunt insertion for cerebral protection during prolonged cross-clamping. Primary stenting via the dacron graft was performed using a flexible balloon-expandable 4 millimeter coronary stent (length 4 centimeters). After the procedure the patient recovered remarkably well without infarction on CT. Six months later, CT angiography revealed a patent extracranial and intracranial ICA.

Discussion

The natural history of patients who suffer from a profound neurological deficit due to acute extracranial carotid occlusion is unsatisfactory, with a stroke rate varying from 40% to 69% and a mortality rate ranging from 16% to 55% [9]. Comparable mortality in patients with intracranial ICA occlusion and/or occlusion of the MCA reaches 53% [26, 34,35]. In our experience, 16 of 20 patients presented with clinical signs of a major ischemic carotid-related stroke. Stroke was caused by acute carotid occlusion in 11 of 16 patients and due to occlusions of the MCA (mainstem and major branches respectively) in all 16 patients. Five remaining patients suffered from intracerebral embolization during elective CEA. All together these 16 patients represent a prognostic unfavorable group, justifying every effort to recanalize brain-supplying arteries.

In highly selected patients, both emergency CEA and thrombolysis may be beneficial in the management of an ischemic carotid-related stroke [9,12-14]. Up to now a combined procedure consisting of CEA and thrombolysis, either staged or simultaneously, has only been reported in case reports [31-33]. The 16 patients reported here represent the first consecutive series in a single-center-experience. Six patients recovered completely, 6 patients suffered from a minor stroke, 2 patients suffered from a major stroke, and 2 patients died postoperatively. After 6 months, 8 patients are functionally independent, 5 patients still have a mild or moderate deficit, and 1 patient still has a severe deficit.

Several prognostic factors may be relevant for a satisfactory result following thrombolysis and emergency surgery. In the surgical literature good outcome is reported in 61% if carotid desobliteration is performed within three hours, indicating that *time* is a major predictor for clinical outcome [10]. In our series restoration of blood flow was achieved within a wide range: thrombolysis was initiated within 2.5 to 5 hours, emergency surgery was performed within 50 minutes to 12 hours. Our data indicate that time can be a limiting factor as an unsatisfactory clinical outcome occurred in two patients in whom emergency CEA was performed after an interval of 12 hours although one patient improved significantly within six months. On the other hand two patients died postoperatively although emergency surgery was performed within a short interval of three hours after onset of stroke. Due to the small number of patients, no definite time window for emergency surgery can be concluded from our data.

Angiographically controlled studies indicate that poor collateral blood flow is associated with a poor or even fatal clinical outcome in patients with an ischemic stroke treated conservatively or with thrombolytic agents [22,26,36,37]. In this series one patient with collateral ICA occlusion suffered from a postendarterectomy stroke due to acute ICA thrombosis. Surgical re-exploration was performed within an interval of 50 minutes, revealing no technical failure. MCA branch embolism and insufficient collateral flow might have been responsible for the development of cerebral infarction in this patient (no.14, Table II).

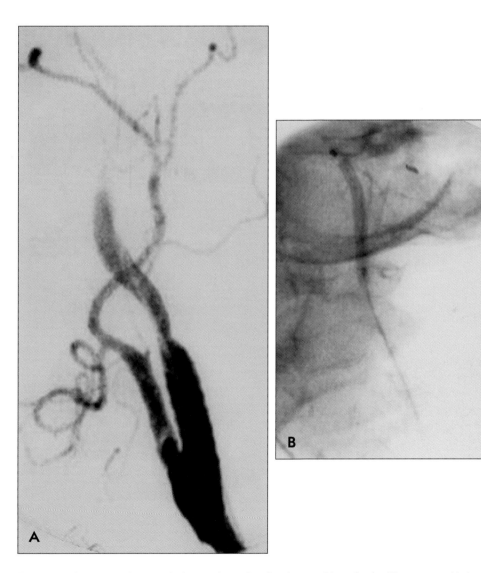

Figure A - Intra-operative completion angiography after interposition of a 6 millimeter carotid dacron graft: proximal and distal graft anastomoses without any problem or stenosis but no flow into the intracranial ICA. Unexpected root cause analyses: contrast stop about 5 centimeters above the distal anastomoses with collapsed true lumen. After revision no sign of dissection at the suture line. Via the prosthesis, successful recanalization of the occluded distal petrous ICA was achieved. B - Implantation of a premounted 4 millimeter balloon-expandable coronary stent at the base of the skull in the petrous ICA. Deployment with 8 atmospheres. The stent length of 4 centimeters was chosen to gain a long overlap with the intimal flap. The exact length of the dissection membrane could not be determined intra-operatively. ▸

Simultaneous occlusion of the MCA is another important factor. Meyer et al. [9] operated on 34 patients with a profound neurological deficit due to an acute carotid occlusion; they achieved a good outcome in 38.3%, a fair outcome in 29.4%, a poor outcome in 11.8%, and a fatal outcome in 20.5%. Co-existence of MCA embolism or exclusion is a risk factor for poor outcome. It was concluded that an associated MCA embolus, detected angiographically, is a relative contra-indication to surgery. Accordingly, angiographically controlled studies with intravenous or intra-arterial administration of thrombolytic agents have shown a strong correlation between recanalization and neurological improvement in acute ischemia, in the vertebro-basilar and the carotid territories [19,21,22,24,27-30]. The efficacy and safety of thrombolysis in acute stroke has recently been demonstrated in selected patients by two large double-blind randomized studies. Both the *European Cooperative Acute Stroke Study (ECASS)* and the *North American National Institute of Neurological Disorders and Stroke rt-PA Stroke Study Group* (NINDSrt-PASSG), although not angiographically controlled, indicated that regression of neurologi-

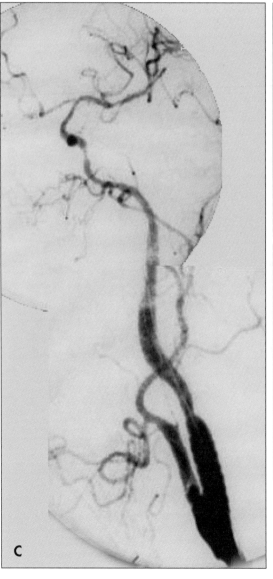

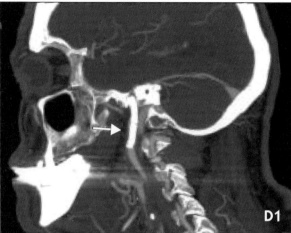

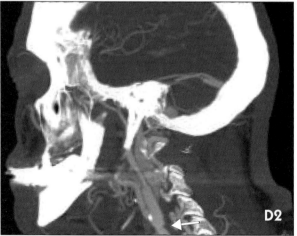

C - Completion angiography: recanalized extracranial and intracranial ICA with open intracranial carotid bifurcation, MCA, and A. communicans anterior. D - Two-year follow-up with 2-dimensional multislice CT angiography: Patent dacron interposition graft and carotid stent at the base of the skull. The patient recovered without neurological complications.

cal deficits is probably related to re-establishment of perfusion to the ischemic brain without any excess mortality [17,20].

Thrombolytic therapy is able to recanalize acute intracranial occlusions; however, the embolizing carotid focus cannot be treated sufficiently if the stenosing plaque remains in-situ. The combination of thrombolysis and CEA offers the possibility to treat the embolus and focus simultaneously. This is also true for patients with a postendarterectomy stroke due to acute carotid thrombosis and cerebral embolization. Intra-operative angiography of the intracranial major arteries should be considered as a *conditio sine qua non* in neurologically unstable patients. In our experience we were able to detect embolic occlusions in the vascular bed of the MCA in all patients with a carotid-related stroke and in all patients with a postendarterectomy stroke. Intracranial on-table angiography should also be performed in cases of unexpected changes in neuromonitoring during CEA [32,33]. Significant SSEP changes indicated intra-operative MCA embolizations in three patients (no. 9-11, Table II), prompting angiography and subsequent application of urokinase in the carotid artery.

Although no study has been undertaken to test the superiority of any kind of administration, it can be assumed that the recanalization rate is higher in intra-arterial as compared to intravenous application. According to the literature, intravenous thrombolysis of MCA occlusions within six hours achieves a recanalization rate between 38% and 59%, whereas intra-arterial infusion results in 45% to 90% patency [27,30]. Microcatheter techniques for selective thrombolysis are probably best to apply a high concentration of thrombolytic agent into the thrombus. In our series selective thrombolysis resulted in (partial) recanalization in three of five patients.

In eight of our patients, urokinase was administered intra-operatively by puncture of the ICA or via an indwelling shunt. It can be disputed that part of the agent is diverted to less relevant arteries (for example ophthalmic artery). Complete or partial recanalization was achieved in six patients. It can therefore be assumed that also other mechanisms than direct intra-thrombus infusion might be effective, like re-opening of collateral pathways or salvage of the ischemic penumbra. As shown by Barr et al. [32], intracarotid thrombolysis represents a therapeutic option that is immediately available during opera-

tion and that can also be effective in elective endarterectomy complicated by intracerebral embolism. Larger doses may be required with proximal ICA infusion, but at present no exact regimens for intrathrombus and/or proximal intracarotid infusion do exist.

The role of spontaneous recanalization of intracranial emboli will maximally be 20% at 24 hours [27,30] but may depend on the location of the occlusion (ICA or MCA), its composition (fibrin embolus, platelet embolus, or thrombus), and its age. Since the majority of our thrombolyzed patients had evidence of recanalization and recovered or improved, we suppose that spontaneous recanalization did not play the major role in this series.

Intracerebral bleeding is a major concern following thrombolysis for acute ischemic stroke. According to the literature, the risk of asymptomatic intracerebral petechial hemorrhage or intracerebral hematoma with clinical deterioration is about 10% and 5%, respectively [30]. The natural course of an ischemic infarction is complicated by a symptomatic hemorrhagic transformation with formation of space-occupying hematomas in approximately 5%. In 15% to 45%, an asymptomatic (petechial) hemorrhagic transformation may occur [30,38-40]. In our series, no parenchymal intracerebral bleeding occurred and hemorrhagic transformation without clinical deterioration could be detected in one patient (CEA and simultaneous thrombolysis three hours after onset of symptoms). Both patients operated on with a delay of 12 hours showed no signs of bleeding on the postoperative CT scan. According to the results of the ECASS study a pre-operative CT scan of the brain must be performed to exclude patients with signs of an already established cerebral infarction for emergency surgery and/or thrombolysis because these patients are exposed to a significantly higher risk for cerebral bleeding than patients without ischemic infarction [17]. All three patients who were pre-operatively thrombolyzed did not suffer from any clinical worsening. Due to the small number of patients, further experiences are necessary to assure that those patients are not at a higher operative risk of intracerebral postoperative hemorrhage as compared to patients not treated by thrombolysis pre-operatively. Larger doses than 1 million IU urokinase should be avoided intra-operatively because dose dependency between thrombolytic agents and intracerebral bleeding is proven [24].

Conclusion

Intracerebral thrombolysis and CEA, either as a staged or as simultaneous procedure, is a new therapeutic approach in the treatment of carotid-related ischemic strokes. Although the individual course is not predictable, major cerebral infarction might be prevented in a significant number of patients. Intraoperative intracerebral angiography is a *conditio sine* *qua non* to reveal intracerebral embolism, and should be performed routinely in CEA for neurologically unstable patients and in patients with loss of SSEP during elective CEA. Although the exact risk of intracerebral bleeding in thrombolysis and emergency surgery (staged or simultaneously) is not determined by our data, absence of any major hemorrhagic complication indicates that this approach should be a subject of further interdisciplinary investigation.

REFERENCES

1 De Weese JA. Management of acute stroke. *Surg Clin North Am* 1982; 62: 467-472

2 Moore WS, Mohr JP, Najafi H, et al. Carotid endarterectomy: practice guidelines. Report of the Ad Hoc Committee to the Joint Council of the Society for Vascular Surgery and the North American Chapter of the International Society for Cardiovascular Surgery. *J Vasc Surg* 1991; 1S5: 469-479.

3 Anonymous. European Carotid Surgery Trialist's Collaborative Group. MRC European carotid surgery trial: interim results for symptomatic patients with severe (70-99%) or with mild (0-29%) carotid stenosis. *Lancet* 1991; 337: 1235-1243.

4 Anonymous. North American Symptomatic Carotid Endarterectomy Trial Collaborators. Beneficial effect of carotid endarterectomy in symptomatic patients with high-grade carotid stenosis. *N Engl J Med* 1991; 1325: 445-453.

5 Wylie EJ, Hein MF, Adams JE. Intracranial hemorrhage following surgical revascularization for treatment of acute strokes. *J Neurosurg* 1964; 21: 212-218.

6 Blaisdell WF, Clauss RH, Gailbraith JG, et al. Joint study of extracranial carotid artery occlusion IV: a review of surgical considerations. *JAMA* 1969; 209: 1889-1895.

7 Fields WS. Selection of stroke patients for arterial reconstructive surgery. *Am J Surg* 1973; 125: 527.

8 Rob CG. Operation for acute completed stroke due to thrombosis of the internal carotid artery. *Surgery* 1969; 65: 862.

9 Meyer FB, Sundt TM Jr., Piepgras DG, et al. Emergency carotid endarterectomy for patients with acute carotid occlusion and profound neurological deficits. *Ann Surg* 1986; 203: 82-89.

10 Gertler JP, Blankensteijn JD, Brewster DC, et al. Carotid endarterectomy for unstable and compelling neurologic conditions: do results justify an aggressive approach. *J Vasc Surg* 1994; 19: 32-42.

11 Thompson JE, Austin DJ, Patman RD. Endarterectomy of the totally occluded internal carotid artery for stroke. results in 100 operations. *Arch Surg* 1967; 95: 791-801.

12 Goldstone J, Effeney DJ. The role of carotid endarterectomy in the treatment of acute neurological deficits. *Prog Cardiovasc Dis* 1980; 6: 415-422.

13 Goldstone J, Moore WS. A new look at emergency carotid artery operations for the treatment of cerebrovascular insufficiency. *Stroke* 1978; 9: 599-602.

14 Mentzer RM, Finkelmeier, BA, Crosby IK, Wellons HA. Emergency carotid endarterectomy for fluctuating neurological deficits. *Surgery* 1981; 89: 60-66.

15 Walters BB, Ojemann RG, Heros RC. Emergency carotid endarterectomy. *J Neurosurg* 1987; 66: 817-823.

16 Boysen G. Overview on thrombolysis in acute ischemic stroke. *Fibrinolysis* 1995; 9: 28-32.

17 Hacke W, Kaste M, Fieschi C, et al., for Acute Stroke Study (ECASS) Group. Intravenous thrombolysis with recombinant tissue plasminogen activator for acute hemispheric stroke. *JAMA* 1995; 274: 1017-1025.

18 Del Zoppo GJ, Pessin MS, Mori E, Hacke W. Thrombolytic interventions in acute thrombotic and embolic stroke. *Semin Neurol* 1991; 11: 368-384.

19 Higashida RT, Van Halbach V, Barnwell SL, et al. Thrombolytic therapy in acute stroke. *J Endovasc Surg* 1994; 1: 4-15.

20 Anonymous. The National Institute of Neurological Disorders and Stroke rt-PA Stroke Study Group. Tissue plasminogen activator for acute ischemic stroke. *N Engl J Med* 1995; 333: 1581-1587.

21 Clark WM, Barnwell SL. Endovascular treatment for acute and chronic brain ischemia. *Curr Opin Neurol* 1996; 9: 62-67.

22 Frey JL, Greene KA, Khayata MH, et al. Intrathrombus administration of tissue plasminogen activator in acute cerebrovascular occlusion. *Angiology* 1995; 46: 649-657.

23 Nesbit GM, Clark WM, O'Neill OR, Barnwell SL. Intracranial intraarterial thrombolysis facilitated by microcatheter navigation through an occluded cervical internal carotid artery. *J Neurosurg* 1996; 84: 387-392.

24 Mori E, Tabuchi M, Yoshida T, Yamadori A. Intracarotid urokinase with thromboembolic occlusion of the middle cerebral artery. *Stroke* 1988; 19: 802-812.

25 Komiyama M, Nishio A, Nishijima Y. Endovascular treatment of acute thrombotic occlusion of the cervical internal carotid artery associated with embolic occlusion of the middle cerebral artery: case report. *Neurosurgery* 1994; 34: 359-363.

26 Jansen O, von Kummer R, Forsting M, et al. Thrombolytic therapy in acute occlusion of the intracranial internal carotid artery bifurcation. *Am J Neuroradiol* 1995; 16: 1977-1986.

27 Del Zoppo GJ, Pessin MS, Mori E, Hacke W. Thrombolytic intervention in acute thrombotic and embolic stroke. *Semin Neuroradiol* 1991; 11: 368-384.

28 Trouillas P, Nighogossian N, Getenet JC, et al. Open trial of intravenous tissue plasminogen activator in acute carotid territory stroke. *Stroke* 1996; 27: 882-890.

29 Hacke W, Zeumer H, Ferbert A, et al. Intraarterial thrombolytic therapy improves outcome in patients with acute vertebrobasilar occlusive disease. *Stroke* 1988; 19: 1216-1222.

30 Wardlaw JM, Warlow CP. Thrombolysis in acute ischemic stroke: does it work? *Stroke* 1992; 23: 1826-1839.

31 Eckstein HH, Hupp T, Allenberg JR, et al. Carotid endarterectomy and local intraarterial thrombolysis: simultaneous procedure in acute occlusion of the internal carotid artery and middle cerebral artery embolism. *J Vasc Surg* 1995; 22: 196-198.

32 Barr JD, Horowitz MB, Mathis JM, et al. Intraoperative uroki-nase infusion for embolic stroke during carotid endarterec-tomy. *Neurosurgery* 1995; 36: 606-611.

33 Comerato AJ, Eze AR. Intraoperative high-dose regional uroki-nase infusion for cerebrovascular occlusion after carotid endar-terctomy. *J Vasc Surg* 1996; 24: 1008-1016.

34 Moulin DE, Lo R, Chiang J, Barnett HJM. prognosis in middle cerebral artery occlusion. *Stroke* 1985; 16: 282-284.

35 Saito I, Segawa H, Shiokawa Y, et al. Middle cerebral artery occlusion: correlation of computed tomography with clinical outcome. *Stroke* 1987; 18: 863-868.

36 von Kummer R, Forsting M. Effects of recanalization and col-lateral blood supply on infarct extent and brain edema after mid-dle cerebral artery occlusion. *Cerebrovasc Dis* 1993; 3: 252-255.

37 Bozzao L, Fantozzi LM, Bastianello S, et al. Early collateral blood supply and late parenchymal brain damage in patients with middle cerebral artery occlusion. *Stroke* 1989; 20: 735-740.

38 DeBakey ME. Successful carotid endarterectomy for cerebrovas-cular insufficiency. Nineteen-year follow-up. *JAMA* 1975; 233: 1083-1085.

39 Hornig CR, Dorndorf W Agnoli AL. Hemorrhagic cerebral infarction: a prospective study. *Stroke* 1986; 17: 179-185.

40 Hart RG, Easton JD. Hemorrhagic infarcts. *Stroke* 1986; 17: 586.

4

CAROTID ENDARTERECTOMY ASSOCIATED WITH PTA OF THE SUPRA-AORTIC ARTERIES

JEAN-PIERRE FAVRE, MARIANGELA DE MASI
DIDIER BOURRA, MARCO VOLA, XAVIER BARRAL

This hybrid technique combines conventional surgical endarterectomy of one of the two carotid bifurcations (CBs) with a proximal endovascular treatment, in the same axis, of the common carotid artery (CCA) or the brachiocephalic trunk (BCT). This excludes the combined treatment of revascularization of the internal carotid artery (ICA) with repair of a supra-aortic artery (SAA) other than the one feeding the CB.

Whereas CCA lesions treated by a hybrid technique do not have a specific morphology, the lesions of the SAAs will generally be short and proximally located. Therefore the hybrid procedures are not applicable to long stenoses or occlusion of the supra-aortic vessels.

Generalities

CAROTID LESIONS

Lesions of the CB are generally caused by atherosclerosis, representing a substantial part of vascular surgery activity. The randomized trials, published more than ten years ago, have clearly defined the indication for surgery in symptomatic, severely stenosed carotid lesions. The recently published meta-analysis [1] has confirmed and even extended these surgical indications. The treatment of asymptomatic stenoses has followed a similar evolution, with even more strict criteria regarding the degree of stenosis and the general condition of the patients to be candidates for this prophylactic procedure.

Surgery remains the method of choice if, in the presence of a carotid stenosis, an indication for anatomical repair is evident [2]. However, endovascular treatment associated with stent placement, often combined with a cerebral protection device, seems to modify our surgical habits [3]. This minimally invasive modality might even become the gold standard in the upcoming years but not before its superiority, or at least equal quality on the short and long-term, has been proven.

LESIONS OF THE SAAS

The incidence of SAA stenotic lesions is much lower than that of carotid artery pathology. SAA lesions can occur as an isolated stenosis and only affect one of the three arteries (most often the left subclavian artery), or involve all three arteries, generally depicted as calcified ostial stenoses (Fig. 1), and is atherosclerotic in the majority of cases, as initially described by Martorell and Fabre [4]. Surgical correction of these lesions was reported in the

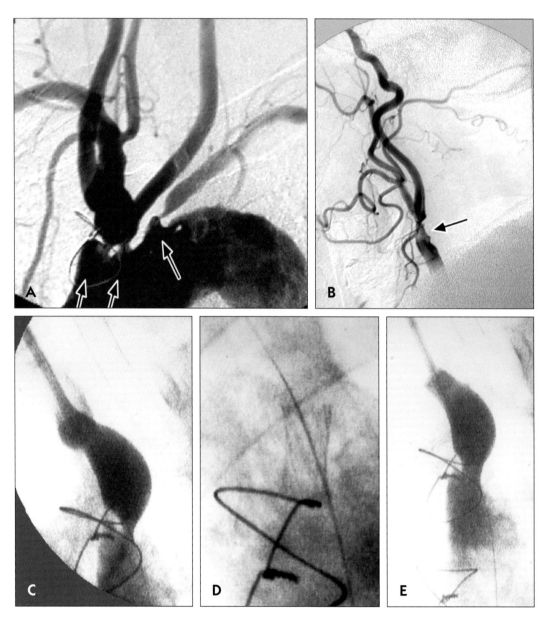

FIG. 1 Proximal diffuse lesions of the supra-aortic arteries associated with stenosis of the left carotid bifurcation. A - Angiography of the aortic arch. B - Selective angiography of the carotid bifurcation. As a first treatment, the brachiocephalic trunk was dilated via cervical access. C - Arteriography before dilatation. D - Stent of 10 mm diameter. E - Completion angiography after dilatation. A hybrid procedure of the left carotid axis was performed as a second treatment.

1960s, originally by means of endarterectomy, which was rapidly replaced by bypass grafting. The first series including substantial volume of patients was reported by Debakey et al. in 1965 [5]. Several series have confirmed these good early and late results of intrathoracic and cervical reconstructions, however, at the price of considerable morbidity and mortality [6-8]. Because of these risks, considered as major surgical trauma, endovascular techniques have been introduced as an appealing and attractive alternative. Although likely to offer less favorable patency rates, overall morbidity and mortality are significantly reduced [9,10].

BIFOCAL LESIONS

Lesions at two different levels rarely occur. While each lesion will carry the risk of embolization, hemodynamic consequences are more important because of the summation of the tandem lesions. The risks of treatment are probably also increased because of the summation of both interventions.

It is not conceivable to treat a lesion of the CB and ignore an upstream stenosis. Vice versa, treating a proximal stenosis only and neglecting a lesion of the ICA will not offer hemodynamic improvement.

Treatment of bifocal lesions can consist of the "classical" attitude, being completely surgical, or the "modern" approach, by means of endoluminal repair. A hybrid procedure, however, combining surgical repair of the CB with endoluminal treatment of the lesion in the SAA, can be an attractive alternative.

The most suitable lesions for these hybrid procedures are proximal stenoses of a SAA (BCT, CCA) associated with a stenosis of the CB. Extensive lesions of the CCA are generally treated by surgery.

Surgical technique

The first case combining carotid endarterectomy with endoluminal treatment of the ipsilateral CCA was published by Kerber et al. [11]. The dilatation was performed just before finishing closure of the endarterectomy by means of catheters with increasing diameters (8F to 14F), according to the technique of Dotter [12]. Several years passed before the first publications on balloon angioplasty of SAA appeared [13]. We describe the hybrid procedure as applied in the most published series [14-18], which actually is the technique we have used in our center (Figs. 2,3).

The intervention comprises a conventional surgical approach and is therefore performed in an operating room. The surgical suite should be equipped with high standard imaging facilities to obtain optimal visualization of the aortic arch [19]. Under local, loco-regional, or general anesthesia, the CCA is surgically exposed, as is the internal and external carotid artery. Following heparinization, with a dose depending on the surgeon's choice (5.000 to 10.000 UI), the carotid artery is clamped, either at the ending of the CCA or at the level of the ICA in such a way that embolization is avoided. An introducer is retrogradely positioned in the CCA by means of a simple puncture or arteriotomy. Arteriography is performed to depict the target lesion. A wire is passed through the lesion and a balloon catheter is placed in the stenosis and subsequently inflated. The diameter of the balloon varies according to the diameter of the target artery: in general 8 millimeters for the CCA and 10 millimeters or greater for the BCT. If a residual stenosis (more than 30%) is observed, if the stenosis springs back following deflation or if a dissection occurs, a stent can be placed. Some authors recommend performing primary stenting, sometime preceded by pre-dilatation by means of a small diameter balloon. Short stents of two to three centimeters are used. We prefer balloon expandable stents because they allow accurate placement and prevent the risk of loosing the stent in the aorta during release of a self-expandable stent. For the treatment of ostial stenosis, the stent should ideally protrude approximately two millimeters into the lumen of the aortic arch [19]. Introduction of a stiff guidewire into the aortic arch by femoral access has been proposed because it aligns itself to the convexity of the arch, thereby depicting the outer layer and making accurate positioning of the stent easier. Another technique consists of passing the lesion assisted by the introducer before withdrawing the occluder. The stent can be correctly positioned inside the introducer whereafter the latter is withdrawn to allow expansion of the stent. This technique has the advantage that predilatation is not required and it avoids the risk of moving the stent when passing a tight or calcified lesion [20]. Completion angiography is performed through the introducer. Some authors assess arterial pressures before and after dilatation. A significant stenosis must have a gradient over 15 mmHg, which should be resolved after treatment [20].

Following removal of the introducer, endarterectomy of the CB is performed according to standard

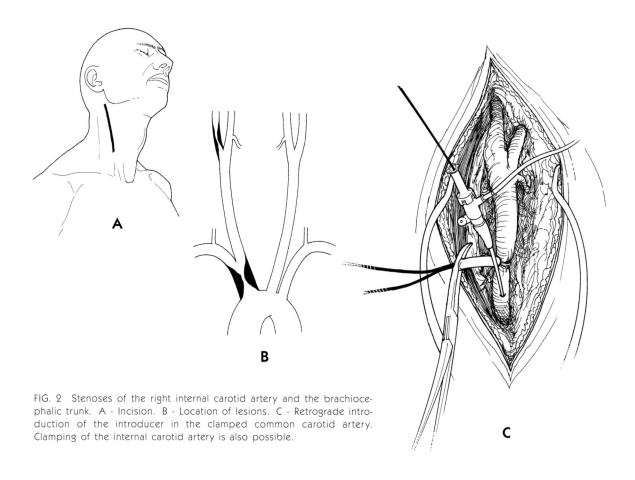

FIG. 2 Stenoses of the right internal carotid artery and the brachioce-phalic trunk. A - Incision. B - Location of lesions. C - Retrograde intro-duction of the introducer in the clamped common carotid artery. Clamping of the internal carotid artery is also possible.

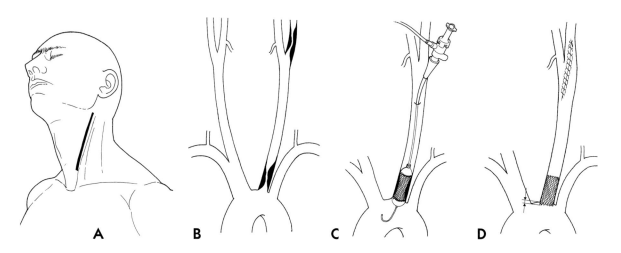

FIG. 3 Stenoses of the left common and internal carotid arteries. A - Incision. B - Location of lesions. C - Angioplasty with stent of the proximal lesion (under carotid clamping). D - Final result following proximal angioplasty with stent and endarterectomy of the carotid bifurcation.

techniques. Some authors use a shunt systematically [17], others only selectively [15,18]. If the endarterectomy is performed after the dilatation, shunt insertion can be considered in order to prevent circulatory arrest in the dilated segment during several minutes: platelet aggregates might develop and embolize after declamping [21]. This risk of thrombosis during clamping has led Macierewicz et al. [18] to increase the amount of anticoagulation; however, postoperative bleeding complications might occur more frequently. For bifocal carotid artery lesions we prefer to perform the endarterectomy prior to the dilatation. For combined pathology in the CB and the BCT we consider the sequence of procedures unimportant.

This technique of dilatation by carotid access offers the advantage of controlling the risk of embolization with a simple and fast treatment of the proximal stenosis. However, this technique is not exempt from complications. Sullivan et al. [21] have observed 3 dissections among 14 cases treated by means of retrograde carotid catheterization and dilatation of the CCA. The first dissection occurred during passing of the guidewire and required transposition of the CCA to the subclavian artery. The other two dissections developed after dilatation and extended into the aortic arch but could be treated by stent placement.

Analysis of the literature

INCIDENCE

Combined occlusive lesions of the SAA and CB that are suitable for hybrid techniques do not frequently occur. Between 1993 and 2000, only five publications addressing this subject were published [14-18], reporting on a total of 61 hybrid treatments. One of these comprises 44 cases, representing 72% of all treated patients. Other authors have cited the use of this type of hybrid technique in publications on endoluminal treatment of the SAAs and for the carotid arteries [21-23]; the data in these publications are not detailed enough to analyze.

Our personal experience consists of seven cases between 1997 and 2002. During this period we operated on 980 CBs and performed percutaneous angioplasty of 39 SAAs. The hybrid approach, in our experience, represents 0.6% of the CB interventions and 15% of the endoluminal SAA repair.

In the experience of Arko et al. [17] the combined treatment represents 1% of all carotid endarterectomies. Rouleau et al. [24] performed an angiographic study and showed, in 672 patients with a carotid stenosis greater than 70%, that 14 (2.1%) had a tandem lesion of the ipsilateral CCA greater than 50% and 14 a stenosis of the contralateral CCA. Koskas et al. [25] operated on 4.672 CBs, and in 150 cases (3%) the feeding SAA was simultaneously repaired by surgical reconstruction. Berguer et al. [7,8] revascularized 282 SAAs (100 via intrathoracic access and 182 via extrathoracic access) and performed simultaneous repair of the CB in 89 cases (32%).

ANALYSIS OF CASES

This assessment combines the 61 reported cases and the 7 patients from our personal experience. The age of these 68 patients varied between 51 and 78 years (mean 64 years): 55% male, 60 patients (88%) were symptomatic, 34 presented with a transient ischemic attack, 16 amaurosis fugax, 6 with a cerebral vascular accident, and 4 with a non-hemispheric accident compatible with a low cerebral flow (Table I). In all cases the suspected tandem

Table I	CHARACTERISTICS OF PATIENTS WHO UNDERWENT A HYBRID PROCEDURE FOR LESIONS OF THE CAROTID BIFURCATION AND ONE OF THE SUPRA-AORTIC ARTERIES [14-18 AND 7 PERSONAL CASES]
Number of patients	**68**
Men (%)	55
Symptomatic (%)	88
Symptomatology	
Transient ischemic attack	34
Stroke	6
Amaurosis	16
Non-hemispheric accident	4
Location of proximal lesion	
Brachiocephalic trunk	30
Left common carotid artery	33
Right common carotid artery	5

pathology as diagnosed by duplex scanning was confirmed by angiography. In 35 patients the right carotid axis was affected, associated with a stenosis of the CB: 30 stenoses in the BCT (Fig. 4) and 5 in the proximal CCA. In 33 cases, left CB pathology was associated with proximal left CCA stenosis (Fig. 5). In the majority of cases the degree of CB stenosis was greater than 70%, except in the series of Levien et al. [16], in which some lesions of the CB were between 50% and 70%. The degree of stenosis in the SAAs varied between 50% and 95%. No occluded BCT has been treated. All patients but one [14] have been operated on in an operating room. General and loco-regional anesthesia were

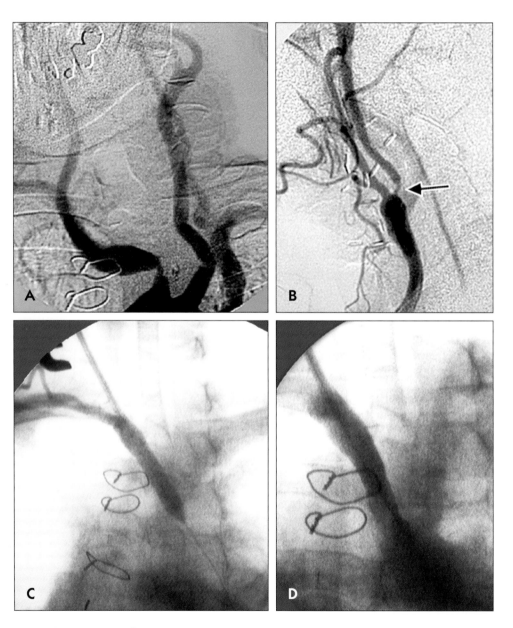

FIG. 4 Tandem lesion of the brachiocephalic trunk (A) and right carotid bifurcation (B). Note the delayed circulation at the right side as compared to the left side. C - Dilatation of the brachiocephalic trunk via the common carotid artery after endarterectomy of the bifurcation. D - Completion angiography after angioplasty and stent placement.

applied in 63 and 5 patients, respectively. Regarding surgical techniques, some differences could be appreciated. Levien et al. [16] clamped the ICA first, followed by arteriotomy and placement of the introducer by retrograde access in order to perform the dilatation of the CCA or BCT. With a purge string around the CCA the endarterectomy was performed with a shunt in-situ. Cerebral monitoring was not used. The technique of Arko et al. [17] is comparable to the one of Levien. Endarterectomy was also done with shunt protection and the arteriotomy was systematically closed with a patch. Macierewicz et al. [18] clamped the ICA first in seven of eight patients. If transcranial doppler showed adequate cerebral hemodynamics, the entire procedure was realized with continuous clamping. A shunt was placed after the proximal dilatation. In the last patient, clamping was hemodynamically not tolerated and dilatation was performed without clamping. Endarterectomy was established with a shunt. Iannone et al. [14] treated his patient in a radiology suite. The CB endarterectomy was performed first and prior to complete closure of the arteriotomy the BCT was dilated by femoral access. Following dilatation the right CCA was purged and flushed before closing the arteriotomy.

We started with the endarterectomy and in our experience a shunt was not necessary because the residual pressure in the ICA was higher than 60 mmHg. Before complete closure of the arteriotomy, an introducer was positioned in the CCA to allow dilatation and primary stent deployment.

RESULTS

The combined procedure could be executed in 67 patients, indicating a technical success rate of 98.5%. In one case, Levien et al. [16] was unable to pass a severely calcified tight stenosis of the BCT: the carotid endarterectomy was still performed and remained patent during the 2-year follow-up.

In 22 cases a stent was placed. In the series of Levien et al. [16] comprising 44 patients, dilatation was performed without stent placement. During follow-up five restenoses occurred, all before 18 months postoperatively, of which four after angioplasty without stent. Restenosis rate is therefore 9% in the absence of stent placement and 5% after. Three of five restenoses were symptomatic. One patient underwent re-dilatation of the BCT by brachial access with excellent outcome after five years. Two patients with BCT restenosis received a graft from the ascending aorta and one left CCA stenosis was

4

41

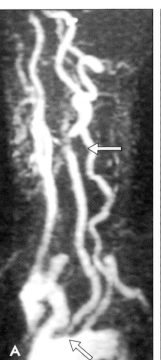
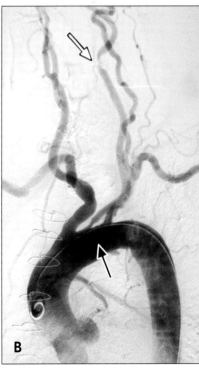

FIG. 5 Bifocal stenosis of the left carotid axis: ostial stenosis of the common carotid artery and left carotid bifurcation. A - Magnetic resonance angiography. B - Arteriography.

managed with a subclavian-carotid bypass. The last stenosis (right CCA) was not operated on and remained stable during follow-up. Two restenoses occurred in the endarterectomized segment and were asymptomatic. Among other complications, four hematomas required surgical drainage and three intra-operative cardiac arrhythmias were noted.

In another series comprising 87 lesions of the SAA treated by means of angioplasty in 83 patients, Sullivan et al. [21] reported five simultaneous interventions by SAA dilatation and CB surgery. Three cases concerned patients who had already undergone endarterectomy (n = 2) and bypass (n = 1). In two patients severe complications were encountered: one CB occlusion caused a massive cerebral vascular accident and subsequent death, and one embolus associated with an intimal flap at the endarterectomy was responsible for a transient neurological deficit.

Alternatives for hybrid procedures

The results obtained by hybrid techniques appear to be beneficial and interesting. By means of an access comparable to the standard carotid endarterectomy, it is feasible to correct a proximal lesion for which surgery, if employed, would require a more aggressive approach. It should be emphasized, however, that the total number of patients is limited, even when pooling different studies. Restenosis rate of the proximal lesion is less than 10% at two years' follow-up. Will series with longer follow-up provide equivalent results, and will favorable outcome remain? Can other, classic or more innovative techniques stabilize or improve these results?

We will address the conventional surgical technique and the endoluminal treatment as exclusive modalities, being the alternatives for the hybrid technique. Regarding management of the proximal lesion, two types of access can be distinguished: intrathoracic or cervical [7,8].

INTRATHORACIC ACCESS

By means of an intrathoracic approach, most often a sternotomy, the proximal lesion can be managed by endarterectomy or aorto-carotid bypass and subsequently combined with a CB endarterectomy. A bypass from the ascending aorta to the ICA can be considered, especially if the CCA is diseased along the whole axis. Using this access, peri-operative mortality varies between 0% and 14.7%, mainly caused by cardiac events. Simultaneously performed coronary bypass grafting aggravates the outcome [7]. Morbidity is also considerable with 8% stroke, 7% pulmonary complications, 3% myocardial infarctions, and 3% mediastinitis. Long-term patency, however, is excellent, associated with a low incidence of stroke (Table II). Surgical revascularization by intrathoracic access, despite the favorable results, is obviously a traumatic intervention and requires extensive pre-operative cardiac risk assessment.

Tandem lesions (SAA and CB) referred for intrathoracic surgery are different and not comparable with lesions for which a hybrid procedure might be considered. It most frequently concerns diffuse pathology in the SAAs with extensive stenotic disease. Therefore, both techniques cannot really be compared as far as surgical risks and mid-term and long-term results are concerned. Furthermore, intrathoracic access is usually indicated if coronary revascularization is required or if multivessel disease has to be managed by several aortic-distal bypasses. In all other cases, less invasive techniques might be preferred.

Table II	RESULTS OF REVASCULARIZATION OF SUPRA-AORTIC ARTERIES VIA INTRATHORACIC AND CERVICAL APPROACH [7,8]						
	Number	*Follow-up - %*		*Primary patency - %*		*Stroke-free event - %*	
		5 years	*10 years*	*5 years*	*10 years*	*5 years*	*10 years*
Intrathoracic access	100	73	52	94	88	87	81
Cervical access	182	72	41	91	82	92	84

CERVICAL ACCESS

The cervical approach allows direct re-implantation of the CCA in the subclavian artery. More frequently the CCA is revascularized by means of a bypass from the ipsilateral subclavian artery or contralateral vessels [26-31]. Subsequently, endarterectomy of the CB can be accomplished. Direct bypass grafting of the ICA, originating from one of the SAAs, is also an option. The surgical risk of this strictly cervical approach is considerably lower than the intrathoracic access, accounting for a combined neurological morbidity-mortality between 0% and 3.5%. Access of the mid and proximal subclavian artery can cause severe local complications: injury of the phrenic nerve, thoracic duct, and brachial plexus [26-28]. Archie [29] recommended avoiding these surgical problems by revascularizing the carotid axis from the proximal axillary artery with a long graft instead of a short subclavian bypass. Despite the excellent results obtained in this series, it seems difficult to prevent compression of the bypass behind the clavicle.

The patency rates of cervical SAA repair are well known and are excellent. Using different techniques, Berguer et al. [8] reported on primary patency rates of 91% and 82% at 5-year and 10-year follow-up, respectively. Stroke-free rate at 5 and 10 years was 92% and 84%, respectively. In a series of 29 axillo-carotid bypasses, Archie [29] reached patency rates of 93% and 87% at 1-year and 10-year follow-up, respectively. No immediate or secondary neurological deficit was encountered. Subclavian-carotid and carotid-carotid crossover grafts [26-28,30] offer similarly good results with regard to long-term patency and stroke-free outcome.

Bypass procedures to the CB or ICA are mainly restricted for completely occluded or multilevel diseased CCAs. These extensive lesions are not accessible for hybrid treatment. An attractive and elegant alternative for a proximal and limited CCA lesion is a short bypass between the subclavian and CCA or re-implantation of the latter in the subclavian artery. Re-implantation of the CCA in the subclavian artery is performed less frequently than re-implantation of the subclavian artery in the CCA. Results are quite similar [8] with a lower morbidity and a patency rate/stroke-free event rate close to 100% [31].

ENDOLUMINAL TREATMENT

Besides surgical treatment as a sole and hybrid procedure, one can imagine that bifocal stenoses in a carotid axis can be treated with a double endoluminal angioplasty. Access can be achieved via percutaneous cervical puncture, as proposed by Diethrich [32], with retrograde puncture to dilate the proximal CCA, followed by a second antegrade puncture to dilate the CB. This technique comprises a double risk of cervical hematoma and increases embolic events of two consecutive angioplasties. Few interventionalists apply the cervical access for this purpose because the femoral artery approach is technically much safer and easier.

Via femoral artery access, the proximal lesion can be managed first, followed by the cranial stenosis [33-35]. From a technical point of view, cerebral protection by means of an occluding balloon or filter has almost become mandatory in the endoluminal treatment of ICA stenosis. Proximal lesions in the SAA are not yet subject to this statement. The embolic risk at this level is probably smaller but to date no evidence can confirm this assumption. The diameters of the cerebral protection devices (occlusive balloon, filter) are adjusted to the diameter of the ICA. Recently, two filter systems have become available with diameters greater than 7.5 to 8 millimeters. For bifocal lesions it is necessary to successively position two cerebral protection devices, the first in the distal CCA and the second in the ICA. Alternatively, one protection system can be placed in the ICA; however, only amenable anatomical lesions can be treated with the latter technique, since maneuverability of the protection system will be limited.

In the absence of substantial experience with bifocal lesions, the results of endoluminal treatment can only be assumed by pooling the results of SAA and ICA angioplasties. The feasibility of SAA angioplasty has now been established but the long-term results are still unknown. All authors agree on the fact that only short stenoses should be treated. Certain anatomical features are considered risk factors: a distinct angulation between the aortic arch and the BCT, severe tortuosity of the CCA, a severely calcified aortic arch, extensive, ulcerated calcified and multilevel lesions. The presence of a thrombus contra-indicates angioplasty by femoral artery access and cannot be managed by cervical approach and carotid clamping [23].

In the most recent studies the success rate of BCT (tight stenoses or occlusions) or CCA angioplasty varies between 92% and 100% [23,36,37]. Neurological events and peri-operative mortality occur in 0% to 4%. Beside the recent series by Dzsinich et al. [36] comprising 112 dilatations of the BCT, other published series only contain some 30 to 40 cases. The series indicate the significant risks associated with the learning curve. Two studies allow assessment of mid-term results of BCT angioplasty [36,37]. In the experience of Dzsinich et al. [36], the patency rate of BCT angioplasty by femoral access was 93% at 33 months. Unfortunately, the substantial number of patients lost to follow-up (36%) limits the importance of this study. Queral and Criado [37] performed BCT angioplasty with primary stent placement (retrograde approach) in 37 patients and achieved a patency of 91.7% at 27 months.

The number of treated CCA is even less. Bergeron et al. [35] have performed 22 angioplasties of the CCA, 20 of which with stent placement. One patient died at the third postoperative day due to cerebral bleeding. Two restenoses occurred during a mean follow-up of 43 months. No secondary neurological events were observed. Watelet et al. [23] consider this technique the primary choice for short atherosclerotic stenoses. A late failure with restenosis does not compromise the options of secondary surgery.

Endoluminal treatment of the CB is performed much more frequently than SAA angioplasty. The published series show favorable outcome, similar to the results of conventional surgery [3,38-40]. Comparative studies assessing surgical and endoluminal techniques are easy to perform. Several have been published and others will soon appear. One study [40] has shown more favorable outcome after endoluminal repair, as compared to surgery; however, this study has been criticized because of methodological issues. Another study [41] has been stopped because of unacceptably poor outcome after carotid angioplasty. Mid-term and long-term restenosis rate appears to be higher after angioplasty compared to endarterectomy. Even if early results are similar to those of surgery, knowledge of the long-term results is absolutely mandatory before the efficacy of endoluminal treatment can be established.

At present, in specific and anatomically selected cases, it seems possible to treat bifocal lesions in one carotid axis by endoluminal techniques, using one or two cerebral protection devices, with or without stent placement at the CB and/or the proximal lesion. Although stent placement during CB dilatation seems to be an accepted policy, there is no study that provides information that would justify the same strategy for SAA lesions. However, according to recent studies [23,32-34], it is expected that stenting of the SAA will increasingly be applied. Regarding the hybrid procedures collected for this chapter, the incidence of restenosis was higher in patients who did not receive a stent. This difference was not statistically different.

Conclusion

At present, combined carotid endarterectomy and SAA angioplasty seem to establish an ideal hybrid strategy to treat bifocal lesions in one carotid axis, specifically addressing short and proximal stenoses of the SAA. The technique requires a radiologic-surgical environment and offers acceptable short-term and mid-term results. As compared to surgery as a sole strategy, this technique implies the advantage of a limited surgical access at the CB, associated with reduced morbidity. If treatment fails, conventional surgery can still be performed via cervical access, provided that one of the other SAAs are not affected. For diffuse and extensive lesions, if age and general condition of the patient allow, revascularization from the ascending aorta is preferred. Compared to endoluminal treatment as a sole modality, the hybrid technique offers the advantage of controlling the embolic risks and limiting the restenosis risk, especially at the level of the CB.

REFERENCES

1 Rothwell PM, Eliasziw M, Gutnikov SA, et al. Analysis of pooled data form the randomised controlled trials of endarterectomy for symptomatic carotid stenosis. *Lancet* 2003: 361: 107-116.

2 Zarins CK. Carotid endarterectomy: the gold standard. *J Endovasc Surg* 1996; 3: 10-15.

3 Wholey MH, Wholey MH, Jarmolowski CR, et al. Endovascular stents for carotid artery occlusive disease. *J Endovasc Surg* 1997; 4: 326-338.

4 Martorell F, Fabre J. El sindrome de obligato de los troncos supraaorticos. *Med Clin* 1944; 2: 26-30.

5 Debakey ME, Crawford ES, Cooley DA, et al. Cerebral arterial insufficiency: one to eleven-year results following arterial reconstructive operation. *Ann Surg* 1965; 161: 921-945.

6 Kieffer E, Sabatier J, Koskas F, et al. Atherosclerotic innominate artery occlusive disease: early and long-term results of surgical reconstruction. *J Vasc Surg* 1995; 21: 326-337.

7 Berguer R, Morasch MD, Kline RA. Transthoracic repair of innominate and common carotid artery disease: immediate and long-term outcome for 100 consecutive surgical reconstructions. *J Vasc Surg* 1998; 27: 34-42.

8 Berguer R, Morasch MD, Kline RA, et al. Cervical reconstruction of the supra-aortic trunks: a 16 year experience. *J Vasc Surg* 1999; 29: 239-248.

9 Motarjeme A. Percutaneous transluminal angioplasty of supra-aortic vessels. *J Endovasc Surg* 1996; 3: 171-181.

10 Schroth G, Remonda L, Dai Do D, et al. Stents in the treatment of supra-aortic vessel stenosis. *Ther Umsch* 2003; 60: 190-198.

11 Kerber CW, Cromwell LD, Loehder OL. Catheter dilatation of proximal carotid stenosis during distal bifurcation endarterectomy. *AJNR* 1980; 1: 348-349.

12 Dotter CT, Judkins MP. Transluminal treatment of arterio-sclerotic obstruction. Description of a technique and preliminary report of its application. *Circulation* 1964; 30: 654-670.

13 Lowman BG, Queral LA, Holbrook WA, et al. The correction of cerebrovascular insufficiency by transluminal dilatation: a preliminary report. *Am Surg* 1983; 49: 621-624.

14 Iannone LA, Toon RS, Rayl KL. Percutaneous transluminal angioplasty of the innominate artery combined with carotid endarterectomy. *Am Heart J* 1993 Dec; 126: 1466-1469.

15 Sidhu PS, Morgan MB, Walters HL, et al. Technical report. Combined carotid bifurcation endarterectomy and intra-operative transluminal angioplasty of a proximal common carotid artery stenosis: an alternative to extrathoracic bypass. *Clin Radiol* 1998; 53: 444-447.

16 Levien LJ, Benn CA, Veller MG, Fritz VU. Retrograde balloon angioplasty of brachiocephalic or common carotid artery stenoses at the time of carotid endarterectomy. *Eur J Vasc Endovasc Surg* 1998; 15: 521-527.

17 Arko FR, Buckley CJ, Lee SD, et al. Combined carotid endarterectomy with transluminal angioplasty and primary stenting of the supra-aortic vessels. *J Cardiovasc Surg* 2000; 41: 737-742.

18 Macierewicz J, Armon MP, Cleveland TJ, et al. Carotid endarterectomy combined with proximal stenting for multilevel disease. *Eur J Vasc Endovasc Surg* 2000; 20: 572-575.

19 Queral LA. Traitement endovasculaire des lésions focalisées des troncs supra-aortiques. *Ann Chir Vasc* 1998; 12: 396-403.

20 Criado FJ, Twena M. Techniques for endovascular recanalization of supra-aortic trunks. *J Endovasc Surg* 1996; 3: 405-413.

21 Sullivan TM, Gray BH, Bacharach JM, et al. Angioplasty and primary stenting of the subclavian, innominate, and common carotid arteries in 83 patients. *J Vasc Surg* 1998; 28 1059-1065.

22 Diethrich EB, Ndiaye M, Reid DB. Stenting in the carotid artery: initial experience in 110 patients. *J Endovasc Surg* 1996; 3: 42-62.

23 Watelet J, Douvrin F, Clavier E, Gallot JC. Traitement endoluminal des lésions occlusives des artères carotides primitives. In Kieffer E (ed). *Chirurgie des troncs supra-aortiques*. Paris, AERCV, 2003: pp 183-196.

24 Rouleau PA, Huston J, Gilbertson J, et al. Carotid artery tandem lesions: frequency of angiographic detection and consequences for endarterectomy. *AJNR* 1999; 20: 621-625.

25 Koskas F, Gomes D, Losy F, et al. Chirurgie associée des lésions athéromateuses des bifurcations carotidiennes et des troncs supra-aortiques. In Kieffer E (ed). *Chirurgie des troncs supra-aortiques*. Paris, AERCV, 2003: pp 197-207.

26 Fry WR, Martin JD, Clagett GP, Fry WJ. Extrathoracic carotid reconstruction: the subclavian-carotid artery bypass. *J Vasc Surg* 1992; 15: 83-88.

27 Salam TA, Smith RB, Lumsden AB. Extrathoracic bypass procedures for proximal common carotid artery lesions. *Am J Surg* 1993; 166: 163-166.

28 Sullivan TM. Subclavian-carotid bypass to an "isolated" carotid bifurcation: a retrospective analysis. *Ann Vasc Surg* 1996; 10: 283-289.

29 Archie JP. Axillary-to-carotid artery bypass grafting for symptomatic severe common carotid artery occlusive disease. *J Vasc Surg* 1999; 30: 1106-1112.

30 Ozsvath KJ, Roddy SP, Darling III C, et al. Carotid-carotid crossover bypass: is it a durable procedure? *J Vasc Surg* 2003; 37: 582-585.

31 Cinà CS, Safar HA, Lagana A, et al. Subclavian carotid transposition and bypass grafting: consecutive cohort study and systematic review. *J Vasc Surg* 2002; 35: 422-429.

32 Diethrich EB. Indications for carotid artery stenting: a preview of the potential derived from early experience. *J Endovasc Surg* 1996; 3: 132-139.

33 Bergeron P, Chambran P, Benichou H, Alessandri C. Recurrent carotid disease: will stents be an alternative to surgery? *J Endovasc Surg* 1996; 3: 76-79.

34 Kachel R. Results of balloon angioplasty in the carotid arteries. *J Endovasc Surg* 1996; 3: 22-30.

35 Bergeron P, Bafort AC, Pietri PA, et al. Long-term results of carotid angioplasty and stenting. In Amor M, Bergeron P, Mathias K, Raithel D (eds). *Carotid artery: angioplasty and stenting*. Torino, Minerva medica, 2002: pp 246-253.

36 Dzsinich C, Hüttl K. Traitement endovasculaire des lésions occlusives du tronc artériel brachiocéphalique. In Kieffer E (ed). *Chirurgie des troncs supra-aortiques*. Paris, AERCV, 2003: pp 109-116.

37 Queral LA, Criado FJ. The treatment of focal aortic branch lesions with Palmaz stents. *J Vasc Surg* 1996; 23: 368-375.

38 Yadav JS. Stenting and angioplasty with protection in patients at high risk for endarterectomy: the SAPPHIRE study. American heart association late breaking clinical trials (abstract). *Circulation* 2002; 106-109.

39 Whitlow PL, Lylyk P, Londero H. Carotid artery stenting protected with an emboli containment system. *Stroke* 2002; 33: 1308-1314.

40 Cavatas Investigators. Carotid and vertebral artery transluminal study (CAVATAS). *Lancet* 2001; 357: 1729-1737.

41 Naylor AR, Bolia A, Abbott RJ, et al. Randomized study of carotid angioplasty and stenting versus carotid endarterectomy: a stopped trial. *J Vasc Surg* 1998; 28: 326-334.

4

45

5

FIRST RIB RESECTION ASSOCIATED WITH PTA, THROMBOLYSIS OR VASCULAR RECONSTRUCTION

PATRICK FEUGIER, OLIVIER ROUVIÈRE
DENIS LYONNET, JEAN MICHEL CHEVALIER

Thoracic outlet syndrome (TOS) is one of the anatomical neurovascular compression syndromes, for which therapy has progressed substantially during the past years. The pathophysiology of this syndrome is usually complex, while its vascular complications are well known. Modern therapeutic options, such as thrombolysis and endovascular treatment, have expanded the therapeutic possibilities. Combination with already existing surgical therapies offers hybrid solutions that may be greatly beneficial to the patients.

Vascular compression is usually the result of costoclavicular compression, so that first rib resection appears to be the common denominator for the treatment of complicated TOS. Even combined with anticoagulant therapy, first rib resection is not sufficient to treat all complications involved. It does, however, play an important role, next to endovascular treatment and arterial or venous surgical reconstructions, in the treatment of complicated TOS by means of hybrid vascular procedures.

Arterial complications

Arterial complications are present in only 2% of cases of TOS. As they compromise the functional prognosis of the upper limb, they are the most serious complications [1]. Arterial vessel wall complications, graded in four stages according to Veith and Wengerten, are most often accompanied by an axillosubclavian thrombosis or symptoms of peripheral embolization [2]. Finding an arterial stenosis or an aneurysm should lead to preventive treatment. In case of acute ischemia, revascularization of the profound humeral artery and more distally in the limb requires emergency treatment and sometimes combined endoluminal and surgical procedures. Under these two circumstances the treatment of the subclavian compression should be discussed.

PERSONAL EXPERIENCE

From 1992 to 2003, 62 patients presenting with arterial symptoms due to TOS were treated (41% of the operated TOS). Of these, 36 were males and 19 females (7 bilateral cases), with a mean age of 42±5.1 years. Among these 55 patients, 14 presented with local or distal complications requiring specific surgical management, the details of which are shown in Table I. The dominating upper limb was affected in 76% of the cases. Eleven patients showed a lesion of the subclavian artery. Six of them required emergency surgery because of a thrombosis of the brachial artery in 1 case, and chronic digital embolization in 5 cases. Emergency fibrinolytic treatment was given in one patient with acute ischemia of the forearm (clinical case n° 2). All patients ben-

efited from arterial decompression by means of first rib resection. Additional removal of a cervical rib and thoracic sympathectomy was performed in 20 cases and 5 cases, respectively. An arterial reconstruction was performed in 9 cases (15%) during the same operation. This comprised resection of an arterial segment in 6 cases, aneurysm closure in 2 cases, and a venous graft in 1 case. Postoperative mortality was nil. One patient secondarily underwent a distal amputation of a finger. In 18 patients (28%) complications were seen due to the surgical approach. Mean follow-up duration was 3.2 years. Fifty patients became asymptomatic and could return to their jobs. Five still had their chronic digital ischemia. Seven patients maintained invalidating neurological symptoms, despite a complete decompression of the plexus. Ultrasound or angiographic investigation did not show any anomalies or progression at the arterial reconstruction sites.

In two patients endoluminal treatment was combined with conventional surgery. We will present these cases before discussing our conclusions.

Table I	ARTERIAL COMPLICATIONS OF TOS: CLINICAL ASPECTS, TREATMENT AND RESULTS IN OUR EXPERIENCE		
	Poststenotic dilatation	*Aneurysm and intima lesion*	*Thrombo-emboli and Raynaud's phenomenon*
Patients	4	1	9
Male/Female	3/1	1/0	4/5
Mean age (years)	37.5	39	39
Dominating limb	4	1	7
Surgical access			
Axillary	-	-	1
Supraclavicular	-	-	1
Supra- and infraclavicular	4	1	7
Treatment			
First rib resection	4	1	9
Cervical rib resection	3	1	4
Fibrinolysis	0	0	1
Sympathectomy	0	0	5
Arterial reconstruction	4	1	4
Results			
Asymptomatic	3	1	4
Distal ischemia	-	-	5
Invalidating complications	1	-	-

Clinical case n° 1. A 30-year-old, left-handed patient was urgently hospitalized in November 2000 because of an episode of severe ischemia of her dominant hand. Ultrasound and angiography confirmed the absence of palmar blood flow and thrombosis of the ulnar artery on the basis of an embolus. An aneurysm of the axillosubclavian junction with a diameter of 13 millimeters was found with an adherent heterogeneous thrombus. Provocation tests showed complete arterial compression in the costoclavicular region. For two years she had been complaining of pain in the left upper limb. A cervical X-ray showed a cervical rib. After a 5-day vasodilatory and anticoagulant treatment, the ischemic symptoms had decreased and it was decided to treat the aneurysm by means of a covered stent (Wallgraft 7 x 7 millimeters, *Boston Scientific Vascular, Natick, MA, USA*) via a femoral approach, and surgery in a second session to remove the first and the extra rib. After the endovascular procedure the endoprosthesis was found to be thrombosed completely without distal embolic complications; this was treated with vitamin K antagonists and vasodilating agents.

The patient was referred to us several weeks later, because of persisting invalidating ischemia of the hand. A new angiogram confirmed thrombosis of the subclavian artery beyond the vertebral artery, with a considerable collateral filling of the thyrocervical trunk, causing a palpable radial pulse and a pressure difference of 10 mmHg. A subclavian compression on the right side was diagnosed simultaneously. For these isolated distal symptoms a thoracic sympathectomy was performed. Three years after the initial embolic event, the patient was able to return to her job. She had persistent peripheral symptoms during cold weather and continuous muscular exercise that responded well to vasodilating treatment. The patient has started a legal procedure.

Clinical case n° 2. A 48-year-old woman visited the emergency room with acute ischemia of the left hand of three days. She smoked moderately and had not experienced this before. Physical investigation showed severe ischemia of the dominating hand and forearm, with a palpable brachial pulse, but no peripheral pulsations. A cardiac ultrasound did not reveal a cardiac reason for emboli. Duplex scanning showed thrombosis of the left brachial and ulnar artery with severely damped signals over the palmar vessels, as well as a dilatation of the subclavian artery with a diameter of 11

millimeters. Angiography via the femoral artery confirmed peripheral embolization from a subclavian wall thrombus in an aneurysm, complicating a unilateral TOS (Fig. 1), and the presence of a cervical rib. Local fibrinolysis with urokinase (UK) was started using a multiperforated catheter in the brachial artery. After 48 hours of uncomplicated treatment the complete distal runoff to the forearm and hand was restored. Two weeks after this event, the patient underwent resections of the aneurysm, the cervical and the first rib, via a subclavicular and supraclavicular approach. The patient was followed regularly for 18 months. She had no peripheral emboli and had returned to work in good condition. Duplex surveillance showed no anomalies at the site of the operation.

FIBRINOLYTIC TREATMENT

Fibrinolytic treatment has already been proposed for acute severe ischemia due to peripheral embolization [3]. We prefer systemic, in-situ injection of the fibrinolytic agent, which has, however, already led to a lethal hemorrhagic complication for this indication [4]. We have applied this once, with an excellent clinical and angiographic result without the need for peripheral thrombectomy. The procedure is identical to that described in peripheral arterial ischemic situations. It should not be considered if the angiogram shows no distal outflow. If a recent thrombus is found in the axillary artery, a primary surgical revascularization of the brachial artery via the upper arm should be considered. A peroperative bolus injection of UK may accompany the proximal revascularization. When fibrinolytic treatment is given, the decompression and/or arterial revascularization procedure needed to treat the TOS should be delayed.

SURGICAL DECOMPRESSION

Even if the nerve or vessel compression is not merely due to the narrow osseous opening between the first rib and clavicle, resection of the first rib remains necessary for an effective decompression of the neurovascular structures. This procedure is even more important when an osseous anomaly exists. In the treatment of a TOS associated with an arterial complication, this procedure should be combined with an anterior and medial scalenotomy and the resection of a cervical rib, if any [5]. Because of the fibromuscular anomalies that are nearly always present, single resection of a cervical rib is associated with a high failure or recurrence

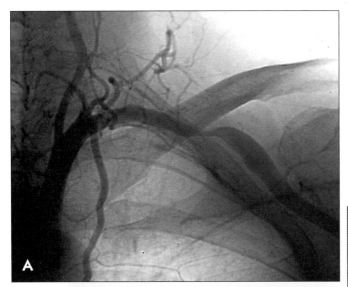

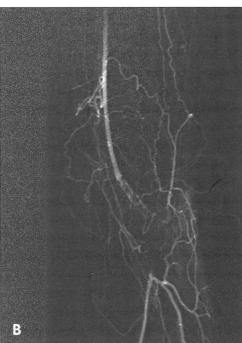

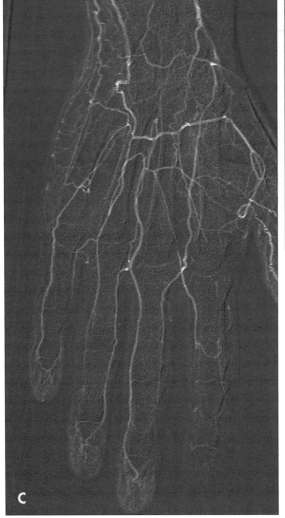

FIG. 1 Stenosis of the subclavian artery at the level of a cervical rib, associated with a poststenotic dilatation (A) causing ischemia of the forearm and hand because of thrombosis of the brachial and digital arteries and distal embolization (B, C). Fibrinolytic treatment led to arterial recanalization. Secondarily, the patient was treated by means of resection of the first and cervical rib.

rate [4]. This extended procedure may be performed by means of a supraclavicular or axillary approach, or through a sub- and supraclavicular incision. We prefer the latter approach if an arterial reconstruction is indicated, if also a venous compression exists, or if thoracic sympathectomy is indicated. This allows for resection of the subclavian muscle or the tendon of the minor pectoral muscle. The results are good, with a low recurrence rate and few major complications [6]. We do not have any experience with the transclavicular approach, which, by resecting the clavicle, offers a wide operation field, but has considerable cosmetic and functional consequences.

ARTERIAL RECONSTRUCTION

A stenosis that is symptomatic or shows poststenotic dilatation, a proximal occlusion, a subclavian aneurysm, or emboligenic lesions, is a good candidate for a curative or preventive arterial reconstruction. The proximal arterial lesion may be treated by resection of the aneurysm, aneurysmorrhaphy, or a venous bypass. The primary removal of the compressing fibromuscular and osseous elements is a requirement that has been clearly shown [7]. The two procedures, arterial reconstruction and decompression, are usually performed in one operation. For this purpose the combined sub- and supraclavicular approach is best.

To date, no studies have been published in favor of endovascular treatment of arterial subclavian lesions. Subclavian artery stenoses due to TOS are rarely clinically significant. Arterial decompression usually suffices to regain the arterial lumen. If needed, these can always be dilated conventionally during the arterial reconstruction. We have presented one direct complication after placement of a covered stent. Phipp et al. reported three cases of early clinical relapse after stent placement [8]. In one case, the endoprosthesis that covered a subclavian aneurysm showed a clear fracture. Although this comprised only three cases, there seems to be no place for arterial stenting for this indication, particularly without preceding arterial decompression. Despite their flexibility, the present stent characteristics do not meet the extrinsic mechanical demands. Moreover, given the good short- and long-term results of conventional surgical revascularizations, the reported complications, which often require a delicate re-intervention, seem unacceptable [9].

In conclusion, the treatment of arterial complications of TOS is well defined, although few studies are published. Surgical decompression of the subclavian artery is an indispensable intervention to cure the arterial lesion and the patency of the revascularization. Local fibrinolysis is a valuable additional therapy in the treatment of peripheral embolization that does not hamper an early proximal intervention. The role of endoluminal angioplasty seems limited for this indication when taking into account the possible failure and the good results of arterial surgery.

Combined treatment of venous complications

With an incidence estimated at 11 per 100.000 hospital admissions, thromboses of the subclavian vein (SVT) represent 1% to 4% of the deep venous thromboses [10,11]. They are the most frequent complication of TOS. Because they occur after exercise, they are also called "exercise-induced phlebitis" or the Paget-Schroetter syndrome [12]. Although these SVTs represent only 3.5% of the complications of a TOS, they form the eventual complication of intermittent venous compression with sometimes substantial functional sequelae, which require a therapeutic as well as preventive approach [13]. Traditionally, the treatment of SVT is based on long-term anticoagulation therapy with elevation and elastic compression of the arm. In nearly 75% of cases this results in more or less invalidating post-phlebitic symptoms [14]. The young age of the patients and the desire to improve the functional results have led several groups to propose a combined treatment, consisting of fibrinolysis and as comprehensive as possible surgical treatment: osseous decompression, venous reconstruction, and/or endovascular intervention [15-17]. Numerous encouraging clinical results have been reported, but the absence of prospective studies does not allow for a uniform therapeutic approach [18-20]. Various opinions exist about the timing of proposed treatments and the value of some prophylactic surgical interventions, which should balance the aggressiveness of the treatment with the severity of the possible consequences. Here, we will present our experience with the treatment of the venous complications in TOS, using a simplified therapeutic scheme and taking into account the prognostic factors.

PATIENTS AND METHODS

Between 1992 and 2003, 48 consecutive patients (29 males, 19 females) were treated for a TOS with a venous complication in the Edouard Herriot Hospital in Lyon, France. Eighteen patients, with a mean age of 37.3 years, presented with an intermittent venous compression syndrome, and 30 patients, with a mean age of 38.1 years, suffered from an SVT (Table II). The symptoms were bilateral in 21 cases (Table III). The diagnosis was confirmed by means of an ultrasound exam in 65% of the cases.

Treatment of the SVT was related to the delay before treatment started: if the delay was less than seven days and no common contra-indications were present, local thrombolysis was performed; if the delay was more than seven days, the patients was given an effective dosage of heparin. Thrombolysis was started directly following a phlebography of the affected arm. A short introducer (5F) was positioned in a superficial arm vein. Under angiographic control a bolus of 100.000 IU of UK (*Laboratoire Sanofi-Synthélabo, France*) was injected at the site of the thrombus through a multiperforated guided catheter placed at the thrombus. The thrombolytic agent was then infused with a dosage of 2.500 IU/kg/h, monitored by the complete coagulation status, including fibrinogen and fibrinogen degradation products. Simultaneously, heparin was administered systemically at a dosage of 100 IU/kg/h. Every 24 hours, radiological monitoring was performed, which allowed for repositioning of the catheter if necessary. Thrombolysis was stopped in case of hemorrhagic complications, if the fibrinogen level dropped below 1 g/L, in case of complete recanalization of the subclavian vein, or if no improvement was seen after two successive phlebographies. In none of the cases was the thrombolytic treatment continued more than 72 hours. After thrombolysis a dynamic bilateral phlebography was performed, taking images of the axillohumeral juncture. When venous compression and/or a residual venous stenosis were found, decompression surgery with phlebolysis or venous reconstruction (thrombectomy, endophlebectomy, angioplasty) was performed. This intervention was performed directly following thrombolysis, when a venous reconstruction had to be performed. If not, surgical decompression by means of first rib resection was postponed for several weeks, while giving curative anticoagulant treatment. When thrombolysis failed, anticoagulant treatment was given for three months. The patients were followed up regularly, both clinically and by means of ultrasound. Surgical decompression was planned when venous recanalization was found. In those who retained invalidating symptoms of a post-thrombotic syndrome, the subclavian vein reconstruction was combined with resection of the first rib and other compressing elements. All patients were followed-up one month postoperatively and subsequently after 6 and 12 months, including an ultrasound exam. The venous patency was checked in 15 cases by means of another phlebography after one year. All operated patients were contacted.

RESULTS

The 18 patients suffering from a venous compression without thrombosis ultimately benefited from surgical decompression including first rib resection in all cases, once a resection of an accessory muscle, and 18 times a complete fibrinolysis.

Table II	VENOUS COMPLICATIONS OF TOS: CLINICAL FINDINGS IN OUR EXPERIENCE		
		Compression (%)	*Thrombosis (%)*
Number of patients		18	30
Female/Male		11/7	8/22
Mean age (years)		37.3 ± 13.7	38.1 ± 13.8
High-level athletes		5 (28)	19 (63)
Dominating limb		13 (72)	18 (60)

Table III	VENOUS COMPLICATIONS OF TOS IN OUR EXPERIENCE: RESULTS OF VENOUS EXPLORATION OF ASYMPTOMATIC CONTRALATERAL SIDE		
Other side \ *Symptomatic side*		*Symptomatic venous compression*	*Thrombosis*
Asymptomatic compression		6	12
Symptomatic compression		2	0
Thrombosis		0	1

The surgical procedure was performed via an axillary approach in nine cases and through an infraclavicular approach in the remaining nine. The early and long-term results are shown in Table IV. After a mean follow-up duration of seven months, no venous thrombosis was observed despite a known stenosis in the subclavian vein, which was not treated in four patients. The functional results were excellent and permanent in the intermediate and long term.

While 17 TOS cases underwent only anticoagulant treatment, 13 benefited from thrombolysis. The mean delay before intervention was 4.6 days ± 1.6. Thrombolysis could be performed in time in all cases, without systemic complications. These thrombolyses led to six complete recanalizations, 4 incomplete recanalizations (residual stenosis or wall thrombus), and three failures.

Similarly, the anticoagulant treatments resulted in eight recanalizations and nine failures. Phlebography was performed in 18 patients in whom the vein was recanalized. Of these, 17 showed compression at the site of the thrombosis. In one case no compression was present and here the thrombosis could be explained by a coagulation anomaly. At the contralateral side, phlebography showed 13 asymptomatic venous compressions in 18 patients.

Among the 12 patients who presented with a TOS and could not be recanalized, only 7 showed invalidating consequences after one month of follow-up.

Surgical decompression of the thoracic outlet was performed 24 times after the occurrence of an SVT (80% of the cases). These 24 patients benefited from first rib resection; 9 cases via an axillary approach, and 15 via a combined supraclavicular and infraclavicular approach. Six patients, in whom the venous system could not be recanalized, did not undergo any decompression procedure. First rib resection was performed between 5 and 10 days after thrombolysis, 4 times in combination with venous thrombectomy, 2 times with an endophlebectomy-angioplasty, and once with an axillo-jugular bypass. We do not have any experience with endoluminal venous angioplasty for this indication.

Apart from the axillo-jugular bypass mentioned earlier, we performed a secondary venous reconstruction in seven patients who kept invalidating symptoms of a post-phlebitic syndrome three months after the first episode. These comprised five axillo-jugular bypasses, for which we used a split saphenous graft, which allowed us to make an autologous graft with an adequate caliber (Fig. 2), and two axillo-jugular transpositions. The venous reconstruction was always combined with a decompression procedure. Five patients who did not have any complaints after the SVT were treated with long-term anticoagulants.

Table IV	VENOUS COMPLICATIONS OF TOS: TREATMENT AND RESULTS IN OUR EXPERIENCE		
		Compression	Thrombosis
Number of patients		18	30
Treatment			
Anticoagulants only		0	6
Surgical techniques			
First rib resection		18	24
Phlebolysis		18	10
Thrombectomy		0	1
Muscle resection		1	0
Endophlebectomy		0	2
Venous reconstruction		0	8
Clinical results *			
Asymptomatic		17	27
Minor complications		1	3
Invalidating complications		0	0

* Mean follow-up: 7 years

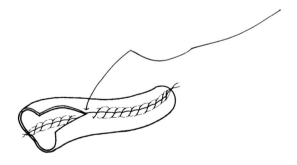

FIG. 2 Drawing showing the construction of a tailored venous graft by means of splitting the saphenous vein.

The in-situ fibrinolytic therapy was complicated by two hemorrhages at the puncture site and one aggravation of the thrombosis at the catheter tip. No postoperative deaths were seen. One patient was re-operated for a localized hematoma. The other complications we observed were three lymph fistulas and four cases with temporary neural root damage of C8-Th1. None of the patients who underwent surgery directly following the thrombolysis suffered from a complication, in particular a hemorrhage. All recanalized venous systems as well as all the venous reconstructions were checked by means of duplex ultrasound before dismissal from the hospital and all were found to be patent. A 30% residual stenosis was seen in five patients after recanalization. These patients later underwent surgical decompression.

Twenty-eight patients were followed-up during a mean period of 7 years ± 3.2. Their initial symptoms had disappeared. They had been able to return to their professional and sport activities after a mean period of 86 days (23 days – 5.5 months). Treatment with vitamin K antagonists was continued in patients after a venous reconstruction or awaiting a contralateral intervention. In six patients a non-invalidating edema persisted. In 1 patient a thrombosis of the basilar vein was observed 10 months after fibrinolytic therapy. Ninety percent of the treated patients had become asymptomatic. Three patients stated to suffer occasionally from edema, which in one patient was associated with persisting paresthesiae in the region of the internal cutaneous brachial nerve. Duplex ultrasound and/or phlebography confirmed the patency of the vein in all operated patients. In two patients who practiced muscle training continually, a persisting stenosis was seen related to the tendon of the lesser pectoral muscle.

Literature data

ANTICOAGULANT TREATMENT
This is identical to that for deep venous thrombosis of the lower extremities. It comprises direct intravenous administration of heparin or low molecular weight heparins. This therapy should be effective quickly in order to limit the growth of the thrombus, to prevent possible pulmonary embolization (1% to 10%), and to enhance local fibrinolysis [21]. After a few days this treatment is replaced by vita-

min K antagonists for 3 to 12 months. This therapy should always be given, either as single treatment or in addition to fibrinolysis. In our experience, this accompanies every decompression procedure or venous reconstruction performed after the acute phase. The results of this treatment only are less satisfying than the treatment of a secondary axillo-subclavian thrombosis. Invalidating edema is the most common complication and causes functional limitations in more than 70% of the patients treated [22-24]. Post-phlebitic syndromes complicated by ulcers or gangrene are exceptional [25].

FIBRINOLYTIC TREATMENT
Because of these limited results, several authors have promoted thrombolytic therapies to restore venous patency in TOS that exist a few days [26-28]. This more aggressive technique uses protocols based on streptokinase (SK), UK, or rt-PA (Table V). Because of the absence of antigenic properties, based on its low systemic complication rate, its management, and its good results in arterial disease, UK appears the product of choice. The results vary depending on the method of administration and the dosage, which can vary between 750 IU/kg/h and 4.400 IU/kg/h [18,34]. In-situ fibrinolysis has the advantage to act directly on the thrombus in order to accelerate the recanalization and to prevent systemic complications. No series has reported a serious hemorrhage after in-situ fibrinolysis. Minor complications observed using streptokinase were hematomas, prolonged bleeding from the puncture site, hematuria, and fever [27,32]. In-situ injection enables direct phlebographic control and to prove the external compression at the end of the procedure (Fig. 3). Although the reported protocols differ and the series are small, fibrinolytic treatment leads to recanalization in 36% to 100% of the cases and a clinical improvement in 42% to 100% [15,31]. Of the three failures in our series, two failures were secondary to local hemorrhage and termination of the procedure after 72 hours. Retrospectively, the delay between onset of the symptoms and the administration of the fibrinolytic agent was unclear. A delay of less than seven days is a good prognostic factor [32,35]. Some authors even advocate a delay of less than five days, but do not specify which fibrinolytic agent is to be used [22,26].

VENOUS THROMBECTOMY
Direct surgical thrombectomy was performed for the first time in 1926 by means of phlebotomy. This

Table V   RESULTS OF FIBRINOLYTIC THERAPY IN SVT ACCORDING TO THE LITERATURE

1st author [ref.]	Number of patients	Delay (days)	Agent used	Dose	Failure %	Residual lesions %	Asymptomatic %	Follow-up
In-situ								
Becker [26]	4	4.3	UK	1500 UI/kg/h	0	50	75	2 months
Sanders [29]	11	< 5	SK	NS	36	NS	64	NS
Molina [30]	28	-	UK	3000 UI/kg/h	14	53	83	1-3 years
Meier [16]	11	NS	UK	1800 UI/kg/h	0	72	27	NS
Adelman [18]	18	NS	UK	1250 UI/kg/h	29	27	78	1,5 years
Kreienberg [31]	23	9.4	UK rt-PA	2500 UI/kg/h 4 mg/h	0	8.6	-	4 years
Personal experience	13	4.6	UK	2500 UI/kg/h	23	31	90	7 years
Systemic								
Zimmermann [32]	13	32	UK	1000 UI/kg/h	15	54	46	6 months
Sanders [29]	14	< 5	SK	NS	15	NS	75	NS
Urschel [33]	33	NS	UK, SK	1500 UI/kg/h	6	6	88	0-7 years
Machleder [15]	11 / 17	2	SK UK	NS	64 23	NS	100 76.5	3.1 years

rt-PA: recombinant tissue plasminogen activator
SK: streptokinase
SVT: subclavian vein thrombosis
UK: urokinase
NS: not specified

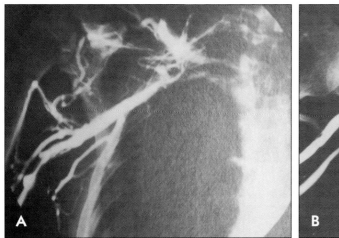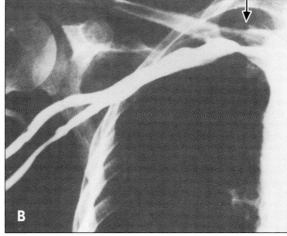

FIG. 3   A - Acute thrombosis of the right subclavian vein, as seen on day four in a 16 year-old patient.   B - After in-situ fibrinolytic treatment, a residual costoclavicular compression was found during minor abduction.

can be performed via a peripheral vein or directly through the subclavian vein. Nowadays it is acknowledged that thrombectomy is more effective when performed before the fifth day after the start of the symptoms. To avoid a possible recurrence, it should be accompanied with a venous decompression and complete phlebolysis [17]. Some prefer to always create a temporary arteriovenous fistula, which we have not done in the two cases of our series [29]. The early results appear to be excellent, but the number of reported cases is limited and the follow-up is poor (Table VI).

VENOUS RECONSTRUCTION

When the patency is not completely restored after fibrinolysis or after surgical venous thrombectomy, correction of the endoluminal venous anomaly (synechia, valve) may be performed by means of an endophlebectomy. This intervention, advocated by Beaujean, is rarely reported in the literature [6,39]. It is performed via a large infraclavicular incision or combined approach (claviculotomy and mediastinotomy) after resection of the first rib. The longitudinal phlebotomy is closed by a venous patch. A secondary surgical venous reconstruction may be justified in case of a post-phlebitic syndrome (edema, chronic pain), which always depends on the severity of the symptoms and the influence of the position of the arm on the collateral circulation. The most frequently used surgical techniques are transposition of the internal jugular vein or a venous bypass using the technique described above (Fig. 2). The venous reconstruction is performed together with the first rib resection. A temporary humeral or axillary arteriovenous fistula may be

added [20,30,40]. Drawbacks are the risk of acute thrombosis, the sacrifice of an internal jugular vein, the possibility of compression of the bypass by the clavicle, and the cosmetic aspects.

The use of a vascular prosthesis is accompanied by a considerably high failure risk [41]. Too few series have been reported on these interventions to show exact results. If no autologous venous material is available, endophlebectomy seems to be preferable rather than a prosthesis.

FIRST RIB RESECTION

At present, the pathophysiological mechanisms leading to an SVT are well known [10]. The repetitive or continuous damage to the subclavian vein due to costoclavicular compression is the main factor. Hence, it seems logical to perform a surgical decompression of the neurovascular subclavian trunk whenever a compression is diagnosed. A recanalization after surgery or thrombolysis does not make a secondary surgical decompression redundant, as it reduces the early risk of thrombosis and leads to better long-term results [17]. In contrast, several other authors reserve this indication only for those patients who remain functionally inadequate after three months [42]. Lokanathan et al. found 3 out of 11 patients after a long follow-up period with a re-thrombosis with progressive clinical symptoms [43]. First rib resection and transsection of the subclavian muscle alleviate the external venous compression. It should be combined with a complete phlebolysis and be added to a venous reconstruction, if performed. If this is done as a single procedure, the axillary approach according to Roos seems preferable [1]. The combined infraclavicular

Table VI	RESULTS OF VENOUS THROMBECTOMY IN SVT ACCORDING TO THE LITERATURE				
1st author [ref.]	*Number of patients*	*Delay (days)*	*Asymptomatic %*	*Follow-up*
Drapanas [36]	2	1	100	6 months
De Weese [37]	20	NS	100	6 months
Grüss [38]	49	NS	86	NS
Sanders [29]	33	NS	94	NS

SVT: subclavian vein thrombosis
NS: not specified

and supraclavicular approach allows for a safe decompression and revascularization in the same session. We have never needed a claviculotomy, which can induce serious functional troubles with the shoulder [13].

Initially, surgical decompression was planned some months after thrombolytic treatment [15]. However, several authors have shown the value and safety of performing this surgical procedure directly after the venous recanalization in order to reduce the short-term risk of re-thrombosis [45,46]. A persisting venous lesion or compression may be responsible for 10% of the early thrombotic recurrences, despite adequate anticoagulant treatment [15]. With a 13% postoperative hematoma rate, Kreienberg et al. found direct decompression to be an effective treatment [31], with the advantage of an early return to normal activities and a reduced treatment period with vitamin K antagonists [47].

It is difficult to evaluate the results of surgical decompression per se. On the basis of a literature review, Sanders and Hang estimated the success rate to be 80% [29]. Except for Etheredge et al. [48], the majority of authors found no effect of decompression in case of longstanding thrombosis. Because of the risk of thrombosis after stopping the anticoagulant treatment, we always advise patients with an asymptomatic contralateral compression to undergo surgical decompression. This prophylactic attitude is particularly indicated for high-level athletes.

ENDOLUMINAL TREATMENT

Percutaneous transluminal angioplasty (PTA) has been proposed to treat residual stenoses. Some perform a PTA at the time of the last phlebographic follow-up before any surgical decompression [49]. However, its intermediate and long-term effect is disputable when the real cause of the thrombosis is not removed. Surgical failures do occur and short-term results of isolated PTA are mediocre. Obviously, the efficacy of simply dilating a residual lesion due to a synechia or elastic fibrous tissue is poor. Beygui et al., and later Lee et al., did not observe any phlebographic improvement after 12 and 11 cases of PTA, respectively [34,42]. No publications have stated the use of the newer generations of balloons such as cutting balloons for this indication.

Performing venous stenting seems a natural consequence of the protocol as proposed by Machleder [15]. The indication is a remaining residual stenosis of more than 50% after PTA. The necessity of using stents with a large diameter (10 to 14 millimeters) at a very mobile anatomical area requires the use of an auto-expanding, flexible stent. The few results show intermediate-term patencies between 64% and 75% (Table VII). When no previous venous decompression is performed, several authors consider the risk of an early venous re-thrombosis or stent fracture to be important [8,50]. Meier et al. found a constant deformation of stents after forced abduction, related to the first rib, but in one case also

Table VII	RESULTS OF ENDOVASCULAR TREATMENT OF SVT ACCORDING TO THE LITERATURE				
1st author [ref.]	*Number of patients*	*Follow-up (years)*	*Residual symptoms %*	*Complications*	*Patency %*
PTA only					
Lokanathan [39]	12	2.9	71	None	83
Kreienberg [31]	9	4	0	NS	100
PTA + stent					
Meier [16]	8	1	25	2 fractures 2 restenoses	75
Kreienberg [31]	14	3	43	-	64

PTA: percutaneous transluminal angioplasty
SVT: subclavian vein thrombosis
NS: not specified

to the second rib [16]. Stent fractures have been observed before eight months of follow-up. If one can wait for adequate treatment of the intrinsic venous lesions, the placement of a stent per se will not treat the external compression. However, the risk and consequences of a possible restenosis due to hyperplasia are unknown.

Algorithm of combined procedures

For an uncomplicated stenosis, a combined treatment comprising angioplasty and surgical decompression is not indicated. Most often, surgical release of the vein will prevent a thrombotic event and will adequately treat the venous claudication. It is for symptomatic recurrences of a stenosis of the subclavian vein that we reserve angioplasty with or without stenting when the surgical decompression seems adequate.

In case of a SVT, the treatment algorithm has changed substantially after the first description of this syndrome [12] (Table VIII). The primary goal is to improve the functional outcome of these patients, who usually are young and active. We propose a therapeutic scheme, which is based on our experience and literature data (Fig. 4). Venous desobstruction by means of in-situ fibrinolysis or thrombectomy should be performed when the SVT is recent. Once the TOS is confirmed, recanalization of the vein is followed by a decompression procedure, which can be performed shortly after or several weeks later. We prefer direct surgical treatment when an indication for venous thrombectomy or additional endophlebectomy exists.

Even though several authors recognize endoluminal treatment as an innovative treatment option for stenoses of the axillosubclavian vein, the early and long-term results, which are even more dubious, should make its place doubtful for this indication. We prefer to perform a venous reconstruction together with the surgical decompression. This therapeutic policy seems even more justified when the patient is a high-level athlete, presenting with a long venous stenosis or an extended thrombosis of the brachial vein.

In case of a post-phlebitic syndrome of the upper limb, complex surgical venous reconstructions remain exceptional and limited to invalidating postphlebitic symptoms. Isolated surgical decompression may sometimes be indicated, either to decompress the collateral circulation, or in case of additional neurological or arterial symptoms.

5
58

| Table VIII | RESULTS OF COMBINED TREATMENTS OF SVT ACCORDING TO THE LITERATURE |

1st author [ref.]	*Number of patients*	*Initial treatment*	*Curative surgery*			*Patency %*	*Follow-up*	*Functional result*	
			First rib resection	*%*	*Venous reconstruction (%)*			*Asymptomatic %*	*Complications %*
Urschel [47]	67	F,ac,T	Yes	81	-	NS	7-25 years	60	40
Machleder [15]	50	F,ac,T,PTA	Yes	72	-	64	3.1 years	80	12
Meier [16]	11	F,ac,PTA	Yes	45	-	64	1 year	72	18
Adelman [18]	18	F,ac	Yes	65	-	100	20.8 months	71	29
Kreienberg [31]	23	F,ac,PTA	Yes	70	-	78	4 years	66	13
Personal experience	30	F,ac,T	Yes	80	8 (37)	83	7 years	90	0

ac: anticoagulants
F: fibrinolysis
PTA: percutaneous transluminal angioplasty
SVT: subclavian vein thrombosis
T: surgical thrombectomy
NS: not specified

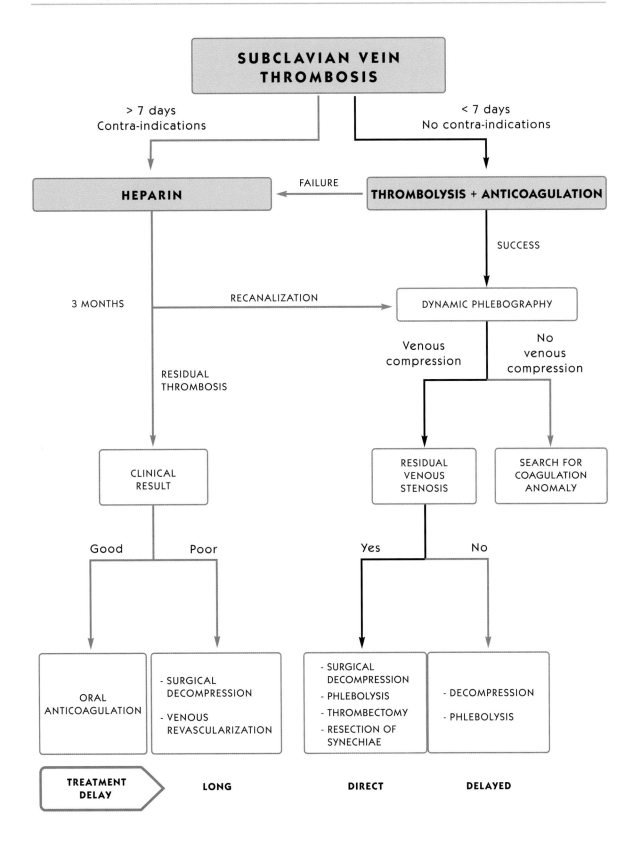

FIG. 4 Algorithm for the treatment of acute subclavian vein obstructions.

5
59

Conclusion

It has been established that the initial treatment of a SVT should be treated as early as possible, comprising fibrinolysis, complete removal of the external compression, and the treatment of any intrinsic venous stenoses. For this indication, surgical decompression remains the mainstay of clinical success and to avoid an early venous re-thrombosis. In direct combination with fibrinolytic treatment and venous decompression, residual stenoses may be treated with a surgical reconstruction or a stent. However, the long-term patency of PTA for this indication awaits further assessment. Multicenter studies will be necessary to evaluate this therapeutic strategy.

REFERENCES

1 Roos DB. Historical perspectives and anatomic considerations. Thoracic outlet syndrome. *Semin Thorac Cardiovasc Surg* 1996; 8: 183-189.

2 Veith FJ, Wengerten KR. Aspect cliniques des manifestations artérielles du syndrome de la traversée thoracobrachiale. In: Kieffer E (ed). *Les syndromes de la traversée thoracobrachiale.* Paris, AERCV 1989: pp 159-164.

3 Hood DB, Kuehne J, Yellin AE, Weaver FA. Vascular complications of thoracic outlet syndrome. *Am Surg* 1997; 63: 913-917.

4 Cormier JM, Amrane M, Ward A, et al. Arterial complications of the thoracic outlet syndrome: fifty-five operative cases. *J Vasc Surg* 1989; 9: 778-787.

5 Scher LA, Veith FJ, Samson RH, et al. Vascular complications of thoracic outlet syndrome. *J Vasc Surg* 1986; 3: 565-568.

6 Salo JA, Varstela E, Ketonen P, et al. Management of vascular complications in thoracic outlet syndrome. *Acta Chir Scand* 1988; 154: 349-352.

7 Roos DB. The place for scalenectomy and first-rib resection in thoracic outlet syndrome. *Surgery* 1982; 92: 1077-1085.

8 Phipp LH, Scott DJ, Kessel D, Robertson I. Subclavian stents and stent-grafts: cause for concern? *J Endovasc Surg* 1999; 6: 223-226.

9 Kieffer E, Jue-Denis P, Benhamou M, et al. Arterial complications in the thoracobrachial outlet syndrome. Surgical treatment of 38 cases. *Chirurgie* 1983; 109: 714-722.

10 Hurlbert SN, Rutherford RB. Primary subclavian-axillary vein thrombosis. *Ann Vasc Surg* 1995; 9: 217-223.

11 Coon WW, Willis PW 3rd. Thrombosis of axillary and subclavian veins. *Arch Surg* 1967; 94: 657-663.

12 Paget J. Clinical lectures and essays. London, Longmans Green 1875.

13 Gloviczki P, Kazmier FJ, Hollier LH. Axillary-subclavian venous occlusion: the morbidity of a nonlethal disease. *J Vasc Surg* 1986; 4: 333-337.

14 Tilney ML, Griffiths HJ, Edwards EA. Natural history of major venous thrombosis of the upper extremity. *Arch Surg* 1970; 101: 792-796.

15 Machleder HI. Evaluation of a new treatment strategy for Paget-Schroetter syndrome: spontaneous thrombosis of the axillary-subclavian vein. *J Vasc Surg* 1993; 17: 305-317.

16 Meier GH, Pollak JS, Rosenblatt M, et al. Initial experience with venous stents in exertional axillary-subclavian vein thrombosis. *J Vasc Surg* 1996; 24: 974-983.

17 Thompson RW, Schneider PA, Nelken NA, et al. Circumferential venolysis and paraclavicular thoracic outlet decompression for *effort thrombosis* of the subclavian vein. *J Vasc Surg* 1992; 16: 723-732.

18 Adelman MA, Stone DH, Riles TS, et al. A multidisciplinary approach to the treatment of Paget-Schroetter syndrome. *Ann Vasc Surg* 1997; 11: 149-154.

19 Rutherford RB, Hurlbert SN. Primary subclavian-axillary vein thrombosis: consensus and commentary. *Cardiovasc Surg* 1996; 4: 420-423.

20 Sanders RJ, Cooper MA. Surgical management of subclavian vein obstruction, including six cases of subclavian vein bypass. *Surgery* 1995; 118: 856-863.

21 Eklof B. Les thromboses veineuses axillo-sous-clavières. In: Kieffer E (ed). *Les syndromes de la traversée thoracobrachiale.* Paris, AERCV 1989: pp 189-194.

22 Aburahma AF, Sadler D, Stuart P, et al. Conventional versus thrombolytic therapy in spontaneous (effort) axillary-subclavian vein thrombosis. *Am J Surg* 1991; 161: 459-465.

23 Ameli FM, Minas T, Weiss M, Provan JL. Consequences of "conservative" conventional management of axillary vein thrombosis. *Can J Surg* 1987; 30: 167-169.

24 Adams JT, DeWeese JA. *Effort* thrombosis of the axillary and the subclavian veins. *J Trauma* 1971; 11: 923-930.

25 Donayre CE, White GH, Mehringer SM, Wilson SE. Pathogenesis determines late morbidity of axillosubclavian vein thrombosis. *Am J Surg* 1986; 152: 179-184.

26 Becker GJ, Holden RW, Rabe FE, et al. Local thrombolytic therapy for subclavian and axillary vein thrombosis. Treatment of the thoracic inlet syndrome. *Radiology* 1983; 149: 419-423.

27 Druy EM, Trout HH 3rd, Giordano JM, Hix WR. Lytic therapy in the treatment of axillary and subclavian vein thrombosis. *J Vasc Surg* 1985; 2: 821-827.

28 Taylor LM Jr, McAllister WR, Dennis DL, Porter JM. Thrombolytic therapy followed by first rib resection for spontaneous *(effort)* subclavian vein thrombosis. *Am J Surg* 1985; 149: 644-647.

29 Sanders RJ, Hang C. Subclavian vein obstruction and thoracic outlet syndrome: a review of etiology and management. *Ann Vasc Surg* 1990; 4: 397-410.

30 Molina JE. Surgery for effort thrombosis of the subclavian vein. *J Thorac Cardiovasc Surg* 1992; 103: 341-346.

31 Kreienberg PB, Chang BB, Darling RC 3rd, et al. Long-term results in patients treated with thrombolysis, thoracic inlet decompression, and subclavian vein stenting for Paget-Schroetter syndrome. *J Vasc Surg* 2001; 33 (2 Suppl): S100-105.

32 Zimmermann R, Morl H, Harenberg J, et al. Urokinase therapy of subclavian-axillary vein thrombosis. *Klin Wochenschr* 1981; 59: 851-856.

33 Urschel HC Jr, Razzuk MA. Improved management of the Paget-Schroetter syndrome secondary to thoracic outlet compression. *Ann Thorac Surg* 1991; 52: 1217-1221.

34 Beygui RE, Olcott C 4th, Dalman RL. Subclavian vein thrombosis: outcome analysis based on etiology and modality of treatment. *Ann Vasc Surg* 1997; 11: 247-255.

35 Wilson JJ, Zahn CA, Newman H. Fibrinolytic therapy for idiopathic subclavian-axillary vein thrombosis. *Am J Surg* 1990; 159: 208-211.

36 Drapanas T, Curran WL. Thrombectomy in the treatment of *effort* thrombosis of the axillary and subclavian veins. *J Trauma* 1966; 6: 107-119.

37 DeWeese JA, Adams JT, Gaiser DL. Subclavian venous thrombectomy. *Circulation* 1970; 41 (5 Suppl): II158-164.

38 Gruss JD. Thrombectomie veineuse axillo-sous-clavière. In: Kieffer E (ed). *Les syndromes de la traversée thoracobrachiale.* Paris, AERCV 1989: pp 195-198.

39 Beaujean MA. Reconstruction directe de la "veine axillo-sous-clavière entravée" dans le cadre de la pathologie du défilé cervico-scapulo-thoracique. In: Kieffer E (ed). *Les syndromes de la traversée thoracobrachiale.* Paris, AERCV 1989: pp 207-217.

40 Feugier P, Aleksic I, Salari R, et al. Long-term results of venous revascularization for Paget-Schroetter syndrome in athletes. *Ann Vasc Surg* 2001; 15: 212-218.

41 Bergan JJ, McCarthy WJ, Vogelzang R, Peck JJ. Thromboses Veineuses Axillo-sous-clavières: place de la thrombolyse et de l'angioplastie. In: Kieffer E (ed). *Les syndromes de la traversée thoracobrachiale.* Paris, AERCV 1989: pp 199-206.

42 Lee WA, Hill BB, Harris EJ Jr, et al. Surgical intervention is not required for all patients with subclavian vein thrombosis. *J Vasc Surg* 2000; 32: 57-67.

43 Lokanathan R, Salvian AJ, Chen JC, et al. Outcome after thrombolysis and selective thoracic outlet decompression for primary axillary vein thrombosis. *J Vasc Surg* 2001; 33: 783-788.

44 Devin R. Aspects médico-légaux de la chirurgie des syndromes de la traversée thoracobrachiale. In: Kieffer E (ed). *Les syndromes de la traversée thoracobrachiale.* Paris, AERCV 1989: pp 329-333.

45 Lee MC, Grassi CJ, Belkin M, et al. Early operative intervention after thrombolytic therapy for primary subclavian vein thrombosis: an effective treatment approach. *J Vasc Surg* 1998; 27: 1101-1108.

46 Angle N, Gelabert HA, Farooq MM, et al. Safety and efficacy of early surgical decompression of the thoracic outlet for Paget-Schroetter syndrome. *Ann Vasc Surg* 2001; 15: 37-42.

47 Molina JE. Need for emergency treatment in subclavian vein effort thrombosis. *J Am Coll Surg* 1995; 181: 414-420.

48 Etheredge S, Wilbur B, Stoney RJ. Thoracic outlet syndrome. *Am J Surg* 1979; 138: 175-182.

49 Glanz S, Gordon DH, Lipkowitz GS, et al. Axillary and subclavian vein stenosis: percutaneous angioplasty. *Radiology* 1988; 168: 371-373.

50 Bjarnason H, Hunter DW, Crain MR, et al. Collapse of a Palmaz stent in the subclavian vein. *AJR Am J Roentgenol* 1993; 160: 1123-1124.

6

HYBRID PROCEDURES FOR TYPE B AORTIC DISSECTION

ROBERTO CHIESA, YAMUME TSHOMBA
EFREM CIVILINI, GERMANO MELISSANO
LUCA BERTOGLIO, FRANCESCO SETACCI

Type B aortic dissection is an insidious, multifocal, and evolving disease. Regardless of the acute organ and/or extremity ischemia, it generally involves the whole thoraco-abdominal aortic wall leading to progressive and chronic weakening. For this reason, a complete and definitive therapy is improbable and, during follow-up, redo-operations or adjunctive procedures are often required.

The therapeutic armamentarium of the vascular surgeon has evolved during the last years for both open repair and endovascular techniques; the results of the treatment of thoraco-abdominal disease are improved, yet current prognosis of type B aortic dissection still remains poor, particularly in the complicated acute phase.

Acute type B dissection: an unsolved problem?

In the case of uncomplicated pattern, careful follow-up and aggressive hypotensive treatment are generally considered the therapy of choice [1]. Nevertheless, aortic-related mortality of medical patients reported in *the International Registry of Acute Aortic Dissection* is significant [2]. A "complication-specific" approach is generally carried out to exclusively correct early ischemic complications [3,4], although reported mortality rates associated with visceral ischemia are invariably high with both the open and the endovascular approach [2].

The risk of rupture in the acute phase is low but it exists and, in cases of evident extra-aortic blood leakage, even with rapid diagnosis, both pressing medical treatment and emergency open repair, mortality is high, ranging from 29% to 50% [5].

Sealing by endograft of the dissecting primary entry tear, generally originating in the descending thoracic aorta, is a hazardous procedure in the acute phase, and it may be not effective. Results have already been discussed extensively and indications are debated [5-7].

Chronic type B dissection: an incurable disease?

For patients surviving the acute phase, open repair of evolving dissecting thoracic and thoraco-abdominal aneurysms is required in 20% to 40% of cases. Nowadays, in these patients, aortic replacement is not generally characterized by increased mortality and morbidity rates compared to atherosclerotic aneurysms [8].

Although several positive experiences have been reported, endovascular exclusion of dissecting aneurysms by means of a thoracic endograft is a procedure that is under debate [9]. Following both open and endovascular procedures, further operations are often required for aortic dilatation of untreated aortic segments.

Management of ischemic complications may be required also in the chronic phase, related to visceral or lower limb hypoperfusion or to renovascular hypertension due to renal ischemia [10]. In these cases, less extensive options to restore perfusion are generally adopted and endovascular techniques represent the first-step attempt. If the less invasive repairs fail, more extensive open approaches are required. A careful follow-up is constantly mandatory to monitor the evolving nature of the disease.

In these patients, as long as there is a remnant of native aortic tissue, there is the risk of dilatation and ischemic syndromes; however, morbidity and mortality rates of thoraco-abdominal aortic repair are too high to justify extensive repair in absence of real dilatation or ischemic complications.

Limits of open treatment

Traditional thoracic and thoraco-abdominal open surgery has demonstrated over the years to effectively manage aortic dissection also; however, there is increasing evidence that less invasive alternative approaches are possible. During open repair of the thoracic and thoraco-abdominal aorta, cardiac and renal comorbidities, increased age, presence of aneurysm-related symptoms, surgical access, duration of proximal aortic cross-clamping, extension of the affected aorta, peri-operative hemodynamic changes, and organ ischemia have been determined as the main variables affecting surgical outcome. During repair of type B dissection, further challenges are related to the aortic tissue friability, to the false lumen extension and morphological features, to the site and number of entry tears, and to the presence of a variety of malperfusion syndromes.

Recent literature on open surgical treatment of thoracic and thoraco-abdominal aortic aneurysms (TAAAs) has shown improved results with the systematic use of technical adjuncts like distal aortic perfusion and cerebrospinal fluid drainage [11]. These advantages have also been proven for type B dissection surgery [8]. During emergency thoracic aortic replacement for acute type B dissection, however, the use of these adjuncts may not be possible because of the hemodynamic instability of the patient. Also, during management of chronic dissecting thoracic or thoraco-abdominal aneurysms, distal cannulation may be challenging because of the presence of a false lumen, despite the fact that cannulation of a pulsating femoral artery generally guarantees adequate blood flow through the visceral vessels arising from both the true and false lumen. Furthermore, the extracorporeal circuit currently used for left heart bypass generally consists of a centrifugal pump and, in case of cannulation of the false lumen, the self-limiting pressure reduces the risk of a retrograde dissection of an intimal flap [12].

The extreme fragility of the aortic wall in an acute dissecting aneurysm makes it difficult to control and to clamp the proximal aorta and may require an open proximal anastomosis under hypothermic circulatory arrest. This technique, often complicated by coagulopathy, may also be necessary in the presence of large chronic dissective aneurysms involving the distal aortic arch. In these cases the size of the aneurysm, associated with the peri-adventitial fibrosis typical in aortic dissections, may jeopardize the control of the proximal aortic neck and increase the risk of injury to the nerves (i.e., recurrent laryngeal, phrenic, and vagus nerves), pulmonary vessels, and esophagus, also calling for a hypothermic arrest.

Aortic type B dissection is a typical example of multifocal and multiple stage disease, frequently requiring thoracic redo-operations. In these cases and in the presence of other redo thoracic cardiovascular surgery or a history of pulmonary resection or pleuritis, severe pleuric adhesions may be present. Although in experienced centers previous thoracic aortic repair is not considered as a significant risk factor for the outcome of thoraco-abdominal aortic repair [13], dissection and control of the thoracic aorta may lead to excessive bleeding or pulmonary parenchymal lesions, inducing acute respiratory failure and coagulopathy. In addition, isolated thoracic aortic repair is not always effective in resolving malperfusion syndromes, and some authors have recommended endovascular methods to restore peripheral perfusion as an adjunct after thoracic aortic surgery [14]. In case of end-organ ischemia, some authors propose early endovascular intervention to treat malperfusion syndromes and delayed aortic repair, also in case of type A dissecting pattern [15]. These indications and their timing are a matter under debate and several factors must be considered, including the patient features, the clinical presentation, the extent of dissection, the mechanism of obstruction, the aortic branches involved, and the local experience with open and endovascular methods.

Limits of endovascular treatment

After the first successful endovascular thoracic aneurysm exclusions with custom-made devices, the stent-graft technique with commercially available endografts has become an interesting alternative treatment for selected patients. In 1994 Dake et al. reported successful aortic endovascular grafting, also in aortic dissections [16].

In complex cases, in which surgery may not be feasible due to hazardous proximal aortic control through a left thoracotomy, endovascular grafting of the proximal aortic neck and thoracic aorta represents a real appealing alternative solution, even if the aortic arch is involved, anchoring the endograft proximally between the left carotid and subclavian artery or even covering supra-aortic trunks after extra-anatomical revascularization.

The effectiveness of endografting in aortic dissection and the rule of re-entry sites have not been clarified. Cases of retrograde type A dissection and of ischemic complications have been reported [17].

Retrograde type A dissection represents an alarming complication in these series; it is described after using a variety of endograft models and seems to be related to the damage of the already diseased aortic wall at the level of the proximal endograft landing zone, using endografts that are not specifically designed for acutely dissected aortic tissue. Ischemic complications are related to the coverage of critical intercostal and/or visceral aortic side branches. Furthermore, ischemia can be induced by means of endovascular obliteration of the false lumen. The latter does not occur during open repair if the distal anastomosis is performed to both the true and false channels [18]. Moreover, fixation of the endograft in cases of extremely large type B aortic dissections is difficult. Finally, perigraft leakage, migration, and rupture are also described. Looking for a patient-tailored treatment, some authors have also attempted custom-made devices with lateral fenestration or side branches to preserve medullar and visceral vascularization. Unfortunately, reports are still anecdotal and results remain to be assessed [19].

Also, the endovascular technique may not be feasible in the emergency settings due to the lack of in-hospital availability of the devices [20].

Personal experience

At our department, from March 1988 to September 2003, we treated 622 patients for thoracic and thoraco-abdominal aortic pathology. Among these patients, 62 presented with a type B dissection; 26 patients required operation in the acute phase, 36 patients were treated for chronic aortic dissection (Table).

ACUTE TYPE B DISSECTION

The vast majority of patients evaluated in the acute phase of aortic dissection (75/101 cases, 74.2%) underwent medical therapy. The 30-day aortic-related mortality in these non-operated patients was 17.3% (13 patients). The total mortality rate of 26 patients requiring interventional procedures in the acute phase was 26.9% (7 patients). In these series, thoracic aortic replacement was performed in 38.5% of cases with a mortality rate of 40% and a neurological deficit rate of 20%. The surgical mortality of malperfusion syndromes treated in the acute phase with open or endovascular peripheral procedures without thoracic aortic repair was 36.4%.

Table	PATIENTS REQUIRING INTERVENTION FOR THORACIC AORTIC DISEASE BETWEEN 1988 AND 2003	
Disease		*Patients*
Ascending aortic aneurysm		182
Aortic arch aneurysm		48
Degenerative descending TAA		136
Degenerative TAAA		161
Adult aortic coarctation		13
Traumatic lesion		20
Acute type B dissection		26
Dissective chronic TAAA		20
Dissective chronic descending TAA		16

TAA: thoracic descending aortic aneurysm
TAAA: thoraco-abdominal aortic aneurysm

CHRONIC TYPE B DISSECTION

Among the 81 patients who survived 30 days after the acute phase of type B aortic dissection, 6 patients (7.2%) developed a dissecting aneurysm (4 TAA, 2 TAAA) requiring elective aortic repair after a mean time follow-up of 28.6 months. The total number of patients we treated in the chronic phase was 36; the peri-operative mortality rate was 5.5% (2/36) and the neurological deficit rate was 8.3% (3/36).

In several cases, including type B dissections, we determined that a multistaged treatment is feasible and that a hybrid treatment seems to be effective. Hybrid treatment comprises the advantage of the minor invasiveness of the endoluminal approach, as we initially used in selected, high-risk patients. It also includes the effectiveness of open surgery, like sometimes required in case of failed endovascular treatment or evolving pathology. We describe two case reports drawn from our series, well representing typical hybrid repair of type B aortic dissection.

Case 1. A 68-year-old man with a history of severe hypertension, was admitted to our department for the treatment of critical lower limb ischemia secondary to an acute type B dissection without aneurysmal dilatation, as diagnosed with a contrast enhanced computed tomography (CT) scan.

On admission, the patient was hemodynamically stable and the emergency angiography showed a type B dissection originating at the level of the aortic isthmus, with a myointimal flap causing left renal artery dissection and static occlusion of the distal aorta. After cannulation of the false and true lumen by means of percutaneous right femoral and brachial access (Fig. 1A), the occlusive intimal flap was perforated via a Brockenborough needle, followed by introducing a guidewire trough the two dissection channels and fenestration with an angioplasty balloon catheter (*Ultra-Thin Diamond* ® 14 mm) (Fig. 1B). Despite the large communication created between the two channels (Fig. 1C), the flow in the infrarenal aorta and in the left renal artery was not adequately restored. A Palmaz stent (20 x 60 mm) was then released in the true juxtarenal aortic lumen (Fig. 1D) and another stent (*Corinthian* ® 6 x 20 mm) was released in the true lumen of the left renal artery. Completion angiography documented the good result with adequate flows restored in the distal abdominal aorta and in the left renal arteries without flow compromise in other arteries. No brachial-infrarenal aorta pressure drop was assessed after completion of the procedure. A residual dissection that extended to the right common iliac artery was successfully treated with a direct iliac stent (*Smart* ® 9-40 mm and 12-40 mm). The postoperative course was uneventful.

Fifteen months later the patient was well and asymptomatic. Magnetic resonance angiography (MRA) was performed and revealed an 8 centimeter diameter dissecting aneurysm involving the distal arch and descending aorta. An open aortic replacement under hypothermic circulatory arrest was electively accomplished (*Hemabridge* ® 30 mm) with associated distal fenestration (Fig. 2).

The first postoperative day was characterized by cerebral hemorrhage, which resolved without significant neurological deficits. The following postoperative period was uneventful. The patient was extubated at the sixth postoperative day and discharged at the tenth postoperative day. At 6 months follow-up the patient is alive and well, without radiological changes at CT scanning (Fig. 3).

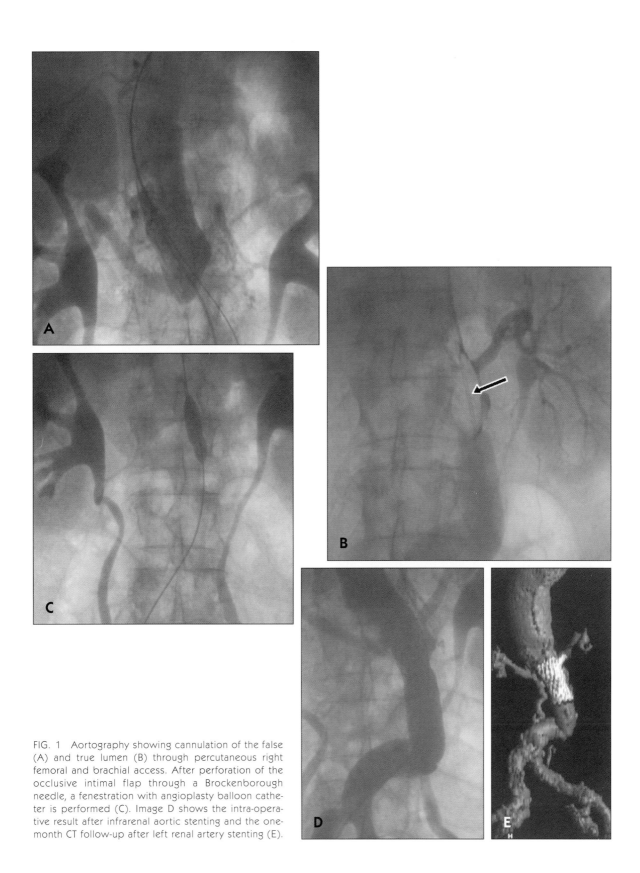

FIG. 1 Aortography showing cannulation of the false (A) and true lumen (B) through percutaneous right femoral and brachial access. After perforation of the occlusive intimal flap through a Brockenborough needle, a fenestration with angioplasty balloon catheter is performed (C). Image D shows the intra-operative result after infrarenal aortic stenting and the one-month CT follow-up after left renal artery stenting (E).

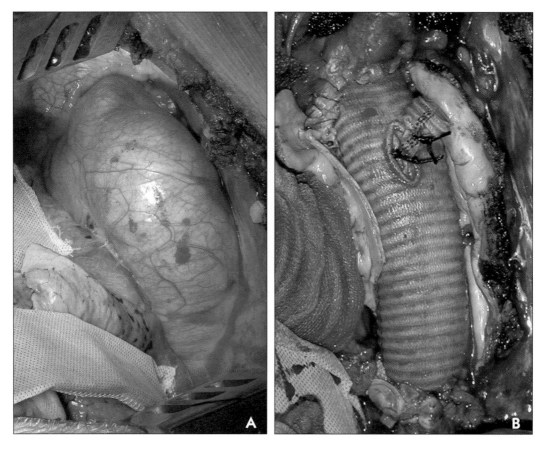

FIG. 2 Intra-operative image of an 8 cm diameter dissecting aneurysm involving distal arch and descending aorta (A). Intra-operative image of the same case following aortic replacement under hypothermic circulatory arrest (B).

Case 2. A 37-year-old man with Marfan syndrome, professional opera singer with previous emergent replacement of the supracoronary ascending aorta with a 28 mm end-to-end polyester graft for acute type A dissection, was admitted to our department for the treatment of a large chronic dissecting aneurysm (diameter 10 centimeters) extending from the distal aortic arch to the infrarenal aorta, as assessed with MRA (Fig. 4) and angiography. The patient was considered for endovascular repair. The intimal tears were located 2 centimeters distal to the left subclavian artery and proximal to the celiac artery. After a complete written informed consent was obtained, the procedure was performed in the operating room under general anesthesia. Via the right common femoral artery, two straight self-expandable endografts 34 x 20 mm Excluder Gore-Tex®, *(W.L. Gore and Associates, Inc., Flagstaff, AZ, USA)* were released to cover the aorta

from the origin of the left subclavian artery to the level of the celiac artery. Completion angiography showed adequate endograft deployment, good patency of the left subclavian and visceral arteries, and a significantly decreased perfusion of the false lumen. The remaining false lumen perfusion was probably sustained by intimal tears localized distally to the celiac artery.

The postoperative course was characterized by the development of acute pulmonary edema secondary to severe aortic valve insufficiency, requiring emergency aortic valve replacement with a Carbomedics® n° 27 *(Sulzer, Carbomedics, Austin, TX, USA)* mechanical valve prosthesis. The patient recovered well and was discharged on the 11th postoperative day under warfarin therapy. The one month follow-up contrast-enhanced CT scan showed that the thoracic false channel was completely collapsed with partial thrombosis of the false lumen down to the level of

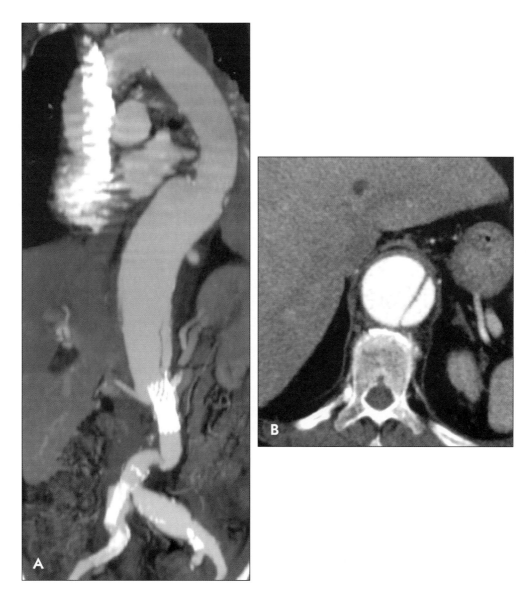

FIG. 3 Six-month follow-up CT-scan shows the good result of thoracic open repair and of the infrarenal aortic, left renal, and right iliac stenting (A). Residual dissection of the suprarenal abdominal aorta without significant dilatation or ischemic complications (B).

the visceral arteries. At this level the aortic false lumen was still perfused (Fig. 5).

Seven months later, after routine contrast-enhanced CT scan, the patient was re-admitted to our department with a diagnosis of a large type III dissecting thoraco-abdominal aneurysm, extending from the lower thoracic aorta to the infrarenal abdominal aorta with a maximum diameter of 9 centimeters (Fig. 5). Aortography confirmed the diag-

nosis at admission. Because of the involvement of the visceral vessels in the aneurysm, the young age of the patient, and the good general conditions, a surgical treatment of the dissecting TAAA was planned. Surgery was performed through a left thoraco-abdominal incision in the sixth intercostal space with a limited phrenotomy (Fig. 6A) employing left heart bypass. A traditional thoraco-abdominal repair with the technique of sequential

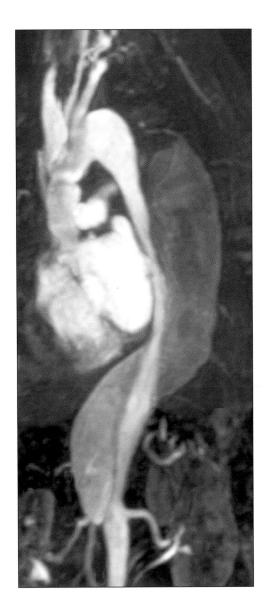

FIG. 4 MRA showing a large chronic dissecting aneurysm (diameter 10 centimeters) extending from the distal aortic arch to the infrarenal aorta.

(Fig. 7A). The postoperative period was uneventful. MRA performed at one month showed adequate exclusion of the thoracic aneurysm without evidence of endoleak, and good results of open surgical reconstruction of the thoraco-abdominal aorta (Fig. 7B). At six months follow-up, following neurosurgical treatment of an anterior cerebral artery aneurysm, the patient is alive and well and has successfully returned to his profession.

Discussion

Hybrid open endovascular repair is an attractive investigational procedure for the treatment of thoracic and thoraco-abdominal pathology, particularly in type B dissection. It exploits both the less invasiveness of endovascular techniques and the direct control of open surgery. Hybrid open endoluminal treatment of thoracic and thoraco-abdominal disease, previously predicted by Hollier in 1998, has already been reported [21].

Our experience shows the particularly successful integration of the two methods in type B aortic dissection treatment. In the presence of an acute onset of malperfusion syndrome without risk of aortic rupture (case 1), the approach with endovascular or open peripheral procedures may represent an effective and less invasive first stage approach to complicated type B dissection.

If thoracic aortic repair is required for the risk of thoracic rupture, as previously described, endovascular control of the proximal aorta is an attractive alternative to a demanding and hazardous open repair. It avoids thoracotomy, surgical aortic dissection, and proximal aortic clamping, and it limits blood loss. Nevertheless, in our opinion, in the acute phase thoracic endografting must avoid aortic rupture. It is well experienced that an acutely dissected aorta is terribly fragile and prone to perforation and retrograde dissection, particularly induced by bare springs (Fig. 8). On the other hand, thoracic endografting in chronic phase type B dissection, in selected patients, may be effective in closing the proximal thoracic tears, offering a lower invasiveness as compared to open repair (case 2). If distal re-entry tears remain open after the proximal procedure (case 2), other distal endovascular grafting may be carefully attempted but the risk exists of covering critical visceral, intercostals, or lumbar arteries. In these cases, the rationale of an open treatment is to preserve visceral and medullar vascularization

clamping was carried out. The proximal clamp was positioned on the descending endografted aorta. The distal portion of the thoracic endograft was cut at the level of the midthoracic aorta (Fig. 6B) and the proximal anastomosis was accomplished with a transaortic suture line including endograft and aortic wall. A Carrel patch was performed for visceral revascularization and the distal anastomosis at the aortic carrefour was performed with the true lumen

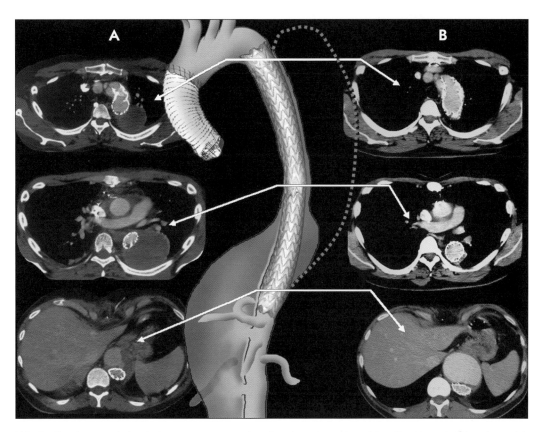

FIG. 5 The thoraco-abdominal aorta seven months after thoracic endografting. The thoracic false channel is completely collapsed and a large type III dissected thoraco-abdominal aneurysm has developed. The outlined contour shows the thoracic aorta diameter at the moment of thoracic endografting. CT scan (A) at one month after endografting, CT scan (B) after seven months.

with an open, conventional repair. This is the policy we adopted in case 2, in which traditional surgery allowed repair of the dissected thoraco-abdominal aorta with re-implantation of the visceral and renal arteries. In these cases previous proximal endografting allows a more distal second stage aortic clamping. The proximal anastomosis, as in case 2, may be directly performed to the endografted aorta achieving satisfactory sealing.

Several combinations of open and endovascular approaches are possible. Open surgical extra- or trans-thoracic revascularizations of the supra-aortic trunks can be performed in combination with endograft deployment to extend the proximal landing zone for the endograft to different segments of the aortic arch.

Also, open visceral revascularization from the infrarenal aorta may be accomplished prior to thoraco-abdominal aortic endografting with coverage of the visceral vessels, (see chapter Wolfe).

We are far from stating that any high-risk patient with a type B dissection should routinely be treated by a hybrid approach. The endovascular stent-grafting of the dissected thoracic aorta itself is still an investigational procedure. Long-term follow-up and adequate devices are still awaited [22]. With wider experience and newer generations of endografts, we believe that endografting in association with open surgery or vice-versa will broaden the range of critical patients that may be treated with reduced invasiveness.

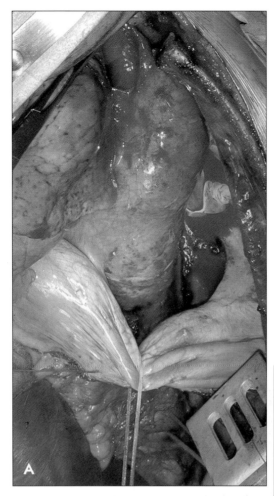

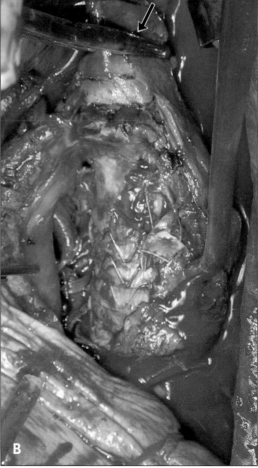

FIG. 6 A - Intra-operative image showing the large dissecting thoraco-abdominal aneurysm and the limited phrenotomy. B - Intra-operative image showing the proximal clamp positioned at the descending endografted aorta (arrow) and the thoracic endograft exposed after mid-thoracic aortotomy.

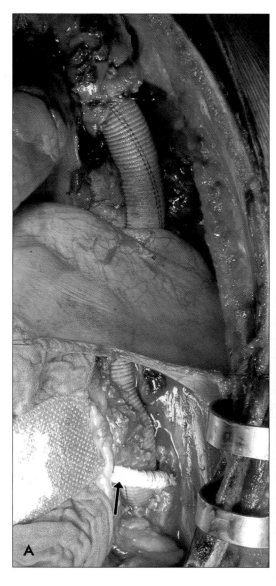

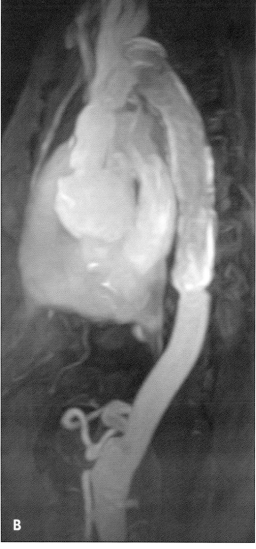

FIG. 7 A - Intra-operative image showing the thoraco-abdominal repair carried out with the technique
of sequential clamping, employing left heart bypass.
Arrow shows a grafted left retro-aortic renal vein.
B - One month follow-up MRA shows the adequate
exclusion of the thoracic aneurysm without evidence
of endoleak and good results of open surgical reconstruction of the thoraco-abdominal aorta.

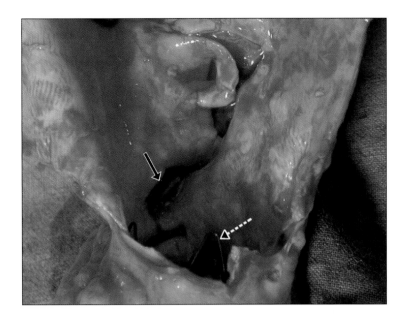

FIG. 8 Autoptic specimen showing the large aortic intimal fracture *(continuous arrow)* at the level of the proximal bare springs *(outlined arrow)* of an endograft inserted for acute type B aortic dissection. The patient developed a retrograde dissection in the aortic arch and died postoperatively due to a massive stroke.

REFERENCES

1 Hata M, Shiono M, Inoue T, et al. Optimal treatment of type B acute aortic dissection: long-term medical follow-up results. *Ann Thorac Surg* 2003; 75: 1781-1784.

2 Hagan PG, Nienaber CA, Isselbacher EM, et al. The International Registry of Acute Aortic Dissection (IRAD): new insights into an old disease. *JAMA* 2000; 283: 897-903.

3 Cambria RP. Surgical treatment of complicated distal aortic dissection. *Semin Vasc Surg* 2002; 15: 97-107.

4 Chiesa R, Melissano G, Tshomba Y, et al. Dissection aiguë de type B: traitement chirurgical. In: Kieffer E, Fabiani JN (eds). *Chirurgie des dissections aortiques.* Paris, AERCV 2002: pp 195-216.

5 Nienaber CA, Ince H, Weber F, et al. Emergency stent-graft placement in thoracic aortic dissection and evolving rupture. *J Card Surg* 2003; 18: 464-470.

6 Dake MD, Kato N, Mitchell RS, et al. Endovascular stent-graft placement for the treatment of acute aortic dissection. *N Engl J Med* 1999; 340: 1546-1552.

7 Kato N, Hirano T, Kawaguchi T, et al. Aneurysmal degeneration of the aorta after stent-graft repair of acute aortic dissection. *J Vasc Surg* 2001; 34: 513-518.

8 Huynh TT, Porat EE, Miller CC 3rd, et al. The effect of aortic dissection on outcome in descending thoracic and thoracoabdominal aortic aneurysm repair. *Semin Vasc Surg* 2002; 15: 108-115.

9 Jing ZP, Feng X, Bao JM, et al. Endovascular stent-graft exclusion for Stanford B type aortic dissections: a report of 146 patients. *Zhonghua Wai Ke Za Zhi* 2003; 41: 483-486.

10 Starnes BW, O'Donnell SD, Gillespie DL, et al. Endovascular management of renal ischemia in a patient with acute aortic dissection and renovascular hypertension. *Ann Vasc Surg* 2002; 16: 368-374.

11 Coselli JS, Conklin LD, LeMaire SA. Thoracoabdominal aortic aneurysm repair: review and update of current strategies. *Ann Thorac Surg* 2002; 74: S1881-1884; discussion S1892-1898.

12 Coselli JS, LeMaire SA, Poli de Figueiredo L, Kirby RP. Paraplegia after thoracoabdominal aortic aneurysm repair: is dissection a risk factor? *Ann Thorac Surg* 1997; 63: 28-36.

13 Coselli JS, Poli de Figueiredo LF, LeMaire SA. Impact of previous thoracic aneurysm repair on thoracoabdominal aortic aneurysm management. *Ann Thorac Surg* 1997; 64: 639-650.

14 Slonim SM, Miller DC, Mitchell RS, et al. Percutaneous balloon fenestration and stenting for life-threatening ischemic complications in patients with acute aortic dissection. *J Thorac Cardiovasc Surg* 1999; 117: 1118-1126.

15 Deeb GM, Williams DM, Bolling SF, et al. Surgical delay for acute type A dissection with malperfusion. *Ann Thorac Surg* 1997; 64: 1669-1677.

16 Dake MD, Miller DC, Semba CP, et al. Transluminal placement of endovascular stent-grafts for the treatment of descending thoracic aortic aneurysms. *N Engl J Med* 1994; 331: 1729-1734.

17 Pamler RS, Kotsis T, Gorich J, et al. Complications after endovascular repair of type B aortic dissection. *J Endovasc Ther* 2002; 9: 822-828.

18 Fukada J, Morishita K, Naraoka S, et al. Significance of distal fenestration in graft replacement for chronic aortic dissection. *J Cardiovasc Surg* 2002; 43: 655-656.

19 Chuter TA, Gordon RL, Reilly LM, et al. An endovascular system for thoracoabdominal aortic aneurysm repair. *J Endovasc Ther* 2001; 8: 25-33.

20 Chiesa R, Castellano R, Lucci C, et al. Traumatic rupture of the thoracic aorta. In: Branchereau A, Jacobs M (eds). *Vascular Emergencies*. Elmsford, Blackwell Publishing Inc - Futura Division 2003: pp 107-123.

21 Hollier LH. Combining endovascular and surgical techniques: the best of both worlds. *J Endovasc Surg* 1998; 5: 333-334.

22 Melissano G, Chiesa R, Tshomba Y, et al. Disappointing results with a novel commercially available thoracic endograft. *J Vasc Surg*. In press.

7

ENDOLUMINAL REPAIR OF THE AORTIC ARCH COMBINED WITH REVASCULARIZATION OF SUPRA-AORTIC ARTERIES

EDOUARD KIEFFER, FABIEN KOSKAS, PHILIPPE CLUZEL
ALBERT-CLAUDE BENHAMOU, AMINE BAHNINI, LAURENT CHICHE

During the last decade several endovascular modalities for the treatment of aortic arch aneurysms have been developed. The required revascularization of the supra-aortic arteries basically comprises two surgical strategies. One or several arteries can be treated with branched endografts; however, this technique is complicated and hazardous. While Inoue et al. [1,2] are the only team performing this procedure, Chuter et al. [3,4] recently published a clever system for branched endovascular repair of aortic arch aneurysms. Alternatively, supra-aortic arteries (left common carotid, left subclavian arteries) can be translocated to a proximal artery (right common carotid artery approached via cervical access) to treat aneurysms of the distal arch [5-8]. Finally, the ascending aorta can be used, via sternotomy, as donor site to revascularize all three supra-aortic arteries in endovascular treatment of aneurysms of the complete arch [9]. The value of this new modality is still poorly defined and we aimed for analysis of our experience by evaluating all aortic arch aneurysm cases treated during the last eight years, since endovascular treatment first became available in our department.

Patients and methods

Between January 1, 1995 and December 31, 2003 we operated on 115 aneurysms involving the aortic arch. We did not include aneurysms of the ascending aorta for which the distal anastomosis required cross-clamping of the brachiocephalic trunk and aneurysms of the descending thoracic aorta for which clamping of the left subclavian artery was necessary. Also, patients operated in emergency settings, like acute dissection, were not enrolled in this analysis. The group of patients consisted of 76 men and 39 women with a mean age of 56.9±16.1 years (range 18 to 83 years). Etiology of the aneurysms was degenerative disease in 45 cases, chronic dissection in 40 (28 chronic type A of which 10 were operated before for urgent ascending aortic repair and 12 retrograde type B), Takayasu arteritis in 12, and miscellaneous in 12 patients [Marfan (n = 4), non-specific inflammation (n = 4), congenital disease (n = 3), syphilis (n = 2), and unknown (n = 5)].

The anatomical lesions could be classified into four groups:
- group A: aneurysms involving the ascending aorta and aortic arch but not extending in the descending aorta (n = 35);
- group B: aneurysms involving the ascending aorta, aortic arch and descending or thoraco-abdominal aorta (n = 28);
- group C: aneurysms of the aortic arch and descending or thoraco-abdominal aorta in which the ascending aorta was not affected or already replaced (n = 29);
- group D: aneurysms only affecting the aortic arch (n = 23) without involvement of the ascending or descending thoracic aorta.

At present, in our opinion, mainly aneurysms of group D are potential candidates for endovascular treatment with proximal transposition of the supra-aortic arteries. We have performed endovascular treatment in 16 patients from Group D (13.9% of the total series, 69.6% of group D). The main reason we chose this less invasive procedure in 13 patients was advanced age, associated with a poor physical condition and cardiopulmonary comorbidity. In contrast, two young patients were considered good candidates because we assumed that their disease would benefit more from endovascular than from conventional repair (one polychondritis, one Behcet disease). The last case concerned a patient with a limited saccular aneurysm at the origin of a bronchial artery. The remaining 7 patients (30.4%) of group D underwent surgical treatment because of young age (n = 4), associated myocardial revascularization (n = 2), and associated aneurysm of a retro-esophageal right subclavian artery.

The demographic and anatomical details of the 16 patients who underwent endovascular repair are summarized in Table I. The group comprised 14 males and 2 females with a mean age of 73.4 ± 12.6 years (range 41 to 83 years). Seven patients complained about symptoms resulting from compression (thoracic pain and/or dysphonia and/or dysphagia), 3 patients suffered from hemoptesis caused by aortobronchial or pulmonary fistula, one patient had an embolic cerebral infarction, and 5 patients were asymptomatic but showed a large arch aneurysm with a diameter extending 6 centimeters. Etiology comprised degenerative disease (n = 12) (Fig. 1), inflammatory disease (one polychondritis, one Behcet) (Fig. 2), dysplastic disease (n = 1), and post-traumatic lesion (n = 1). Eight aneurysms involved the complete aortic arch and eight others affected the posterior arch only, not involving the brachiocephalic trunk.

Prior to endovascular treatment, the supra-aortic arteries were revascularized by means of sternotomy (Fig. 3) and bypass grafting originating from the ascending aorta in 9 patients, cervicotomy and subsequent bypass departing from the right common carotid artery (Fig. 4) in 6 patients, and subcutaneous extra-anatomical bypass (Fig. 5) in one patient. Three of the right common carotid grafts

Table I	DEMOGRAPHIC AND ANATOMICAL DETAILS	
✓ 14 males, 2 females		
✓ Mean age	73.4 ± 12.6 years	
Range	41 - 83 years	
✓ Degenerative aneurysms	12	
Inflammatory aneurysms	2	
Miscellaneous	2	
✓ Posterior wall of aortic arch	8	
Total aortic arch	8	

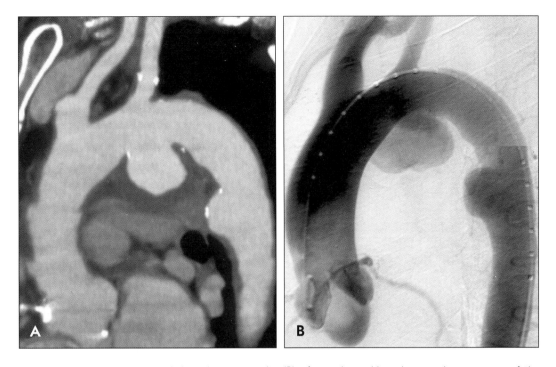

FIG. 1   CT angiography (A) and thoracic aortography (B) of a patient with a degenerative aneurysm of the aortic arch, associated with an aneurysm of the proximal part of the descending thoracic aorta.

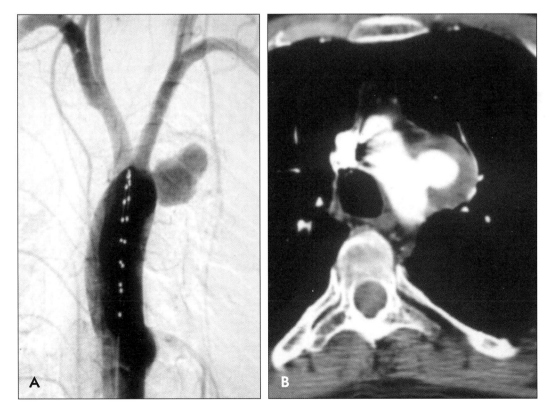

FIG. 2   Thoracic aortography (A) and CT angiography (B) of a patient with a saccular aneurysm of the distal aortic arch (Behcet-disease).

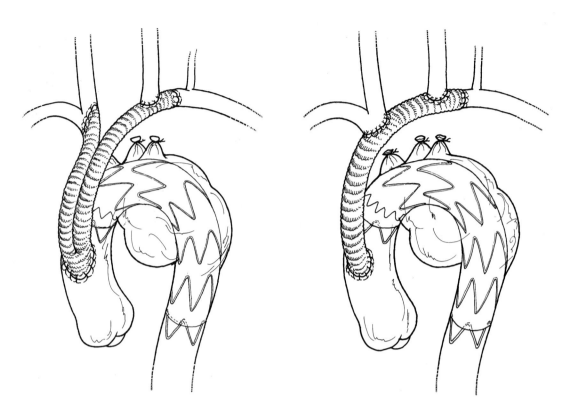

FIG. 3   Drawing showing two types of bypasses from the ascending aorta to the three supra-aortic arteries.   A - Bifurcation graft. B - Sequential bypass.

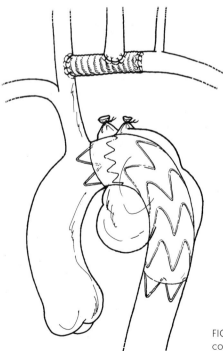

FIG. 4   Drawing showing crossover bypass from the right common carotid artery to the left common carotid and left subclavian arteries.

were saphenous vein conduits and all other grafts were polyester prostheses.

All endografts were tailor made and consisted of polyester grafts with Gianturco stents. Deployment was achieved by means of 20F to 24F introducers with femoral access in 12 patients (Fig. 6), abdominal aortic approach in 2 patients, iliac artery in one patient, and ascending aorta in one patient.

Early results

Early technical complications have been encountered in 10 patients (62.5%), and are indicated in Table II. An 80-year-old patient successfully underwent revascularization of all three supra-aortic arteries. However, during the endovascular procedure, the introducer perforated the left ventricle. Sternotomy confirmed this diagnosis but suturing of the extremely fragile myocardium failed and the patient died during surgery.

Two patients with a distal aortic arch aneurysm were converted to open surgery during the endovascular procedure. Following access via cervicotomy, a bypass was constructed from the right subclavian artery to the left common carotid and subclavian arteries. In the first patient, the pushing maneuver of the endograft occluded the brachiocephalic trunk. In the other patient the endoprosthesis was too short and did not cover the distal part of the aneurysm. Both patients were operated under

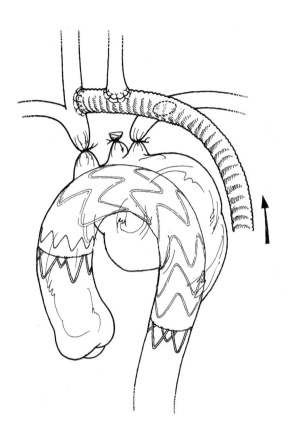

FIG. 5 Drawing showing an extra-anatomical bypass from the iliac artery to the three supra-aortic arteries.

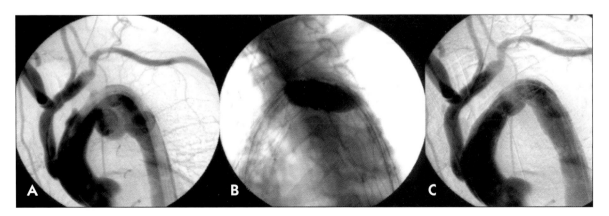

FIG. 6 Intra-operative images visualizing deployment of the endograft via femoral access after sequential bypass from the aorta to the brachiocephalic trunk, left carotid, and left subclavian artery. A - Positioning of the introducer. B - Inflation of a balloon to expand the stents at the level of the aortic angle. C - Deployed endograft.

profound hypothermia and circulatory arrest and recovered without event (Fig. 7).

Four patients suffered from ischemic cerebral vascular accidents, probably due to emboli caused by manipulation of guidewires and introducer in the aortic arch. Two of them died. Two patients developed dissection of the ascending aorta: one patient during intra-aortic maneuvering with the introducer (Fig. 8) and one patient at the twelfth postoperative day. The latter patient died during surgical re-intervention.

In one patient the endoprosthesis migrated distally at the fifth postoperative day, causing acute occlusion of the descending thoracic aorta with subsequent malignant upstream hypertension and intracerebral hypertension. Emergency surgery via sternotomy was performed with simple cross-clamping because of the risk of aggravating the cerebral damage. Clinical outcome was uneventful (Fig. 9).

Finally, in one patient sternotomy was contra-indicated and therefore an extra-anatomical bypass from the iliac artery to the three supra-aortic arteries was constructed. At the 56th postoperative day the patient died from respiratory complications.

In total, five patients (31.2%) died and five (31.2%) required re-operation during the early postoperative period.

Table II	EARLY TECHNICAL COMPLICATIONS		
Complications	*N (%)*	*Re-interventions (%)*	*Mortality (%)*
Left ventricular perforation	1	1	1
Conversion	2	2	0
Embolic stroke	4	-	2
Distal migration and aortic occlusion	1	1	0
Aortic dissection	2	1	1
Total	**10 (62.5)**	**5 (31.2)**	**4 (25.0)**

Mid-term results

The 11 patients who survived the procedure were followed with a mean of 23 months (range 1 to

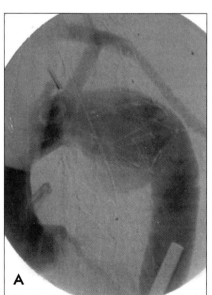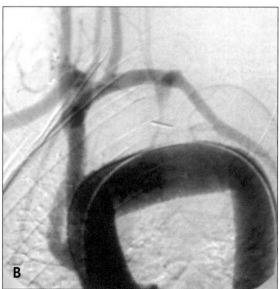

FIG. 7   A - Intra-operative aortography: following deployment the endograft is too short. B - Postoperative aortography following conversion to open surgery.

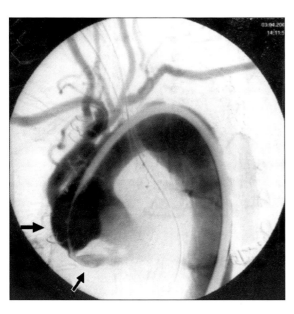

FIG. 8 Intra-operative aortography showing dissection of the ascending aorta caused by the introducer *(arrows)*.

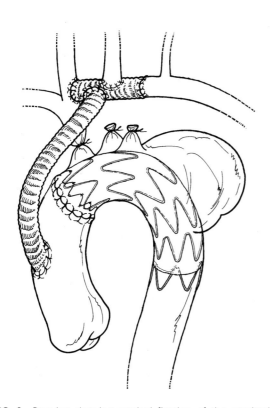

FIG. 9 Drawing showing surgical fixation of the proximal part of an endograft which migrated distally in the aorta as well as the surgical revascularization of the supra-aortic arteries by means of a bypass from the aorta to the previously constructed graft.

58 months). Two patients developed an aortoesophageal fistula at 6 and 29 months, due to the rigidity of the stents at the level of the distal angle in the aortic arch. Both patients died, one during re-intervention via left thoracotomy and one before arrival in the hospital. In the other patients, computed tomography (CT) showed absence of endoleaks. At present, nine patients (56.2%) are alive with an excluded aneurysm, as depicted by CT angiography scanning (Figs. 10,11).

Discussion

The present indications for endovascular treatment of aortic arch aneurysms are limited: patients at high age, poor general condition, and/or absolute or relative contra-indications for conventional surgery. Furthermore, specific anatomical details are required: normal diameter of the ascending aorta and aneurysm only affecting the aortic arch, or with limited extension to the isthmus. Excessive angulation of the distal arch (Fig. 12) is also a limiting factor with regard to plication of the endograft and late occurrence of an aorto-esophageal fistula caused by perforation of the aortic wall by the stent. These general and anatomical issues explain why we only treated 13.9% of patients (16 out of 115) with an aortic arch aneurysm by means of an endovascular procedure.

The currently applied bypass techniques that allow the above-described endovascular procedures are well established. Crossover grafts from the right common carotid artery to the left common carotid and subclavian arteries are simply performed via bilateral cervicotomy or infraclavicular access. The easiest technique consists of performing the end-to-side anastomosis of the graft to the right carotid artery first followed by the end-to-end anastomosis to the left subclavian artery (pre-vertebral) and finally re-implanting the left common carotid artery in the cranial part of the graft. Placement of a clip at the origin of the left common carotid artery will assist exact release of the endograft.

In the event that all three supra-aortic arteries have to be excluded, median sternotomy is the access of choice: only a partial proximal sternotomy, possibly associated with short cervicotomy, is necessary. The ascending aorta serves as the donor site. A bifurcation graft can be used; however, the size of the main body requires a long anastomosis and might obstruct the mediastinum. Alternatives in-

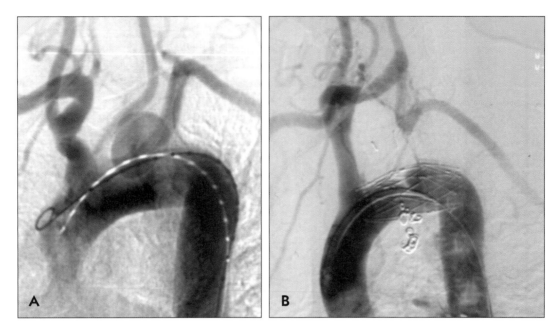

FIG. 10 Pre-operative (A) and postoperative (B) aortography of a crossover graft and endoprosthesis for an aortic arch aneurysm (posterior part).

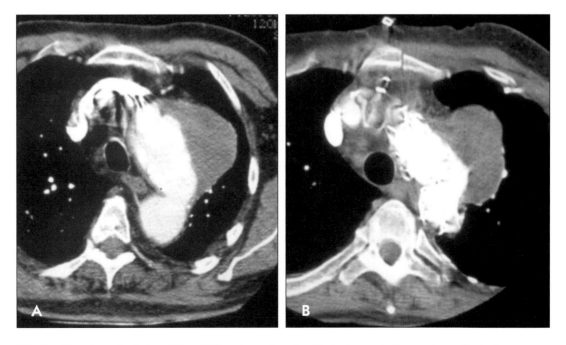

FIG. 11 CT angiography before (A) and CT angiography after (B) deployment of an endoprosthesis for an aneurysm involving the complete aortic arch.

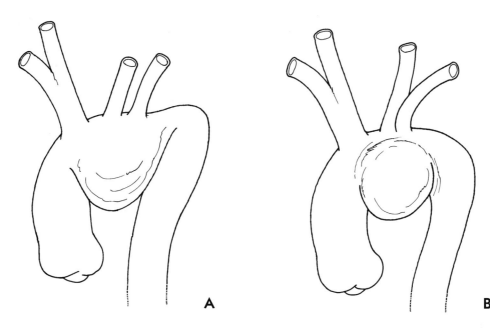

FIG. 12 Drawing showing an angulated aortic arch (A), causing difficult launching of an endograft and an aortic arch with a smooth curve (B), allowing gentle positioning of the prosthesis.

clude a sequential graft or a double bypass: aorto-brachiocephalic trunk bypass, proximally implanted at the right lateral side of the ascending aorta and an aorto-left subclavian artery graft, originating from the left lateral ascending aorta. Only in very exceptional cases in which sternotomy is absolutely contra-indicated it might be considered to revascularize supra-aortic arteries by means of extra-anatomical grafts from iliac or femoral arteries.

In our experience, the results of endovascular treatment of aortic arch aneurysms are relatively disappointing: approximately half of the patients (56.2%) have an adequate clinical and anatomical outcome at mid-term, meaning being alive with a totally excluded aneurysm. Improvement of the endovascular material is necessary, especially its flexibility in order to pass the angled aortic isthmus. However, these improvements will not prevent complications associated with intra-aortic manipulations like cerebral emboli, aortic dissection, and left ventricular rupture, especially occurring in older patients.

A multicenter, prospective randomized study will definitely solve the problem of which technique (endovascular or conventional surgery) should be proposed for the treatment of aortic arch aneurysms. Such a study, however, is difficult to organize because of the limited number of patients and the wide range of anatomical appearances and the diversity of applied techniques, both in endovascular and conventional surgery.

At present, while awaiting technical improvements and observing long-term results, we propose to reserve endovascular treatment of aortic arch aneurysms for patients at high age and poor general condition, suffering from symptomatic and/or large aneurysms.

REFERENCES

1 Inoue K. Branched stent-grafts for complex thoracic aortic aneurysms. In: Branchereau A, Jacobs M (eds). *Surgical and endovascular treatment of aortic aneurysms.* Armonk, Futura Publishing Compagny 2000: pp 35-41.

2 Inoue K, Hosokawa H, Iwase T, et al. Aortic arch reconstruction by transluminally placed endovascular branched stent graft. *Circulation* 1999; 100 (19 Suppl): 316-321.

3 Chuter TA, Schneider DB, Reilly LM, et al. Modular branched stent graft for endovascular repair of aortic arch aneurysm and dissection. *J Vasc Surg* 2003; 38: 859-863.

4 Schneider DB, Curry TK, Reilly LM, et al. Branched endovascular repair of aortic arch aneurysm with a modular stent-graft system. *J Vasc Surg* 2003; 38: 855.

5 Criado FJ, Barnatan MF, Risk Y, et al. Technical strategies to expand stent-graft applicability in the aortic arch and proximal descending thoracic aorta. *J Endovasc Ther* 2002; 9 (Suppl 2): II32-38.

6 Criado FJ, Clark NS, Barnatan MF. Stent graft repair in the aortic arch and descending thoracic aorta: a 4-year experience. *J Vasc Surg* 2002; 36: 1121-1128.

7 Kato M, Kaneko M, Kuratani T, et al. New operative method for distal aortic arch aneurysm: combined cervical branch bypass and endovascular stent-graft implantation. *J Thorac Cardiovasc Surg* 1999; 117: 832-834.

8 Kato N, Shimono T, Hirano T, et al. Aortic arch aneurysms: treatment with extraanatomical bypass and endovascular stent-grafting. *Cardiovasc Intervent Radiol* 2002; 25: 419-422.

9 Buth J, Penn O, Tielbeek A, Mersman M. Combined approach to stent-graft treatment of an aortic arch aneurysm. *J Endovasc Surg* 1998; 5: 329-332.

8

WHEN TO REVASCULARIZE THE SUBCLAVIAN ARTERY IN THORACIC AORTIC STENTING?

VICENTE RIAMBAU, GUSTAVO CASERTA
CESAR GARCÍA-MADRID, CARLOS URIARTE, MANUEL CASTELLÁ
MIGUEL JOSA, JAUME MULET

Thoracic aortic endografting is suggested as a valuable alternative to treat aortic lesions such as aneurysm, dissection, penetrating ulcer, intramural hematoma, trauma, or aortobronchial fistula [1]. It is frequently recommended to cover the ostium of the left subclavian artery (LSA) in order to increase the proximal landing zone or when the aortic lesion involves the LSA itself. The potential consequences of covering the LSA ostium without a previous revascularization include upper limb ischemia and neurological sequella such as subclavian steal syndrome or, more rarely, spinal cord ischemia and paraplegia. Nevertheless, there are several reports suggesting the innocuousness of this intentional procedure. Moreover, subclavian revascularization has been associated with some morbidity and even mortality. This situation leads to a controversial issue: revascularization is mandatory prior to an intentional coverage by endograft or is only necessary in special circumstances. In this chapter we will adress this controversial topic on the basis of the literature and our own experience.

Indications for revascularization of LSA prior to thoracic endografting

At the beginning of the history of aortic endografting, when inexperience was common and the exact consequence of acute coverage of the subclavian artery was unknown, it was always recommended to revascularize the LSA prior to the endovascular treatment [2]. This prudent behavior changed over time due to the observation of inadvertent or unintentional occlusion of the LSA without any serious clinical complications. In addition, subclavian revascularization, carotid-subclavian bypass, and subclavian transposition are associated with secondary problems such as mortality (1.2%), nerve injury (10%), stroke (5%), lymphatic leakage (2%), and graft infection (1.2%), as reported in a recent review [3] (Table I). For these reasons the actual indications for LSA revascularization prior to an endograft coverage should be tailored to special clinical and anatomical situations. The following indications have been identified (Table II).

As a first scenario, it is mandatory to maintain direct blood flow to the LSA and its branches if the patient has a patent left internal mammary-coronary bypass. Coverage of the LSA in these particular circumstances will induce myocardial ischemia. Furthermore, if a patient will be a clear candidate for a left mammary-coronary bypass, it is recommended to perform a preventive LSA revascularization if LSA occlusion by a thoracic aortic stent is indicated.

The next indication is the presence of the anatomical variation in which the right subclavian artery (RSA) arises from the descending thoracic aorta, distally to the LSA ostium (lusoria artery) [4]. The prevalence of this situation is less than 0.5% [5]. In this particular case, it seems mandatory to perform an LSA or RSA revascularization because the intentional occlusion of the LSA will exclude both subclavian and both vertebral arteries with subsequent neurological problems. Subclavian revascularization prior to stent-grafting will reduce this potential risk.

The third clear scenario is related to arteriosclerotic obstructive disease of the right vertebral axis (brachiocephalic trunk, RSA and/or right vertebral artery itself) combined with a dominant left vertebral artery. As in the previous situation, LSA revascularization seems to be a safe procedure preventing

neurological consequences derived from intentional LSA occlusion by endograft and leaving all direct basilar circulation to a diseased vertebral axis. In 1% to 3% of humans, the left carotid artery and the LSA have a common ostium. It is obvious that coverage of the LSA is contra-indicated and that

Table I	MORTALITY AND MORBIDITY OF CAROTID-SUBCLAVIAN BYPASS AND SUBCLAVIAN TRANSPOSITION ACCORDING TO CINA ET AL. [3]	
	Bypass grafting %	*Transposition* %
30 days mortality	1.2	1.2
Mortality during follow-up	14.4	15.4
Nerve injury	9.2	11.2
Stroke	6.6	4.4
Lymphatic leak	2.1	2.4
Postoperative thrombosis	3.5	0.9
Graft infection	1.2	0
Hematoma	0.8	0.9

Table II	INDICATIONS FOR LEFT SUBCLAVIAN ARTERY REVASCULARIZATION PRIOR TO ENDOGRAFT COVERAGE

➤ Left internal mammary-coronary bypass

➤ Lusoria artery

➤ Occlusive disease of innominate, right subclavian, right vertebral artery

➤ Common ostium of left carotid and left subclavian artery

➤ Arteriovenous access shunt for hemodialysis in left arm

➤ Left-handed professionals

carotid-subclavian revascularization prior to endografting is mandatory.

Another indication for LSA bypass or transposition is the presence of an arteriovenous access shunt for hemodialysis.

One additional scenario, which is more controversial and exceptional, is related to left-handed professionals. Since left arm claudication is the most frequent adverse event of LSA occlusion after aortic endografting, it seems prudent to revascularize this artery when the patient is a pianist or painter or another professional with a dominant left arm.

When a prior LSA revascularization is indicated, we prefer to perform the carotid-LSA bypass or LSA transposition some days before the endovascular procedure, like a staged procedure. It is mandatory to keep the left vertebral artery well perfused after this part of the procedure and also after the endograft deployment. That means that left vertebral surgical damage must be avoided. Furthermore, if a proximal ligation of the LSA is performed, this must be done in a prevertebral position.

Intentional occlusion without previous revascularization

Following the observation that unintentional LSA occlusion caused few complications, some authors explored the possibility of intentional occlusion of the LSA without prior revascularization. Some of

these clinical experiences have been published [6-9], and we summarize these ones in Table III.

Hausegger et al. reported their initial experience of intentional LSA occlusion by thoracic aortic stent-grafts without prior revascularization in three patients (two with aortic type B dissection and one with thoracic aneurysm). The reduction of blood pressure in the left arm was the most relevant clinical finding after these procedures [6]. Similar consequences were observed in the series of Gorich et al. [7]. In their experience, 23 patients were operated with thoracic endografting (11 aortic ruptures, 9 type B dissections, and 3 aneurysms). In all patients, the stent-graft was intentionally placed over the LSA. As previously described, the arterial systolic pressure in the left arm dropped in all patients, without proximal endoleaks. In four patients with proximal leakage, a limited reduction of the systolic pressure was encountered. Twenty patients did not report any clinical differences and only three patients complained of minimal discomfort. One patient suffered from exercise-dependent paresthesias, one patient complained of transient non-exercise-related intermittent dizziness, and the third experienced a cooler left hand. No patient needed a secondary LSA revascularization. Similar experience was reported in another series comprising 14 patients treated with thoracic endograft, covering the LSA origin without previous revascularization. Only one patient required a late revascularization due to persistent complaint of claudication in the left arm [8].

Table III	Number of patients	In-hospital Malperfusion (%)		Follow-up Asymptomatic (%)		Late surgery (%)	
1st author [ref.]							
Rehders (*)	13	0		11	(85)	0	
Hausegger [6]	4	0		4	(100)	0	
Görich [7]	23	3	(13)	23	(100)	0	
Palma [8]	14	0		13	(93)	1	(7)
Riambau [9]	20	2	(10)	20	(100)	0	
Total	74	5	(6)	71	(96)	1	(1.3)

CLINICAL EXPERIENCE WITH COVERAGE OF THE LSA WITHOUT PRIOR REVASCULARIZATION

* Personal communication

In our experience [9], stent-graft repair of the thoracic aorta was performed in 88 consecutive patients for different aortic lesions. Intentional coverage of the LSA was necessary in 23 cases: for management of rupture (1), aortobronchial fistula (1), type B dissection (9), aneurysm (8), and penetrating ulcers (4). In the majority of cases, coverage of the LSA was necessary because a greater length of landing zone was mandatory. In only five cases the thoracic lesion involved the origin of the LSA. Carotid-subclavian bypass was previously performed in three cases, one of them because of a left mammary-coronary bypass (Fig. 1) and the other two in left-handed patients. In order to be completely informed about the vascular anatomy of the supra-aortic branches, duplex scanning, angiography, and magnetic resonance angiography were performed

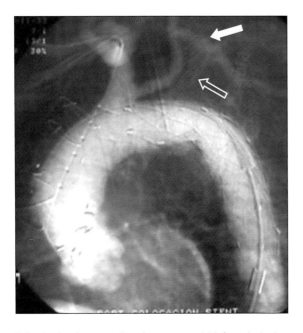

FIG. 1 Angiogram showing a carotid-left subclavian bypass (*white arrow*) prior to a LSA occlusion by endograft. This was indicated because of a previous mammary-coronary bypass (*open arrow*).

in this particular group of patients. Routinely, our anesthesiologists use esmolol during the deployment of the endograft in order to induce a bradycardia and hypotension. Esmolol is a cardiospecific beta-2 blocker with a fast and short effect. In addition, esmolol offers spinal cord protection, as demonstrated in experimental studies [10].

Patients who did not receive any revascularization were observed during the early follow-up in order to identify neurological or arm ischemic phenomena. All patients presented a drop of systolic pressure after the procedure. Only two patients developed a transitory (6 months) left arm claudication, not requiring any additional surgical treatment. No other vertebro-basilar or arm ischemic events were registered. Temperature difference between the both upper extremities was the most common clinical sign, but without any complaint.

After a mean of 28 month follow-up of this particular group of patients, we detected one type I endoleak and one type III endoleak resulting from a fabric perforation, both solved with an additional endograft cuff. A type II endoleak arising from an LSA was treated with a coil embolization using a brachial approach (Fig. 2). From this experience, we now embolize the LSA at its origin after its coverage with the endograft if the lesion involves this artery. Three patients died during the follow-up due to unrelated reasons.

Conclusion

Overstenting the LSA is most often necessary in proximal descending thoracic aortic endografting. In the majority of centers, as in ours, it appears not to be necessary to perform LSA revascularization prior to endografting in all patients. LSA coverage is generally well accepted and morbidity is limited. However, some specific indications exist for which LSA revascularization is recommended, several days before endograft coverage. Secondary revascularization of the LSA following endograft stenting is rarely necessary.

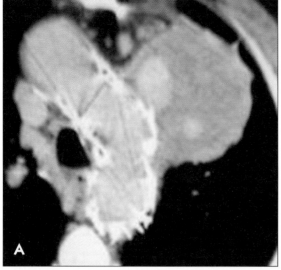

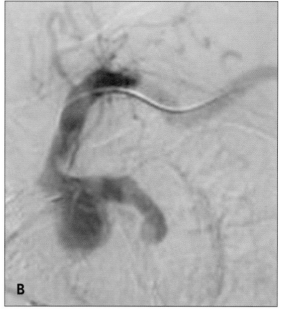

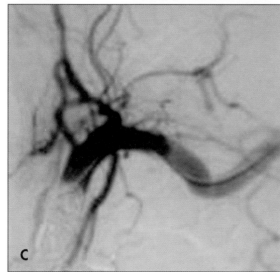

FIG. 2 Computed tomography demonstrating a type II endoleak in a patient who needed a LSA occlusion by the endograft 5 years before (A). A retrograde angiogram via brachial approach shows the subclavian origin of this endoleak (B) and the final angiogram after coil embolization of the first segment of the LSA in the same procedure (C).

REFERENCES

1 Fattori R, Napoli G, Lovato L et al. Descending thoracic aortic diseases: stent-graft repair. *Radiology* 2003; 229: 176-183.

2 Shigemura N, Kato M, Kuratani T et al. New operative method for acute type B dissection: left carotid artery-left subclavian artery bypass combined with endovascular stent-graft implantation. *J Thorac Cardiovasc Surg* 2000; 120: 406-408.

3 Cina CS, Safar HA, Lagana A et al. Subclavian carotid transposition and bypass grafting: consecutive cohort study and systematic review. *J Vasc Surg* 2002; 35: 422-429.

4 Vos AW, Wisselink W, Rijbroek A et al. Endovascular repair of a type B aortic dissection with transposition of a coexistent aberrant subclavian (lusoria) artery. *J Endovasc Ther* 2002; 9: 549-553.

5 Berguer R, Kieffer E. The aortic arch and its branches: anatomy and blood flow. In: Berguer R, Kieffer E (eds). *Surgery of the arteries of the head*. New York, Springer-Verlag 1992: pp 5-31.

6 Hausegger KA, Oberwalder P, Tiesenhausen K et al. Intentional

left subclavian artery occlusion by thoracic aortic stent-grafts without surgical transposition. *J Endovasc Ther* 2001; 8: 472-476.

7 Gorich J, Asquan Y, Seifarth H et al. Initial experience with intentional stent-graft coverage of the subclavian artery during endovascular thoracic aortic repairs. *J Endovasc Ther* 2002; 9 Suppl 2: II39-43.

8 Palma JH, de Souza JA, Rodrigues Alves CM et al. Self-expandable aortic stent-grafts for treatment of descending aortic dissections. *Ann Thorac Surg* 2002; 73: 1138-1142.

9 Riambau V, Garcia-Madrid C, Saldana G et al. We must not translocate the left subclavian artery prior to stent grafting. *J Cardiovasc Surg* 2003; 44 (suppl): 31.

10 Ryan T, Mannion D, O'Brien W et al. Spinal cord perfusion pressure in dogs after control of proximal aortic hypertension during thoracic aortic cross-clamping with esmolol or sodium nitroprusside. *Anesthesiology* 1993; 78: 317-325.

9

ENDOLUMINAL REPAIR OF THORACO-ABDOMINAL ANEURYSMS COMBINED WITH REVASCULARIZATION OF THE VISCERAL ARTERIES

PETER ROBLESS, JOHN WOLFE, MARK COWLING, MARTIN CLARK

Management of patients with complex thoraco-abdominal aortic aneurysms (TAAA) is a formidable challenge. The prevalence of these aneurysms is frequently underestimated and they have a high risk of rupture [1]. Until recently, the only effective treatment was open surgical repair, with high morbidity and mortality [2]. Surgical intervention for TAAA traditionally involves a thoracolaparotomy with medial visceral rotation and in-line grafting using the inclusion patch technique for visceral revascularization. The left renal artery may require either a separate bypass graft or re-implantation with a Carrel patch. Results of these approaches have been satisfactory, however, morbidity can reach 10% to 20% [2], with the most common complications being renal and respiratory failure, bleeding, and spinal cord ischemia. Thoracolaparotomy, phrenotomy, and collapse of the left lung all contribute to impaired postoperative lung function. In Crawford's series of 1414 open operations, 8% of patients had prolonged respiratory support [3]. This complication was associated with mortality rate of 40%.

Prolonged supraceliac aortic cross-clamping is associated with a poor outcome [4,5]. Short supraceliac clamp times have also been associated with neutrophil activation and postoperative inflammatory response syndrome with remote organ dysfunction [6]. This results in a prolonged stay in the intensive care unit [7].

Endovascular aneurysm repair has frequently been used for infrarenal abdominal aortic aneurysms (AAA) [8]. To date thoracic stenting has been used in the treatment of isolated thoracic aortic pathology but has a limited role with extensive TAAA repair [9]. In this setting thoracic stenting has the advantage of avoiding a thoracotomy and cross-clamping of the thoracic aorta. However, endovascular stenting in TAAA is more challenging as the aneurysm usually involves the origins of the visceral and renal arteries. We and others have performed a number of infrarenal or type IV open repairs followed by stenting of the thoracic aorta, if the TAAA has an hour glass *morphology with a relatively normal caliber waist at the level of the visceral and renal arteries. However, a fully aneurysmal TAAA involving the visceral and renal artery origins requires a more imaginative solution. We have sought to overcome these difficulties by using a combination of adjunctive open surgical techniques to enable an endovascular approach in selected patients with significant respiratory comorbidity and complex TAAA. Our initial experience with these hybrid procedures combining endoluminal repair of TAAA with revascularization of the visceral and renal arteries will be discussed in this chapter.*

Hybrid procedures

Two such patients will be discussed to illustrate the approaches used for visceral and renal artery bypass prior to TAAA stenting. These patients posed a challenge in that they were not fit for a full thoracolaparotomy and had aneurysmal disease at the level of the visceral and renal arteries.

This problem is highlighted in this first patient who initially had a chronic type B aortic dissection with extensive aneurysmal disease. He had a pre-vious infrarenal abdominal aneurysm repair followed by a thoracic aneurysm repair. A few years later he was referred to our unit with a large nine centimeter type III TAAA as well as bilateral iliac aneurysms (Fig. 1). His respiratory comorbidity and his previous thoraco-abdominal surgery made his risks for further open TAAA repair prohibitive.

Instead, a combined approach using an abdominal operation to repair his iliac aneurysms, followed by renal and mesenteric artery bypass to allow stenting of his TAAA, was performed. This hybrid procedure avoided a thoracotomy, redo sur-

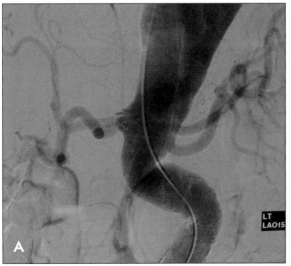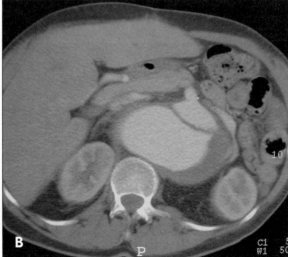

FIG. 1 Large type III TAAA involving origins of celiac axis, SMA, and renal arteries.

gery in the chest, and supraceliac clamping with its high morbidity and mortality rate.

The procedure was performed under general and epidural anesthesia with the patient in the supine position. Spinal drainage, cell salvage, and a rapid infuser were used. Transesophageal echocardiography was also performed. Double lumen endotracheal intubation was not required as a totally intra-abdominal approach was used. Through a transperitoneal approach, a bifurcated 24 by 12 mm Hemashield® *(Meadox, Oakland, NJ, USA)* graft was anastomosed to his previous infrarenal repair in order to deal with his iliac aneurysms. The origins of both renal arteries, celiac axis, and the superior mesenteric artery (SMA) were exposed. Bilateral renal artery bypass grafting was performed with two 6 mm Hemashield® *(Boston Scientific, Wayne, NJ, USA)* grafts in a retrograde configuration using the limbs of the iliac grafts as inflow sites. An inverted 16 by 8 mm graft was used to perfuse the celiac axis and SMA (Fig. 2). This was anastomosed in an end-to-side fashion to the hood of the new bi-iliac graft. Both limbs of the inverted 16 by 8 mm graft were brought along the base of the mesentery for anastomosis, with the SMA (end-to-side) and to the celiac axis (end-to-side) sequentially. The routing of the graft to the celiac axis required a retro pancreatic tunnel. All the anastomoses were performed in nor-

mal arterial segments distal to any aneurysmal segments. The visceral arteries were ligated proximal to each anastomosis to prevent endoleaks. Performance of the visceral or renal anastomoses did not require aortic cross-clamping, thereby decreasing the total visceral ischemic time to a brief period of clamping of the individual visceral vessels.

Following visceral and renal artery bypass, TAAA stent deployment was performed through a pre-sewn 10 mm side graft on the new bifurcated graft. A 5F measuring pigtail catheter *(Cook Australia Pty. Ltd., Queensland, Australia)* was advanced into the ascending aorta over a 0.035" diameter stiff guidewire *(Terumo Corporation, Tokyo, Japan)*. This pigtail catheter was used to exchange the Terumo guidewire for a 0.035" diameter Back-up Meier® *(Boston Scientific Corp., Natick, MA, USA)*. The guidewire was placed in the true lumen of the aneurysm and snared via a right brachial approach. After intravenous administration of 5000 IU of heparin sodium, the Talent® stent-graft system *(Medtronic AVE, USA)* was passed over the Back-up Meier® wire. Four Talent® stent-grafts were then deployed across the TAAA with good result (Fig. 3). Balloon molding was used to further expand the stent-grafts.

Angiography was performed before and after stent-graft deployment to check for position and aneurysm exclusion as well as visceral and renal

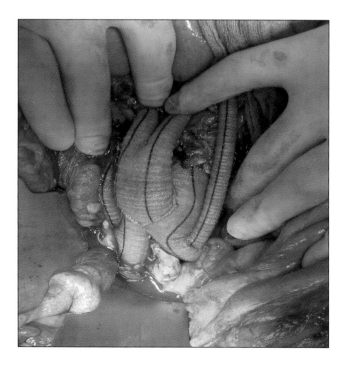

FIG. 2 Bilateral retrograde renal artery bypass grafting was performed with two 6 mm grafts using the limbs of the iliac grafts as inflow sites. An inverted 16 by 8 mm graft was used to revascularize the celiac axis and SMA.

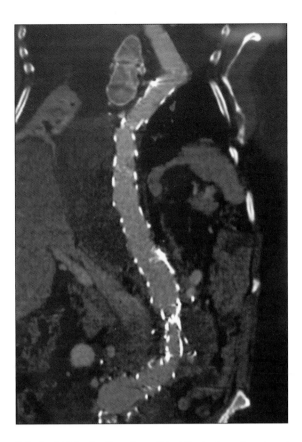

FIG. 3 TAAA stenting. Four Talent® stent grafts placed across the thoracoabdominal aorta to exclude the TAAA and covering the origins of the visceral and renal arteries.

As described above, the operation was performed under general and epidural anesthesia. Spinal drainage, cell salvage, and a rapid infuser were used. Through a transperitoneal approach the origins of the celiac axis, SMA, and renal arteries were exposed. The normal caliber infrarenal aorta and both common iliac arteries were exposed and clamped following the administration of heparin. An aortotomy was performed in the distal infrarenal aorta and an inverted 14 by 7 mm graft was used for a retrograde bypass to both renal arteries (end-to-side). Following this a second 1- by 7 mm graft was "piggy backed" onto the origin of the first graft (Fig. 5). A retrograde bypass was then performed to the celiac axis and SMA as described earlier. Doppler signals were checked in the renal and visceral vessels with the origins clamped. These were satisfactory, and the origins of the visceral and renal vessels were then ligated to prevent endoleaks. The visceral and renal arteries were bypassed sequentially and the mean ischemic time for each bypass was only 12 minutes.

Following successful visceral and renal bypass, an arteriotomy was performed in the right iliac artery for stent deployment. The left iliac artery was punctured and guidewires were introduced in both iliac arteries. An angiogram catheter was placed through the left iliac artery. Through the right iliac artery, 5 Talent® stents (36F to 42F) were deployed sequentially to exclude the TAAA and cover the origins of the visceral and renal vessels.

Both lower limbs were ischemic following the procedure. This was due to dissection of the external iliac arteries presumably from catheter and sheath manipulation. Therefore, a jump graft from the right common iliac artery to both common femoral arteries was performed to revascularize both legs. The entire procedure took 11 hours.

perfusion. After removal of the device, the presewn side graft was ligated. Follow-up spiral computed tomography was performed prior to discharge and at 3- to 6-month intervals. The sequence of surgical procedures are schematically represented in fig. 4. A second patient was treated for a ten centimeter type II TAAA using the same combined approach of endovascular stenting with renal and visceral bypass. She had significant respiratory comorbidity, having had a previous left thoracotomy and partial lobectomy and therefore was not fit for a thoraco-laparotomy and open repair of her type II TAAA. The TAAA extended from the proximal descending thoracic aorta to below the level of the renal arteries. Therefore she had open revascularization of her renal and visceral arteries followed by stent-grafting of the TAAA.

Outcome

Both patients had spinal drains peri-operatively and neither had neurological complications. Due to their pre-existing respiratory comorbidity, both patients required prolonged respiratory support in intensive care. The mean stay in hospital was 29 days. Mean follow-up is 16 months and there were no endoleaks on computed tomography scan.

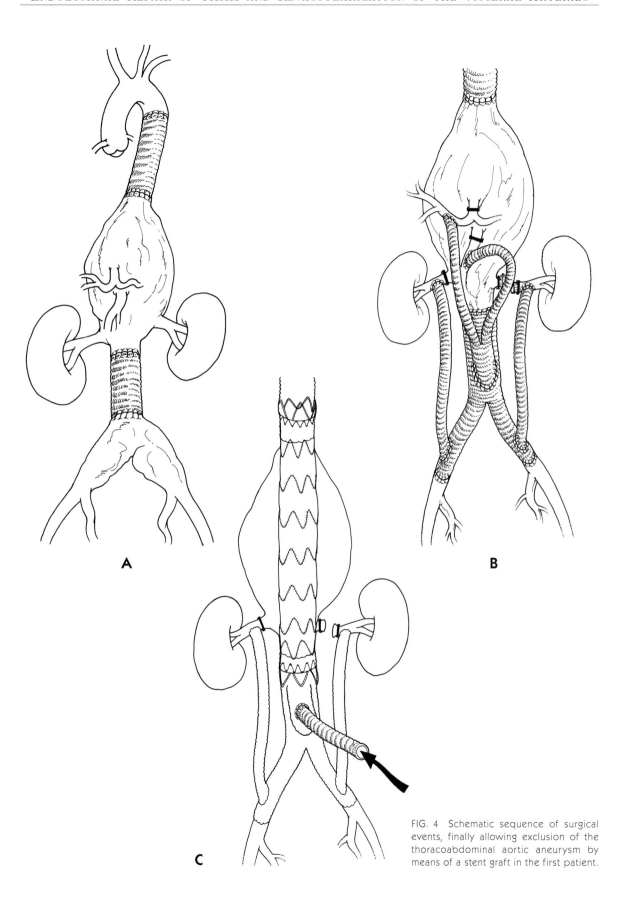

A

B

C

FIG. 4 Schematic sequence of surgical events, finally allowing exclusion of the thoracoabdominal aortic aneurysm by means of a stent graft in the first patient.

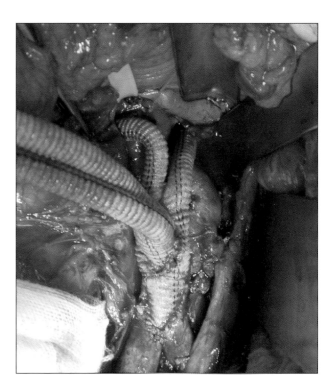

FIG. 5 An inverted 14 by 7 mm graft was used for a retrograde bypass to both renal arteries. Subsequently, a second 14 by 7 mm graft was "piggy backed" onto the origin of the first graft for the retrograde visceral bypass.

Endovascular versus open repair

TAAA as classified by Crawford usually involves the origins of the major aortic side branches. Current aortic stent graft technology is unable to routinely achieve aneurysm exclusion with preservation of the side branches. Some authors have reported successful TAAA stent graft deployment with preservation of side branches using custom made modular stent grafts with side branches [10]. This modular endograft system was first used in a 76-year-old man with a contained rupture of a supraceliac ulcer and a large AAA ending proximally at the celiac artery. The endograft was deployed successfully, but the patient developed paraplegia on day 2. Follow-up imaging showed an excluded aneurysm and good flow through the endograft and all prosthetic side branches.

The Perth group has reported some success using fenestration in endovascular grafts for suprarenal aneurysms [11]. Accurate placement of a fenestration over the orifice of a target vessel is feasible, but long-term maintenance of position is dependent on secure graft fixation. Placement of a Palmaz stent overlapping the fenestration and vessel orifice secures the junction. This may be difficult in a large TAAA where the origins of the visceral and renal arteries are often surrounded by extensive thrombus. Catheter manipulation may result in mesenteric ischemia or renal impairment.

The same group has also described a technique combining endoluminal and open approaches for the repair of TAAA involving the celiac axis [12]. Two patients with type I TAAA and suboptimal cardiac reserve underwent endoluminal stent graft implantation. To achieve a satisfactory distal seal, the distal end of the endograft was circumscribed with a dacron band that was sutured to the aorta and endograft through a midline incision. The patent celiac artery in both patients was ligated to stop retrograde filling of the aneurysm sac. The patients developed no problems peri-operatively, and exclusion of the aneurysms was confirmed by follow-up imaging. Three years after endografting, both patients had excluded aneurysms without evidence of endoleak or device migration.

We have embarked on open revascularization of the visceral and renal arteries instead of fenestration or modular side branched stent devices. This avoids the problems with accurate positioning of the fenestrations and prosthetic side branches with its risks of thrombosis, distal embolization and potentially fatal side branch occlusion. The treatment of these complex TAAA using a hybrid procedure has several advantages. First, it can be performed through a transabdominal approach, avoiding a thoracotomy and retroperitoneal exposure. In addition, because aortic clamping was avoided, ischemic time to each of the visceral arteries was limited to the time of construction of the distal anastomosis, which in this case was less than 15 minutes for each anastomosis. Prolonged simultaneous hepatic, mesenteric, and renal ischemia was avoided. Visceral and renal ischemia are both associated with peri-operative complications and increased mortality [13].

Surgical considerations

This combined approach, however, presents potential hazards. Intraperitoneal routing of the dacron grafts should be avoided and therefore both renal bypass grafts were routed in a retroperitoneal position. The grafts for the SMA and celiac reconstructions were tunneled under the small bowel mesentery and in a retropancreatic route. However, the long-term patency of these grafts remains a cause of concern.

The safety and durability of retrograde mesenteric bypass grafting versus antegrade bypass grafting remains a controversial issue. The advantages of the latter are a usually normal supraceliac aorta for proximal anastomosis with a shorter and more anatomical bypass grafting route. This is not the case in patients with TAAA with significant supraceliac aneurysmal disease.

The retrograde approach is technically easier to perform, avoids supraceliac aortic clamping, and reduces visceral ischemic time. In a review of 24 cases of chronic mesenteric ischemia, Moawad et al. showed no significant differences in long-term results for 17 patients who underwent antegrade bypass grafting and 7 patients who had a retrograde bypass [14]. In contrast, Johnston et al. noted a higher failure rate with the retrograde technique, reporting 3 thromboses in 16 cases and none in 5 patients treated with the antegrade approach [15]. McMillan et al. objectively documented graft patency postoperatively with duplex scanning. They showed that patency rates for antegrade and retrograde bypass grafting procedures were similar [16]. A review and critical analysis of the literature failed to identify a superior technique for mesenteric revascularization and concluded that the choice of operation should be individualized [17].

Mesenteric and renal artery retrograde bypass has a proven track record for long-term patency in large surgical series for mesenteric ischemia [18,19] and in the treatment of renal artery stenosis [20]. Lin et al. from the Baylor group report a case of iliorenal artery bypass grafting to facilitate endovascular abdominal aortic aneurysm repair [21]. They describe a patient with an infrarenal AAA originating three millimeters below the left renal artery with cardiac morbidity that precluded open AAA repair. Left renal artery relocation with retroperitoneal iliorenal bypass grafting was performed to lengthen the proximal landing zone, which facilitated successful endovascular AAA repair. Postoperative surveillance after three years showed aneurysm reduction with a patent iliorenal bypass graft.

The effect of this combined approach on spinal cord ischemia is unknown and will require further investigation. Neither of our patients developed spinal cord ischemia but this complication may occur with either technique. Re-implantation of intercostal arteries alone has not been shown to eliminate spinal cord ischemia [22]. The etiology of this complication is likely to be multifactorial, with prolonged ischemia, hypotension, and reperfusion all contributing [23]. These are all minimized with the hybrid approach described earlier for these aneurysms.

Future perspectives

Dake et al. found that 37% (13/35) of descending thoracic aneurysms were suitable for thoracic stenting [9]. In our series of 229 consecutive patients with TAAA, a retrospective review showed that an endovascular option could have been considered in 25% of type I, 11% of type II, and 5% of type III TAAAs. It is likely that an increasing proportion of patients with extensive thoraco-abdominal aneurysms may be treated by the combination of adjunctive surgical procedures and endovascular stenting. This widens the application of endovascular repair and we shall continue with the hybrid procedure, which may reduce morbidity and mortality in this group of high-risk patients.

REFERENCES

1 Bickerstaff LK, Pairolero PC, Hollier LH, et al. Thoracic aortic aneurysms: a population-based study. *Surgery* 1982; 92: 1103-1108.

2 Svensson LG, Crawford ES, Hess KR, et al. Experience with 1509 patients undergoing thoracoabdominal aortic operations. *J Vasc Surg* 1993; 17: 357-370.

3 Svensson LG, Hess KR, Coselli JS, et al. A prospective study of respiratory failure after high-risk surgery on the thoracoabdominal aorta. *J Vasc Surg* 1991; 14: 271-282.

4 Safi HJ, Harlin SA, Miller CC, et al. Predictive factors for acute renal failure in thoracic and thoracoabdominal aortic aneurysm surgery. *J Vasc Surg* 1996; 24: 338-345.

5 Bicknell CD, Cowan AR, Kerle MI, et al. Renal dysfunction and prolonged visceral ischaemia increase mortality rate after suprarenal aneurysm repair. *Br J Surg* 2003; 90: 1142-1146.

6 Foulds S, Cheshire NJ, Schachter M, et al. Endotoxin related early neutrophil activation is associated with outcome after thoracoabdominal aortic aneurysm repair. *Br J Surg* 1997; 84: 172-177.

7 Harward TR, Welborn MB 3rd, Martin TD, et al. Visceral ischemia and organ dysfunction after thoracoabdominal aortic aneurysm repair. A clinical and cost analysis. *Ann Surg* 1996; 223: 729-736.

8 May J, White GH, Ly CN, et al. Endoluminal repair of abdominal aortic aneurysm prevents enlargement of the proximal neck: a 9-year life-table and 5-year longitudinal study. *J Vasc Surg* 2003; 37: 86-90.

9 Dake MD, Miller DC, Mitchell RS, et al. The "first generation" of endovascular stent grafts for patients with aneurysms of the descending thoracic aorta. *J Thorac Cardiovasc Surg* 1998; 116: 689-704.

10 Chuter TA, Gordon RL, Reilly LM, et al. An endovascular system for thoracoabdominal aortic aneurysm repair. *J Endovasc Ther* 2001; 8: 25-33.

11 Stanley BM, Semmens JB, Lawrence-Brown MM, et al. Fenestration in endovascular grafts for aortic aneurysm repair: new horizons for preserving blood flow in branch vessels. *J Endovasc Ther* 2001; 8: 16-24.

12 Lawrence-Brown MM, Sieunarine K, van Schie G, et al. Hybrid open-endoluminal technique for repair of thoracoabdominal aneurysm involving the celiac axis. *J Endovasc Ther* 2000; 7: 513-519.

13 Gilling-Smith GL, Worswick L, Knight PF, et al. Surgical repair of thoracoabdominal aortic aneurysm: 10 year's experience. *Br J Surg* 1995; 82: 624-629.

14 Moawad J, McKinsey JF, Wyble CW, et al. Current results of surgical therapy for chronic mesenteric ischemia. *Arch Surg* 1997; 132: 613-619.

15 Johnston KW, Lindsay TF, Walker PM, Kalman PG. Mesenteric arterial bypass grafts: early and late results and suggested surgical approach for chronic and acute mesenteric ischemia. *Surgery* 1995; 118: 1-7.

16 McMillan WD, McCarthy WJ, Bresticker MR, et al. Mesenteric artery bypass: objective patency determination. *J Vasc Surg* 1995; 21: 729-741.

17 Shanley CJ, Ozaki CK, Zelenock GB. Bypass grafting for chronic mesenteric ischemia. *Surg Clin North Am* 1997; 77: 381-395.

18 Robless P, Belli AM, Geroulakos G. Endovascular versus surgical reconstruction for the management of chronic visceral ischemia: a comparative analysis. In: Geroulakos G, Cherry KJ Jr (eds). *Diseases of the visceral circulation*. London, Edward Arnold 2002: pp 108-118.

19 Sreenarasimhaiah J. Diagnosis and management of intestinal ischaemic disorders. *Br Med J* 2003; 326: 1372-1376.

20 Murray SP, Kent C, Salvatierra O, Stoney RJ. Complex branch renovascular disease: management options and late results. *J Vasc Surg* 1994; 20: 338-346.

21 Lin PH, Madsen K, Bush RL, Lumsden AB. Iliorenal artery bypass grafting to facilitate endovascular abdominal aortic aneurysm repair. *J Vasc Surg* 2003; 38: 183-185.

22 Safi HJ, Miller CC 3rd, Carr C, et al. Importance of intercostal artery reattachment during thoracoabdominal aortic aneurysm repair. *J Vasc Surg* 1998; 27: 58-68.

23 Lintott P, Hafez HM, Stansby G. Spinal cord complications of thoracoabdominal aneurysm surgery. *Br J Surg* 1998; 85: 5-15.

10

ENDOVASCULAR TREATMENT OF THORACIC ANEURYSMS COMBINED WITH OPEN SURGERY OF THE INFRARENAL AORTA FOR TANDEM LESIONS

GEERT WILLEM SCHURINK, MICHIEL DE HAAN, MICHAEL JACOBS

More than 60% of patients who undergo repair of a descending thoracic aortic aneurysm (TAA) have multifocal aortic disease, half of which involves the infrarenal aorta [1]. In patients with abdominal aortic aneurysms (AAA), 12% also have thoracic aneurysms.

Affected patients frequently have major comorbidities including hypertension, coronary artery disease, obstructive pulmonary disease, and congestive heart failure, all of which have significant impact on recovery following operative repair.

Compared to open repair of the abdominal aorta, open repair of the descending thoracic aorta has a significant higher mortality and morbidity, predominantly associated with the thoracotomy, the use of cardiopulmonary bypass, and postoperative complications including bleeding, paraplegia, stroke, renal, and pulmonary insufficiency.

Endovascular stent-grafts have been used for pathology of the descending thoracic aorta for almost ten years with encouraging early results. In an attempt to decrease the risk associated with either a simultaneous thoracotomy and laparotomy or sequential operations in patients with multilevel aortic disease, endovascular treatment of descending thoracic aortic aneurysms in combination with open repair of abdominal aortic aneurysms has been introduced as an alternative. Furthermore, this combined strategy will offer available treatment for patients with prohibitive comorbidities.

Indications for treatment

Indications for treatment of the combination of an AAA and a descending TAA are the same as for both entities individually. An exception to this rule is the obligatory repair of a small AAA in the absence of adequate femoral or iliac access for stent-graft introduction due to obstructive arterial disease. Also for obstructive aorto-iliac disease alone, the implantation of an aortobifemoral graft can be performed prior to stent-graft placement for TAA. The impact of the access problems resulting from aorto-iliac obstructive disease was shown by Carpenter et al. [2] who demonstrated that 48% of the patients were rejected for endovascular treatment of their AAA because of small iliac arteries. Because of the larger diameter of sheaths for most thoracic stent-grafts, this number will even be higher in the patients with AAA and associated descending TAA.

If both aneurysms have a morphology suitable for endovascular treatment, both can be treated by stent-graft implantation (Fig. 1). Especially in high-risk patients, operative mortality and morbidity can be reduced even further. In the literature, few cases of endovascular treatment of both AAA and TAA are reported [3,4], without significant complications.

Operative technique

If a combined treatment of AAA and descending TAA is chosen, the AAA is addressed first. This can be performed by a midline transperitoneal approach or by a left retroperitoneal approach. Advantage of the latter approach is that the patient can be positioned in a 60 degree right lateral decubitus position rotating the aortic arch in an ideal fluoroscopic position for stent-grafting of the distal arch. Also, draping of the left thoracic side is possible for potential conversion to open repair of the thoracic aneurysm.

The standard technique for abdominal aortic replacement is used. After completion of the distal anastomosis and re-establishing aortic flow, a 10 millimeter dacron tube graft can be anastomosed in an end-to-side fashion to the main trunk of the abdominal graft. This graft is used as a side limb through which the stent-graft will be introduced. Introduction and deployment of the thoracic stent-graft is done by the standard technique with the use of a movable radiographic C-arm image intensifier.

If staged repair of the abdominal and thoracic aneurysm is chosen, the 10 millimeter dacron side limb can be tunneled through the fascia into the subcutaneous plane [5]. For the second stage, no femoral artery cut down is necessary. A subcutaneous dissection allows easy access to the side limb which, after trombectomy, allows routine stent-graft introduction.

Paraplegia

Only a limited number of patients with concomitant treatment of AAA and descending TAA are reported in the literature (Table). Most of the cases are reported in larger series of endovascularly treated descending TAAs. The largest series is from *Stanford University*, describing 103 patients treated for descending TAAs [6]. Within this group, 19 patients underwent simultaneous open repair of their AAA. The most striking difference between the group with isolated TAA treatment and group with the concomitant treatment of AAA and TAA was the difference in paraplegia rate. Two of the 19 patients (11%) suffered from early paraplegia in contrast to one case of paraplegia in the remaining 84 patients (1%). This last patient had undergone aortic aneurysm repair in the past.

In their experience with 27 stent-grafts for descending TAA, Saccani et al. reported four cases with combined open abdominal aortic grafting [7]. They did not experience paraplegia. Cambria et al. performed three cases of simultaneous open AAA and endovascular TAA repair among a total of 18 endovascular TAA cases, without neurological deficit [8]. Gravereaux et al. described three cases of paraplegia in a group of 53 patients with endovascular treatment of the descending TAA [9]. One patient had simultaneous open repair of a small AAA after malpositioning of one thoracic stent-graft over the visceral vessels, which had to be removed through the abdominal aorta. The other two patients had undergone AAA repair in the past. In this publication, neither the total number of patients with concomitant open AAA repair, nor the amount of patient with previous AAA repair was mentioned.

Analysis of other factors that are probably important for developing paraplegia after concomitant AAA and TAA repair, such as extent and level of descending thoracic aorta covered by the stent-graft, cannot be analyzed from the literature because of the scarcity of publications concerning this issue. Nevertheless, the paraplegia rate in the Stanford experience for concomitant repair of

AAAs and descending TAAs is 11%, which is considerably higher than the range from 0% to 6% reported for open repair of the thoracic aorta, but compares to the 10% to 15% paraplegia rate of thoraco-abdominal aortic repair with the use of distal

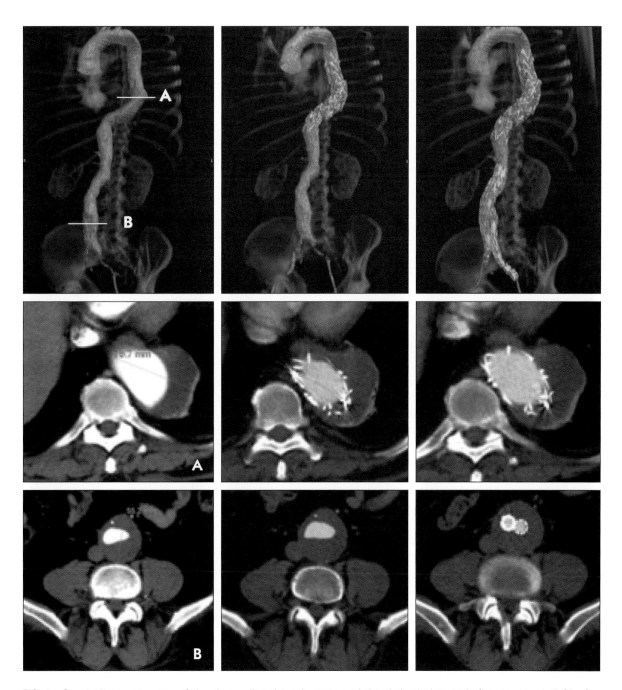

FIG. 1 Concomitant aneurysms of the descending thoracic aorta and the abdominal aorta before treatment *(left)*, after endovascular treatment of the thoracic aneurysm *(middle)*, and after endovascular treatment of the AAA *(right)*. Levels A and B correspond with the axial computed tomography slides of the thoracic aneurysm and abdominal aneurysm, respectively.

Table	TOTAL ENDOVASCULAR TAA CASES, CONCOMITANT AAA AND TAA TREATMENT, AND ENDOVASCULAR TAA AFTER PREVIOUS AAA REPAIR					
1st author [ref.]		Number of endoTAAs		Number of paraplegia		
	Total	*Concomitant open AAA repair*	*Previous AAA repair*	*Concomitant open AAA repair*	*Previous AAA repair*	*Total*
Dake et al. [6]	103	19	47 *	2	1	3
Saccani et al. [7]	27	4	1	0	0	0
Cambria et al. [8]	28	3	9	0	0	0
Gravereaux et al. [9]	53	NA	NA	1	2	3
Personal experience	13	4	1	0	0	0

* Number of previously repaired or co-existing AAAs

AAA: abdominal aortic aneurysm
TAA: thoracic aortic aneurysm
NA: not available

aortic perfusion and cerebrospinal fluid (CSF) drainage [10].

Whether previous AAA repair is a risk factor for paraplegia after endovascular TAA treatment cannot be proven from the published data, although many authors suggest this. On theoretical grounds, the occlusion of lumbar arteries in both concomitant open treatment of AAA and after previous AAA repair reduces the possibility of an adequate collateral circulation to the spinal cord, especially when more important intercostal arteries become occluded by the thoracic stent-graft.

With regard to the latter, assessment of the spinal cord function by means of measuring motor evoked potentials (MEPs) during operation can predict whether the patient will suffer from paraplegia [11]. Although attempted with *homemade* devices [12,13], not one of the commercially available devices is retrievable. Should MEP registration show impaired spinal cord function after stent-graft deployment, conversion to open repair, removal of the stent-graft, and intercostal artery reattachment is the only chance to regain spinal cord function [14]. MEP registration during temporary balloon exclusion of the thoracic aneurysm with axillo-femoral bypass (as distal aortic perfusion) could be a way to predict the spinal cord function outcome in these patients [15,16].

Other methods generally used in open thoraco-abdominal aneurysm repair, such as administration of steroids and CSF drainage, could also reduce the risk of paraplegia in open repair of AAAs and endovascular repair of descending thoracic aneurysms. CSF drainage has been described in endovascular TAA cases as an attempt, sometimes successfully, to reverse paraplegia; however CSF drainage was always initiated after clinical evidence of spinal cord ischemia was detected [9,17,18].

Our endovascular protocol for distal descending TAAs (Th8-Th12) approaches our open TAA protocol, including pre-operative installation of CSF drainage and administration of steroids. Also spinal cord function assessment by registration of the MEPs is performed. If spinal cord function is decreased, one of the strategies includes elevation of blood pressure, inducing return of MEPs as illustrated in Figure 2. In this patient, following stent-graft deployment, MEP amplitudes at both legs decreased to 30% of the initial level. Raising the mean arterial blood pressure returned the amplitudes to more than 50%. The patient had no signs of spinal cord ischemia after surgery.

Planning treatment

Before the era of endovascular treatment, there was debate over whether concomitant aneurysms of the abdominal and descending thoracic aorta should be treated simultaneously through separate incisions or staged several weeks apart.

Crawford et al. observed in a group of 112 patients with descending TAA repair an 11% mortality, of which 30% were due to rupture of infrarenal AAA that was not simultaneously repaired [19]. In 1982, Crawford and Cohen published mortality rates of both simultaneous and staged repair (10% and 16%, respectively) [1].

When discussing open treatment of AAAs and endovascular treatment of descending thoracic aneurysms, the latter will not add significant mortality if performed simultaneously. However, the impact of staged repair on the paraplegia rate might be positive. During staged repair, the endovascular treatment of the TAA will be performed in a more hemodynamically stable situation, without abdominal aortic cross-clamping and reperfusion causing cardiodepression and hypotension. The aortic cross-clamping and lumbar artery closure can potentially cause mild spinal cord ischemia which can deteriorate after simultaneous thoracic stent-graft placement. Also postoperative hypotension can be the cause of delayed-onset spinal cord ischemia due to a marginal collateral blood supply to the spinal cord. Scheduling the endovascular treatment of the TAA after the patient's recovery might reduce the risk of paraplegia.

A disadvantage of staged treatment is the second period of anesthesia and the necessity of an adequate access site for the stent-graft insertion.

Personal experience

Within our series of 28 patients with endovascular treatment of the thoracic aorta, 13 were treated for thoracic aneurysms, 11 for complicated dissections, and 4 for traumatic aortic transsections. Of the patients with a descending thoracic aneurysm, five had concomitant aneurysms of the descending thoracic and abdominal aorta.

The first patient was a 72-year-old man with a midthoracic aortic aneurysm and a juxtarenal AAA. The latter aneurysm was treated first by an open insertion of a tube graft. The thoracic aneurysm was treated endovascularly. During this procedure, MEP registration of the lower legs showed a significant drop after stent-graft deployment (30% of initial amplitude) and returned to 50% after blood

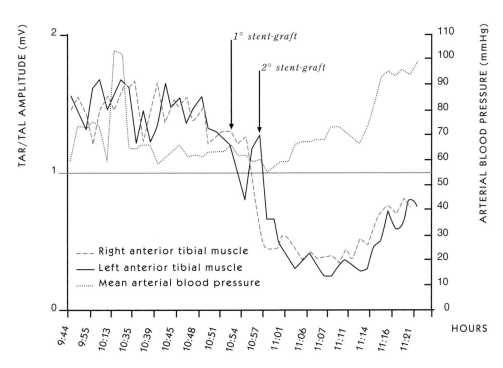

FIG. 2 Monitoring of MEPs during endovascular treatment of descending TAA. Amplitudes of right and left anterior tibial muscle (TAR/TAL amplitudo) decrease after stent-graft deployment and partially return after elevation of the mean arterial blood pressure (ABP).

pressure elevation (Fig. 2). CSF drainage was continued for three days. No clinical signs of paraplegia developed.

The second patient was a 59-year-old man with a rupture of a descending TAA, which was treated endovascularly. His almost 10 centimeter AAA was operated three weeks later by open tube graft reconstruction (Fig. 3). Despite his congestive heart failure, two myocardial infarctions, and repeated coronary artery bypass grafting in his medical history, both procedures had an uneventful outcome.

The third patient was a 62-year-old man who had a distal descending TAA with an infrarenal aortic aneurysm. During the first operation, the thoracic aneurysm was treated by endovascular stent-grafts.

MEP registration of the lower legs showed significant decrease after stent-graft deployment (50% of initial amplitude) and returned to 70% after blood pressure elevation. The infrarenal AAA with a left common iliac aneurysm was also treated endovascularly. Before this second intervention, the left hypogastric artery was embolized after 30 minutes of uneventful hypogastric balloon occlusion to evaluate the support of this artery to the spinal cord circulation (Fig. 1) No paraplegia occurred in this patient.

In the fourth patient, a 65-year-old man, a midthoracic saccular aneurysm with intramural hematoma was treated with a stent-graft. No changes in MEP registration occurred. His infrarenal aneurysm was

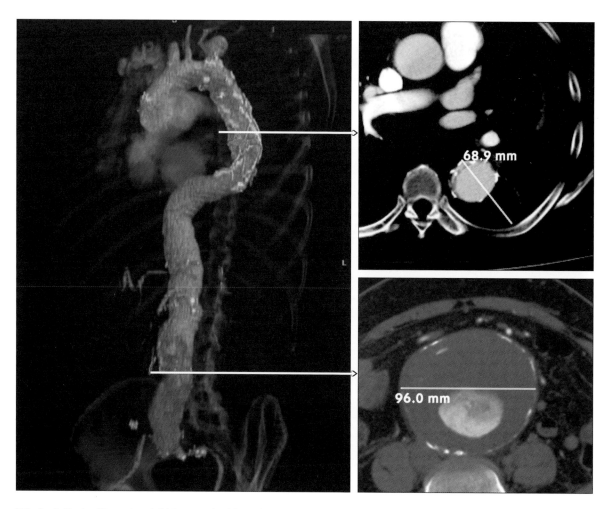

FIG. 3 Patient with ruptured TAA treated with endovascular stent-graft. Three weeks later, the AAA was replaced by a tube graft.

treated in a second operation with an aorto-uni-iliac system because of left iliac artery tortuosity. No complications occurred during and after both procedures.

The last patient, a 56-year-old man, was treated endovascularly for a ruptured midthoracic aneurysm and is still in follow-up for his slowly growing suprarenal aortic aneurysm.

Conclusion

Concomitant aneurysms of the descending thoracic aorta and the abdominal aorta are not a rare problem. Both simultaneous and staged open repair are associated with significant mortality and morbidity, especially in high-risk surgical patients. By performing endovascular treatment of the descending TAA, an attempt is made to lower the peri-operative and postoperative complications. Especially the risk of paraplegia during the combined endovascular and open procedure is still significant. Spinal cord function monitoring during the intervention and peri-operative protective measures like CSF drainage and steroid administration can probably lower the paraplegia rate. Theoretically, staged repair of the concomitant aneurysms will lower the change on paraplegia, because the endovascular treatment of the TAA will be performed in a more hemodynamically stable patient.

REFERENCES

1 Crawford ES, Cohen ES. Aortic aneurysm: a multifocal disease. Presidential address. *Arch Surg* 1982; 117: 1393-1400.
2 Carpenter JP, Baum RA, Barker CF, et al. Impact of exclusion criteria on patient selection for endovascular abdominal aortic aneurysm repair. *J Vasc Surg* 2001; 34: 1050-1054.
3 Wolf YG, Zarins CK, Rubin GD, Fogarty TJ. Concomitant endovascular repair of descending thoracic and abdominal aortic aneurysm. *Circulation* 2000; 102: E36.
4 Meguid AA, Bove PG, Long GW, et al. Simultaneous stent-graft repair of thoracic and infrarenal abdominal aortic aneurysms. *J Endovasc Ther* 2002; 9: 165-169.
5 Moon MR, Mitchell RS, Dake MD, et al. Simultaneous abdominal aortic replacement and thoracic stent-graft placement for multilevel aortic disease. *J Vasc Surg* 1997; 25: 332-340.
6 Dake MD, Miller DC, Mitchell RS, et al. The "first generation" of endovascular stent-grafts for patients with aneurysms of the descending thoracic aorta. *J Thorac Cardiovasc Surg* 1998; 116: 689-703; discussion 703-704.
7 Saccani S, Nicolini F, Beghi C, et al. Thoracic aortic stents: a combined solution for complex cases. *Eur J Vasc Endovasc Surg* 2002; 24: 423-427.
8 Cambria RP, Brewster DC, Lauterbach SR, et al. Evolving experience with thoracic aortic stent graft repair. *J Vasc Surg* 2002; 35: 1129-1136.
9 Gravereaux EC, Faries PL, Burks JA, et al. Risk of spinal cord ischemia after endograft repair of thoracic aortic aneurysms. *J Vasc Surg* 2001; 34: 997-1003.
10 Jacobs M, Elenbaas T, Schurink GW, et al. Complications of descending thoracic aortic surgery. In: Branchereau A, Jacobs M (eds). *Complications in vascular and endovascular surgery (part I).* Armonk, NY, Futura Publishing Company, Inc. 2001: pp 201-209.

11 Jacobs MJ, Elenbaas TW, Schurink GW, et al. Assessment of spinal cord integrity during thoracoabdominal aortic aneurysm repair. *Ann Thorac Surg* 2002; 74: S1864-S1866.
12 Watanabe Y, Ishimaru S, Kawaguchi S, et al. Successful endografting with simultaneous visceral artery bypass grafting for severely calcified thoracoabdominal aortic aneurysm. *J Vasc Surg* 2002; 35: 397-399.
13 Ishimaru S, Kawaguchi S, Koizumi N, et al. Preliminary report on prediction of spinal cord ischemia in endovascular stent graft repair of thoracic aortic aneurysm by retrievable stent graft. *J Thorac Cardiovasc Surg* 1998; 115: 811-818.
14 Reichart M, Balm R, Meilof JF, et al. Ischemic transverse myelopathy after endovascular repair of a thoracic aneurysm. *J Endovasc Ther* 2001; 8: 321-327.
15 Midorikawa H, Hoshino S, Iwaya F, et al. Prevention of paraplegia in transluminally placed endoluminal prosthetic grafts for descending thoracic aortic aneurysms. *Jpn J Thorac Cardiovasc Surg* 2000; 48: 761-768.
16 Bafort C, Astarci P, Goffette P, et al. Predicting spinal cord ischemia before endovascular thoracoabdominal aneurysm repair: monitoring somatosensory evoked potentials. *J Endovasc Ther* 2002; 9: 289-294.
17 Oberwalder PJ, Tiesenhausen K, Hausegger K, Rigler B. Successful reversal of delayed paraplegia after endovascular stent grafting. *J Thorac Cardiovasc Surg* 2002; 124: 1259-1260.
18 Fuchs RJ, Lee WA, Seubert CN, Gelman S. Transient paraplegia after stent grafting of a descending thoracic aortic aneurysm treated with cerebrospinal fluid drainage. *J Clin Anesth* 2003; 15: 59-63.
19 Crawford ES, Walker HSJ, Saleh SA, Normann NA. Graft replacement of aneurysm in descending thoracic aorta: results without bypass or shunting. *Surgery* 1981; 89: 73-85.

11

OPEN PROCEDURES TO ACQUIRE AORTIC ACCESS FOR ENDOLUMINAL GRAFTING

RACHEL BELL, PETER TAYLOR

Endoluminal repair is a popular, minimally invasive technique for the treatment of abdominal and thoracic aortic disease; however, co-existing iliac occlusive disease, tortuosity, or small native arteries can limit the applicability of this technique. A recent study of 307 patients showed that 57% were not suitable for endovascular repair because of iliac occlusive disease or tortuosity [1]. Damage to the access artery occurs in 5.1% to 17% of all endovascular aneurysm repairs [2-5]. In these circumstances it is possible to use adjunctive open and endovascular techniques to allow safe delivery of the device. Good pre-operative imaging is essential to identify potential problems with arterial access and to allow the procedures to be tailored to the individual. Hybrid endovascular and open procedures increase the number of patients who can be offered endoluminal treatment.

Pre-operative imaging

All patients should have contrast-enhanced multislice computerized tomography and calibration digital subtraction angiography with antero-posterior and oblique views of the iliac arteries. If the iliac arteries are tortuous, a stiff wire (Amplatz® super stiff or Lunderquist® wire) can be inserted through the pigtail catheter to see if the artery will straighten. If the wire will not pass or the artery does not straighten, then the stent-graft delivery system is unlikely to pass through. In general, iliac arteries must be greater than 7 millimeters in diameter to accommodate the current delivery systems. Good pre-operative imaging should identify those patients with access problems. If possible, it is preferable to perform any necessary adjunctive procedure prior to the endovascular repair.

Anesthetic techniques

Endovascular procedures can be performed under general, regional, or local anesthesia, and the choice is influenced by the extent of arterial access required. Regional or local anesthesia is preferred in patients undergoing thoracic endoluminal repair, as it allows continual monitoring of distal neurological function. Invasive blood pressure monitoring via an arterial line is essential, as hypotension from undisclosed hemorrhage is usually an indication of a ruptured iliac artery.

Techniques for endovascular device delivery

COMMON FEMORAL ARTERY EXPOSURE

The common femoral artery is the most frequent access site for endovascular procedures. This can be done through a vertical or oblique incision in the groin. An oblique incision is preferred, as it provides adequate exposure and has a lower incidence of postoperative wound complications [6,7] (Fig. 1A). Using a double sling proximally and distally can provide proximal control if there is a persistent leak around the sheath (Fig. 1B). The branches of the external iliac artery underneath the inguinal ligament (the deep circumflex iliac artery and the inferior epigastric artery) can be dissected out and controlled by double ligatures. The proximal sling can then be placed above these with the advantage that it will stay in place and not slide distally. If the common femoral artery is short, then both the superficial and profunda femoral arteries should be controlled separately. The needle to pass the guidewire should be placed in the center of the exposed common femoral artery, so that adequate space is left proximally and distally to apply clamps to repair the artery after removal of the sheath at the end of the procedure. It is not necessary to perform a formal arteriotomy if the device has a smooth tapered nose cone, as advancing the device over a wire splits the common femoral artery transversely. This can be closed with an interrupted or continuous non-absorbable polypropylene suture.

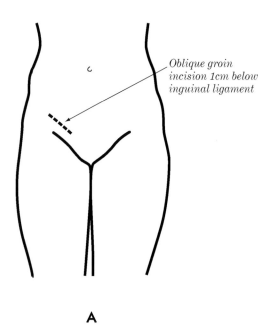

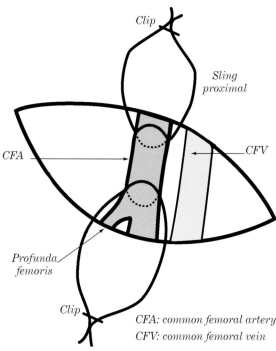

FIG. 1 A - Exposure of the common femoral artery is gained through an oblique incision 1 centimeter below the inguinal ligament and 2 centimeters above the skin crease. B - The common femoral artery can be controlled by using a double sling proximally and distally.

COMMON ILIAC ARTERY EXPOSURE

An extraperitoneal approach through an oblique incision in the iliac fossa gives good access to the common iliac arteries and aortic bifurcation. A 8 to 10 millimeter dacron or polytetrafluoroethylene (PTFE) graft can be sutured end-to-end or end-to-side to the common iliac or distal aorta (Fig. 2). There are theoretical advantages to an end-to-end anastomosis, as this allows easier insertion of the device by obliterating the awkward angle between the conduit and the artery. Some groups have suggested using a 2 centimeter cuff of graft material to re-inforce the end-to-end anastomosis and to reduce bleeding from the suture line. Then the graft can be brought into the groin under the inguinal ligament and the vessels straightened by traction. The graft can then be used as an access conduit to insert the delivery sheath. This graft can be temporary or permanent and can be anastomosed to the common femoral or external iliac artery at the end of the procedure. However, an end-to-end anastomosis will result in distal limb ischemia, which can produce complications in patients with distal occlusive disease. End-to-side anastomoses allow the distal limb to be perfused throughout the procedure and are preferred. The anastomosis to the native artery must be long so as to ensure a smooth passage of the device into the artery. A short anastomosis with an acute angle may cause problems in delivering the device into the vessel.

Some authors have advocated direct puncture of the common iliac artery using a superficial double purse string for hemostasis. The main problem with direct access is the unfavorable angle between the delivery sheath and the common iliac artery, which can be exaggerated in obese patients. To align the delivery sheath and artery, it is possible to create a transabdominal wall tunnel using a puncture site inferolateral to the surgical incision [8,9] (Fig. 3).

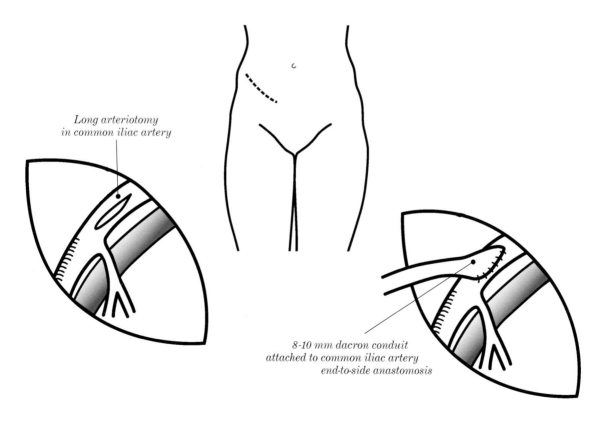

*Long arteriotomy
in common iliac artery*

*8-10 mm dacron conduit
attached to common iliac artery
end-to-side anastomosis*

FIG. 2 An oblique incision is made above the inguinal ligament for access to the iliac arteries. A longitudinal incision is made and a graft sutured to the artery.

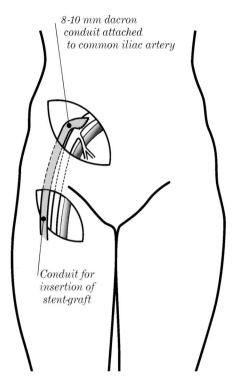

8-10 mm dacron conduit attached to common iliac artery

Conduit for insertion of stent-graft

FIG. 3 A graft is sutured to the common iliac artery and tunneled under the inguinal ligament for insertion of the stent-graft.

DISTAL AORTIC EXPOSURE

In patients with thoracic aortic pathology with occluded or tortuous iliac arteries it may be necessary to introduce the device from the distal abdominal aorta. This can be done via an extraperitoneal approach from an incision in the iliac fossa. Some authorities suggest that it is only necessary to expose a small area on the surface of the aorta in order to attach an 8 to 10 millimeter dacron conduit sewn end-to-side. However, it is safer to have a good exposure for proximal and distal control. A side-biting clamp can be used, but in patients with normal caliber arteries, this usually occludes the aorta. Conventional front-to-back clamping allows a decent view of the lumen and aids surgical technique. In patients with co-existent abdominal and thoracic aneurysms, some surgeons elect to perform open surgery on the abdominal aortic aneurysm (AAA) and stent the thoracic aneurysm at the same time. However, there is evidence that this is associated with a higher risk of paraplegia [10].

Supra-aortic access

SUBCLAVIAN AND AXILLARY ARTERY EXPOSURE

Arterial access via the subclavian and axillary arteries is sometimes necessary for patients with severe aorto-iliac disease. The right subclavian artery allows access to the descending thoracic aorta and the left subclavian artery to the arch and ascending aorta. Access via the subclavian or axillary artery carries a potential risk of vertebral artery embolization, particularly when the device is withdrawn [11].

COMMON CAROTID ARTERY EXPOSURE

The left common carotid artery has been used for access for thoracic endoluminal procedures in patients with severe aorto-iliac disease who were unfit for open surgery. The artery is exposed as for carotid endarterectomy through a longitudinal incision along the anterior border of the sternocleidomastoid muscle but through an incision sited lower in the neck (Fig. 4). A skin crease incision can be used in preference to the longitudinal incision to gain a better cosmetic result, but both tend to heal well. The left common carotid artery has a relatively large diameter and is "in line" with the descending thoracic aorta [12]. However, sometimes the right common carotid artery may provide the best access to the descending thoracic aorta. The final decision as to which artery gives the best access should be based on angiography. The main concern is the potential

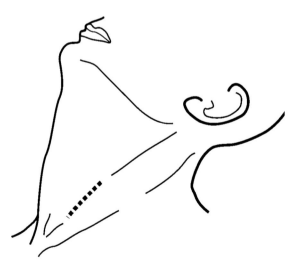

FIG. 4 An incision is made in the lower part of the neck to gain access to the common carotid artery.

risk of stroke from cerebral hypoperfusion or emboli. Pre-operative duplex assessment of the extracranial carotid and vertebral arteries is essential. However, common carotid artery clamping is usually well tolerated because of the continued flow through the external carotid system. Carotid-to-carotid bypass prior to the procedure would further minimize the risk of stroke.

CAROTID-CAROTID BYPASS

Right-to-left carotid-carotid bypass can be used to increase the proximal landing zone in patients undergoing endoluminal repair of thoracic aortic disease. This technique allows the stent-graft to be placed over the origins of the left subclavian and left common carotid arteries. An 8 millimeter PTFE graft is used and anastomosed end-to-side to the right common carotid artery and end-to-end on the distal left common carotid artery with ligation of the proximal left common carotid artery.

CAROTID-SUBCLAVIAN BYPASS AND TRANSPOSITION

It appears to be safe to cover the origin of the left subclavian artery with a thoracic stent-graft without the need for revascularization [13]. However, the potential risks of posterior circulation stroke, acute arm ischemia, type II endoleak, and paraplegia have led some to advise preemptive revascularization of the left subclavian artery. All patients ideally should have carotid and vertebral artery duplex prior to thoracic endoluminal repair if the left subclavian artery is to be deliberately covered. Patients with right vertebral stenosis or occlusion should undergo pre-operative bypass to reduce the risk of a posterior circulation stroke. If acute arm ischemia occurs following deployment of an endoluminal graft, then a bypass procedure can be performed subsequently.

Overcoming access problems

TORTUOUS ILIAC ARTERIES

Use of a stiff wire (Amplatz® super stiff or Lunderquist®). It is possible to straighten the iliac segment with a stiff wire (*Amplatz*® super stiff or *Lunderquist*®). Ideally this should be done at the pre-operative angiogram, because if it fails to straighten the artery, a further adjunctive procedure may be required. Stiff guidewires across tortuous iliac segments can introduce foreshortening

and temporary kinking. The change in geometry caused by the stiff wire may affect critical measurements used for sizing and selection of graft components [14].

Use of a brachiofemoral line. A through-and-through wire introduced from the brachial artery can help with the negotiation of a device through tortuous iliac arteries. However, there is a risk of tearing of the origin of the left subclavian artery or causing a stroke due to manipulation of the guidewire in the aortic arch. The cutting tendency of the wire may be reduced by using a catheter to protect the subclavian artery origin [3].

Pulling down on the common femoral artery. After exposing the common femoral artery, dissection under the inguinal ligament and ligation of the inferior epigastric and deep circumflex iliac branches allows the distal external iliac artery to be mobilized. Once this has been done a sling can be passed around the common femoral artery and pulled down, resulting in straightening of the iliac segment. This technique works well for the external iliac artery but is not so successful for the relatively immobile common iliac artery.

Use of a conduit. As previously mentioned, an 8 to 10 millimeter dacron or PTFE conduit can be attached to the common iliac or distal abdominal aorta to avoid tortuous iliac arteries. The use of iliac conduits can potentially broaden the applicability of endovascular aneurysm repair. However, concerns have been raised that this may increase the morbidity and mortality for these patients. Studies have shown that adjunctive techniques are safe despite a significant increase in operation time and blood loss [15].

OCCLUSIVE ILIAC DISEASE

Percutaneous transluminal angioplasty and stenting. Occlusive disease of the iliac arteries can be treated with percutaneous transluminal angioplasty with or without stenting. Some advise that this is performed several weeks prior to endoluminal grafting to allow for stent incorporation prior to traversing the iliac stent with the delivery system [3]. However, others suggest performing the angioplasty at the time of the procedure with stent placement in the iliac after deployment of the aortic graft [16].

Iliac endarterectomy. This can be performed as an open or endovascular procedure. Open endarterectomy involves exposure of the common iliac artery (as described earlier) and a longitudinal arteriotomy in order to perform a localized endarterectomy. The arteriotomy can then be used to attach a dacron or PTFE conduit for insertion of the delivery system.

Endoluminal balloon endarterectomy involves multiple balloon inflations throughout the occlusive external iliac arterial segment with removal of the atheromatous debris through the femoral arteriotomy site. This should be followed by stenting of the iliac segment after placement of the aortic graft.

Aortomono-iliac and femorofemoral crossover. In patients with AAA and unilateral iliac occlusive disease, an aortomono-iliac device can be used in conjunction with a femorofemoral crossover graft. This technique has increased the number of patients eligible for endovascular repair of AAAs [17,18].

Use of a conduit. As previously mentioned, an 8 to 10 millimeter dacron or PTFE conduit can be attached to the common iliac or distal abdominal aorta to avoid occluded or stenotic iliac arteries.

Supra-aortic access. Axillary, subclavian, or left common carotid arteries have all been used for access in patients with occlusive iliac disease.

SMALL NATIVE ARTERIES

Serial dilators. In patients with small caliber arteries, it can be possible to gently dilate the native artery with serial dilators to allow the passage of the delivery system. This must be done carefully, as there is a risk of rupture.

Prolene suture. A Prolene suture placed in the middle of the proximal edge of the arteriotomy can be used to gently lift the arterial wall over the lip between the nose cone and the sheath of the device (Fig. 5). This can be very helpful when the device keeps taking the artery with it. Occasionally, silicone gel can be a useful lubricant.

Conduit. Conduits can be used in patients with iliac arteries less than 7 millimeters in diameter on pre-operative imaging. This can be done prior to the procedure or at the same time.

Brachiofemoral wire. A brachiofemoral wire can be useful in patients with small native arteries, as it helps negotiate tortuous aortas and iliacs.

Future

Improvements in stent-graft design will produce more flexible devices with lower profile delivery systems that will reduce the problems with arterial access. Eventually the devices will be small enough to be placed percutaneously, removing the need for surgical access. Some centers have reported reasonable results using percutaneous access for 16F to 22F devices in conjunction with the Perclose® system *(Perclose Inc, Redwood City, CA, USA)* with an 85% successful femoral artery closure [19,20]. Usually two sutures are required for such large devices, and these are placed on each side of the arteriotomy puncture before the device is inserted into the artery.

Conclusion

With good pre-operative imaging and adjunctive techniques it is possible to overcome most of the access problems commonly associated with endoluminal aneurysm repair. The ability to modify the standard transfemoral approach for aortic stent-graft placement is particularly important for patients who are unfit for open surgery and require a less invasive approach.

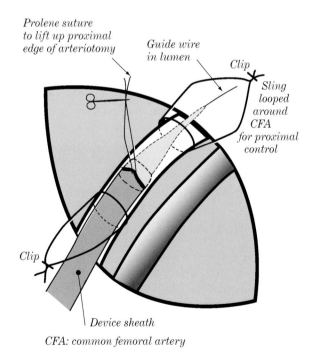

Prolene suture to lift up proximal edge of arteriotomy

Guide wire in lumen

Clip

Sling looped around CFA for proximal control

Clip

Device sheath

CFA: common femoral artery

FIG. 5 A Prolene suture is inserted to lift the proximal edge of the arteriotomy to allow passage of a large device.

REFERENCES

1 Carpenter JP, Baum RA, Barker CF, et al. Impact of exclusion criteria on patient selection for endovascular abdominal aortic aneurysm repair. *J Vasc Surg* 2001; 34: 1050-1054.

2 Blum U, Voshage G, Lammer J, et al. Endoluminal stent-grafts for infrarenal abdominal aortic aneurysms. *N Engl J Med* 1997; 336: 13-20.

3 Henretta JP, Karch LA, Hodgson KJ, et al. Special iliac artery considerations during aneurysm endografting. *Am J Surg* 1999; 178: 212-218.

4 Stelter W, Umscheid T, Ziegler P. Three-year experience with modular stent-graft devices for endovascular AAA treatment. *J Endovasc Surg* 1997; 4: 362-369.

5 Mialhe C, Amicabile C, Becquemin JP. Endovascular treatment of infrarenal abdominal aneurysms by the Stentor system: preliminary results of 79 cases. Stentor Retrospective Study Group. *J Vasc Surg* 1997; 26: 199-209.

6 Chuter TA, Reilly LM, Stoney RJ, Messina LM. Femoral artery exposure for endovascular aneurysm repair through oblique incisions. *J Endovasc Surg* 1998; 5: 259-260.

7 Caiati JM, Kaplan D, Gitlitz D, et al. The value of the oblique groin incision for femoral artery access during endovascular procedures. *Ann Vasc Surg* 2000; 14: 248-253.

8 Carpenter JP. Delivery of endovascular grafts by direct sheath placement into the aorta or iliac arteries. *Ann Vasc Surg* 2002; 16: 787-790.

9 Macdonald S, Byrne D, Rogers P, et al. Common iliac artery access during endovascular thoracic aortic repair facilitated by a transabdominal wall tunnel. *J Endovasc Ther* 2001; 8: 135-138.

10 Dake MD, Miller DC, Semba CP, et al. Transluminal placement of endovascular stent-grafts for the treatment of descending thoracic aortic aneurysms. *N Engl J Med* 1994; 331: 1729-1734.

11 Berguer R, Morasch MD, Kline RA, et al. Cervical reconstruction of the supra-aortic trunks: a 16-year experience. *J Vasc Surg* 1999; 29: 239-248.

12 Estes JM, Halin N, Kwoun M, et al. The carotid artery as alternative access for endoluminal aortic aneurysm repair. *J Vasc Surg* 2001; 33: 650-653.

13 Gorich J, Asquan Y, Seifarth H, et al. Initial experience with intentional stent-graft coverage of the subclavian artery during endovascular thoracic aortic repairs. *J Endovasc Ther* 2002; (9 suppl 2): II39-43.

14 Dawson DL, Hellinger JC, Terramani TT, et al. Iliac artery kinking with endovascular therapies: technical considerations. *J Vasc Interv Radiol* 2002; 13: 729-733.

15 Abu-Ghaida AM, Clair DG, Greenberg RK, et al. Broadening the applicability of endovascular aneurysm repair: the use of iliac conduits. *J Vasc Surg* 2002; 36: 111-117.

16 Yano OJ, Faries PL, Morrissey N, et al. Ancillary techniques to facilitate endovascular repair of aortic aneurysms. *J Vasc Surg* 2001; 34: 69-75.

17 Yusuf SW, Whitaker SC, Chuter TA, et al. Early results of endovascular aortic aneurysm surgery with aortouniiliac graft, contralateral iliac occlusion, and femorofemoral bypass. *J Vasc Surg* 1997; 25: 165-172.

18 Rehring TF, Brewster DC, Cambria RP, et al. Utility and reliability of endovascular aortouniiliac with femorofemoral crossover graft for aortoiliac aneurysmal disease. *J Vasc Surg* 2000; 31: 1135-1141.

19 Rachel ES, Bergamini TM, Kinney EV, et al. Percutaneous endovascular abdominal aortic aneurysm repair. *Ann Vasc Surg* 2002; 16: 43-49.

20 Quinn SF, Duke DJ, Baldwin SS, et al. Percutaneous placement of a low-profile stent-graft device for aortic dissections. *J Vasc Interv Radiol* 2002; 13: 791-798.

12

HAND-ASSISTED LAPAROSCOPIC INFRARENAL AORTIC RECONSTRUCTION

YVES ALIMI, GIOVANNI DE CARIDI, OLIVIER HARTUNG
PIERRE BARTHÉLEMY, MOURAD BOUFI, KARIM AISSI, ANDRES OTERO

The indications of surgical repair of the infrarenal aorta are well defined: occlusive aorto-iliac lesions stages C and D according to the TASC consensus criteria, or aortic aneurysms not amenable to endovascular treatment [1,2]. However, the discomfort and prolonged recovery time following open surgery justify the endovascular and minimally invasive developments during the last ten years in order to reduce the surgical trauma [3-13]. The technical evolution, particularly desired by an aging western population, consists of maintaining the quality and durability of aortic repair, together with significantly reducing the length of the abdominal incision. The acquired progress realized by abdominal surgeons, gynecologists, and urologists since 1987 has demonstrated the value of hand-assistance in laparoscopic surgical techniques. Multiple experimental studies have allowed us to grasp the advantages and difficulties associated with the different aortic approaches by means of laparoscopic access and to develop and design specific surgical instruments [14,15]. Aortic surgery imposes certain constraints such as the risks associated with prolonged clamp times or the difficulties of suturing in a severely calcified aorta. These specific issues justify the application of a hybrid technique, combining laparoscopic dissection of the infrarenal aorta and performance of the aortic suture via a mini-laparotomy of 5 to 9 centimeter length [6-8,12,13].

In the future, the development of surgical techniques and specific aortic instruments will guide us to a completely laparoscopic procedure, especially for the treatment of aorto-iliac occlusive disease.

Hand-assisted laparoscopic surgery (HALS)

PERSONAL TECHNIQUE [12,13]

The procedure is performed under general anesthesia. Placement of an epidural catheter is not necessary because postoperative pain is easily managed with oral medication. The patient is placed supinely on the operating table with a pillow under the lumbar region to raise the aortic area. The operating surgeon and first assistant are positioned to the left of the patient and the second assistant to the right (Fig. 1). A 15 millimeter umbilical incision is made for the insertion of the first 12 millimeter trocar, enabling insufflation with carbon dioxide to a pressure of 8 mmHg and abdominal visualization by means of a 30-degree viewing laparoscope. This trocar is subsequently used by the second assistant for surgical exposure. Three additional 12 millimeter ports are positioned in triangulation in the left abdominal wall for insertion of the camera and two surgical instruments (Fig. 2). The table is temporarily tilted to a 25-degree Trendelenburg and 10-degree to 15-degree right lateral decubitus position to shift the bowel in a cranial and right direction. We have designed a laparoscopic intestinal retractor consisting of a 3 millimeter metal rod, directly introduced through the abdominal wall, below and to the right of the xiphoid process, and threaded along the left side of the fourth duodeno-jejunal angle, the promontory, and the lateral

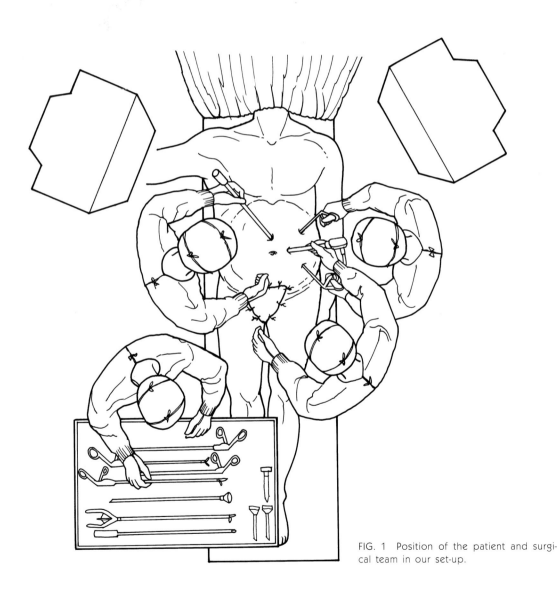

FIG. 1 Position of the patient and surgical team in our set-up.

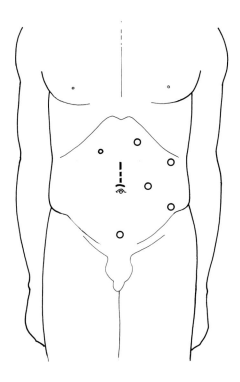

FIG. 2 Position of the trocars in our personal technique.
- Three 10 millimeter trocars are placed in a triangle in the left lower abdominal wall for the 30 degree camera and two laparoscopic instruments.
- Two 10 millimeter trocars in the left subcostal region and one above the symphysis allow introduction of proximal and distal laparoscopic aortic clamps.
- Orifice (3 millimeters) in the right upper abdomen for introduction of our laparoscopic intestinal retractor.
- The 5-9 centimeter mini-laparotomy is used for the aorto-prosthetic anastomosis.

edge of the right iliac axis. Its proximal extend portion is fixed to the operating table (Fig. 3). A polypropylene net with a lapel sewn along one of its long edges is placed in the abdomen. Then the lapel is slipped around the metallic rod to maintain the net on the floor of the abdominal cavity. Then the net is applied to the bowel and fixed with three to four sutures to the right part of the abdominal wall, keeping the intestines out of the working area. Then it is possible to reduce the Trendelenburg-right lateral decubitus positioning of the operating table to 5-degrees. The retroperitoneum is opened, along the duodeno-jejunal angle, which is liberated by transecting the Treitz muscles. The left renal vein is identified. Dissection of the peri-aortic tissue by means of a coagulating scissor allows anterior hemi-circumferential exposure of the infrarenal aorta as well as its lateral walls.

AORTO-ILIAC OCCLUSIVE LESIONS

The aortic dissection is performed from the left renal vein to the aortic level below the inferior mesenteric artery. A laparoscopic aortic clamp *(B/Braun-Aesculap, Tuttlingen, Germany)* is introduced under video guidance into the abdominal cavity through a separate 10 millimeter incision without a trocar, and placed below or, if necessary, above the renal arteries. Another laparoscopic clamp is placed at the aorta, distal to the inferior mesenteric artery in order to prevent aortic and lumbar artery back-bleeding. Next, all trocars are removed and a 5 to 8 millimeter mini-laparotomy is made at the level of the umbilicus. Longer incisions are made in obese patients or in case of suprarenal aortic clamping. The laparoscopic intestinal retractor is still in place and a self-retaining retractor is positioned (Omnitract®, *Surgical, a division of Minnesota Scientific, Inc., USA*). After heparinization (50 IU/kg), an end-to-side or end-to-end aorto-prosthetic anastomosis is performed under direct and camera vision using standard surgical instruments. Following aortic declamping, the prosthetic limbs are tunneled in an anatomical position to the groin by means of digital manipulation in the retroperitoneal space via the mini-laparotomy. The distal anastomoses to the femoral arteries are performed using standard techniques.

AORTIC OR AORTO-ILIAC ANEURYSMS

According to the programmed repair, laparoscopic aortic dissection is performed to allow supra- or infrarenal aortic clamping and common iliac artery control. Before or after the umbilical midline mini-laparotomy of 6 to 9 centimeters, a laparoscopic aortic clamp is placed around the proximal aortic neck, and if an aortic tube or an aortobilateral common iliac artery bypass is to be placed, a releasable laparoscopic clamp is prepared around each common iliac artery *(B/Braun-Aesculap)*. If the distal anastomoses are to be made on the external or femoral arteries through separate incisions, the common iliac artery

is occluded with a ligature or laparoscopic stapler (EndoTA-30 ®; *US Surgical, a unit of Tyco Healthcare group LP, Norwalk, CT, USA)*. A heparin bolus (50 IU/kg) is administered intravenously, and the aorta is clamped. Endo-aneurysmorraphy is then performed by opening the aneurysm, occluding the lumbar arteries, and performing an end-to-end aorto-prosthesis anastomosis with direct vision and camera assistance. Depending on the operation scheduled, the distal anastomosis or anastomoses are made on

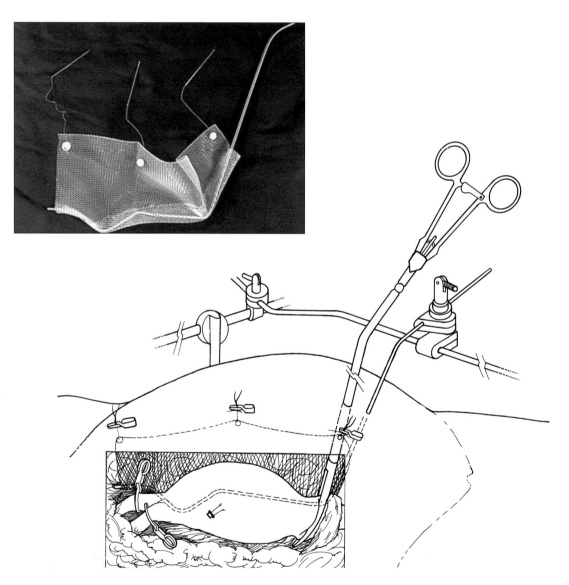

FIG. 3 Drawing showing our laparoscopic intestinal retractor, fixed to the operating table. A laparoscopic aortic clamp is positioned following dissection of the infrarenal aortic aneurysm [12,13]. Photograph showing metallic rod which fixes the polypropylene net to retract the intestines.

the distal aorta and on the iliac or femoral arteries. The aneurysmal sac is closed over the graft in order to prevent direct contact with the bowel. Finally, the retroperitoneum is closed with a running suture, and the port sites, mini-laparatomy, and groin incisions, if necessary, are closed in standard fashion.

Different techniques

HAND-INTRODUCTION WITH MAINTAINING PNEUMOPERITONEUM (THE KOLVENBACH'S TECHNIQUE) [8,16]

The procedure is performed under general anesthesia and gastric decompression by means of nasogastric tube aspiration. Monitoring is assisted with intra-arterial and central venous pressure measurements. The patient is in the supine position at the intervention table, with the surgeon to the left and the assistant to the right of the patient. The first umbilical incision of 10 millimeters is made to create the pneumoperitoneum. A second trocar of 10 millimeters is positioned at the left inferior part of the abdomen. A 30-degree angulated laparoscopic video camera is introduced and intra-abdominal adherences, if any, are released. The marks for creation of the mini-laparotomy are drawn on the abdomen after insufflation, which allows to reduce the length of the incision, to limit gas leakage, and to define the ideal placement of the other trocars (Fig. 4). A 6 centimeter incision is performed and a waterproof sleeve introduced, in which the non-dominant hand of the surgeon enters the abdomen (Fig. 5), all under preserving the pneumoperitoneum (HandPort® *Smith & Nephew Surgical, Andover, Mass., USA*). The retraction system consists of an open cylinder with a flexible ring at each extremity that keeps the incision open: one of the rings is inserted along the incision in the abdominal cavity whereas the other ring remains outside the incision (Fig. 5). More recently, the sleeve has been replaced by a gel sheet (GelPort® *Applied Medical, Rancho Santa Margarita, CA, USA*), which makes taking out and repositioning of the hand or all instruments (trocar, scissors, clamp) easier. Exposure of the aorta is performed with laparoscopic instruments and the surgeon's hand, which retracts the bowels. The table is positioned in a 60-degree Trendelenburg position and a slight turn to the right. The intra-abdominal hand allows digital exploration of the aorta to determine the optimal site of clamping and to assist the proximal anastomosis.

In patients requiring an aortobifemoral bypass for occlusive disease, creation of the tunnel, starting from the groin incisions, under digital and video camera control, should be performed at the end of the laparoscopic phase because these surgical maneuvers are generally accompanied by loss of pneumoperitoneum. Following dissection and exposure, the initial retractor is replaced by two conventional retractor blades of 2.5 centimeters (Omni-tract®, *Surgical, a division of Minnesota Scientific, Inc., USA*). The aortic circulation is interrupted with a standard vascular clamp. The table is left in the Trendelenburg position and the proximal and distal anastomoses are performed with conventional instruments.

In patients with an abdominal aortic aneurysm (AAA), the neck of the aneurysm and both common iliac arteries are dissected with laparoscopic instruments and with assistance of the non-dominant hand of the surgeon. The inferior mesenteric artery is clipped to prevent back-bleeding in the

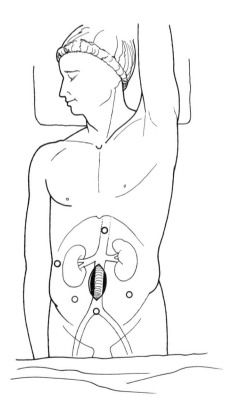

FIG. 4 Position of the patient and insertion of trocars and mini-laparotomy according to Kolvenbach et al.

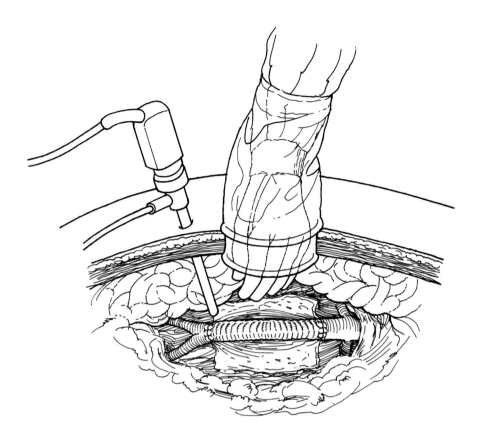

FIG. 5 Drawing showing introduction of the non-dominant hand according to the technique of Kolvenbach et al.

aneurysmal sac. The two common iliac arteries are occluded by traditional oversewing or laparoscopic stapler (TA-30). The aorta is occluded and transsected and, hence, the aneurysm is completely excluded. Before installation of the retractor system, all accessible lumbar arteries are clipped by laparoscopic techniques. An end-to-end aorto-prosthetic anastomosis is performed and the distal anastomoses are created in an end-to-side fashion at the level of the external iliac arteries, which are exposed via small oblique incisions. Finally, the retroperitoneum is closed over the prosthesis by a running suture.

A variant of the hand-assisted technique has been proposed by Da Silva et al., in cooperation with Kolvenbach, consisting of a low transverse mini-laparotomy of 5 to 6 centimeters (modified Pfannenstiel incision). This approach can reduce systemic (respiratory insufficiency) and local (evisceration) complications and offer a better cosmetic result [11].

TECHNIQUE OF KLINE [6]

This technique, published in 1998, has been proposed for selected patients presenting with an aneurysm suitable for aortic tube repair. The patient is in the supine position with both legs in abduction. The surgeon is between the legs of the patient, the first and third assistant to the left and the second assistant to the right of the patient. The video tower is placed to the head of the patient (Fig. 6). The first midline supra-umbilical mini-incision allows introduction of a flexible intraperitoneal retractor (modified Glassman®, *Adept-Med, Diamond Springs, CA, USA*). Next, a 12 millimeter trocar is introduced to create a pneumoperitoneum with a pressure of 15 mmHg. A 30-degree angulated laparoscope is placed and five additional trocars introduced (Fig. 7). With the patient in lateral right supine and Trendelenburg position, transperitoneal laparoscopic dissection of the AAA is performed from the infrarenal aortic neck to the common iliac arteries. Next, the trocars are removed and an 8 to 10 centimeter mini-laparotomy is made at the level of the umbilicus, enabling insertion of a prosthetic graft under direct vision. In a more recent publication, the authors report on a technique with primary aortic access through a mini-laparotomy, without previous laparoscopic dissection [17].

TECHNIQUE OF FABIANI [4]

The patient is in supine position with a pillow under the lumbar region. A Palmer needle placed in the umbilical region is used to obtain a pneumoperitoneum with a pressure of 13 mmHg. The performance of a transperitoneal aortobifemoral bypass for occlusive disease requires three trocars: one right-sided subcostal trocar for the laparoscopic intestinal retractor and two in the left pararectal area to introduce the laparoscope and a surgical instrument. The table is in Trendelenburg with the patient in right lateral supine position. The bowel is retracted, the retroperitoneum opened, and the infrarenal aorta is mobilized over a length of 5 centimeters. A 3 to 5 centimeter midline incision is made to introduce a Satinsky clamp, placed on the aorta under laparoscopic control. The prosthesis is introduced through a trocar and anastomosed in an end-to-side fashion with a 4/0 prolene. The prosthetic limbs are blindly tunneled to the groin and anastomosed to the femoral arteries.

A retroperitoneal unilateral aortofemoral bypass is performed via a 3 centimeter incision at the lateral plane of the rectus muscle. Insufflation of a balloon placed in the retroperitoneum under video camera control allows for the positioning of a telescopic retractor to push the peritoneal sac aside. Two trocars are used for the camera and the instruments. The rest of the operation follows the same steps as described above.

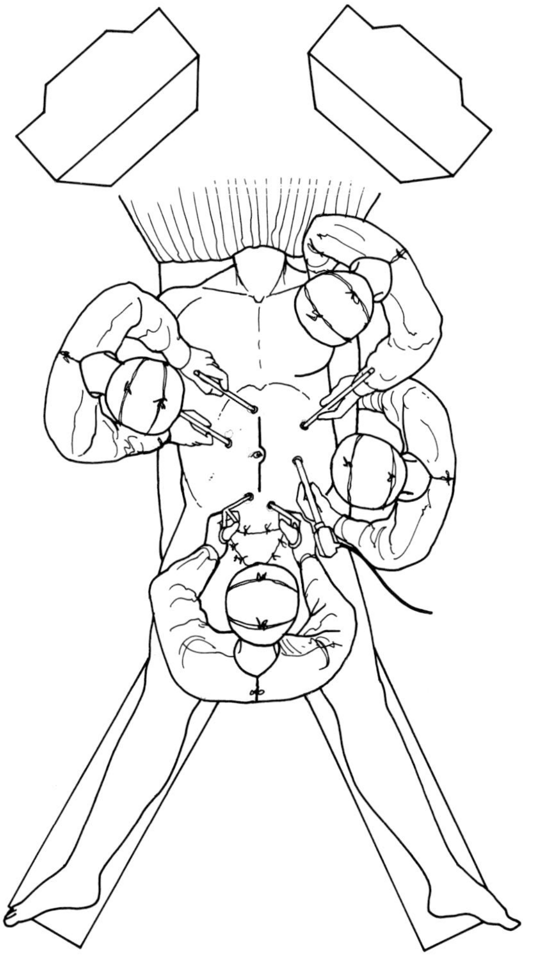

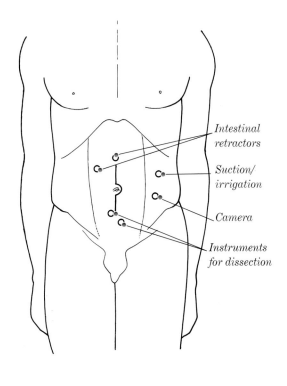

Intestinal retractors

Suction/ irrigation

Camera

Instruments for dissection

FIG. 6   Position of the patient and surgical team according to the technique of Kline et al.

FIG. 7   Position of the trocars for the dissection of the aortic neck and the mini-laparotomy according to the technique of Kline et al.

Transperitoneal AAA repair requires opening of the retroperitoneum and introduction of a laparoscopic aortic clamp under video camera control. Following complete opening of the aorta, the layers are fixed to the edges of the mini-laparotomy. The iliac arteries are controlled with Fogarty balloon catheters.

Discussion

ADVANTAGES OF HALS COMPARED TO CONVENTIONAL SURGERY

Our series comprises 113 patients (103 males, 10 females with a mean age of 64 years, range 37 to 84 years). These patients were operated on since 1998, for severe occlusive aorto-iliac disease (n = 67) or AAA (n = 46). Among these patients, 4 patients underwent thoracoscopic thoracobifemoral bypass for severe occlusive disease and a hostile abdomen.

As our experience progressed, certain contra-indications (morbid obesity, suprarenal clamping), noted in our preliminary study and agreement of the ethical committee (30 first patients), have gradually been abandoned, as summarized in Table I. These changes allowed for inclusion of an increasing number of patients: during the first 34 months of our experience, 54% of all referred patients underwent HALS; this number gradually increased to 91% during the last 34 months [13]. This experience and the data from the literature allow us to describe the following advantages.

Decreased intra-operative surgical trauma. The development of our laparoscopic intestinal retractor enables us to reduce the pressure of the pneumoperitoneum to 8 mmHg, to reposition the patient to the supine position rapidly, and to obtain direct transperitoneal aorto-iliac access, avoiding detachment of the retroperitoneum. Simultaneously, the learning curve has significantly reduced mean operating time from 285 minutes to 192 minutes (p < 0.001) and aortic clamp time from 77 minutes to 32 minutes (p < 0.001) [12,13]. The conversion rate to open surgery varied from 2.5% to 10% [6,8,12].

The absence of a large parietal opening and evisceration diminishes fluid loss and cooling of the patient. Furthermore, the surgical trauma is substantially less. In a prospective study by Kolvenbach et al. [16], the reduction of surgical trauma could be illustrated by a significant decrease of pro-inflammatory proteins (interleukins 6 and 8) in patients treated by HALS as compared to patients operated by means of conventional surgery.

Improved early postoperative outcome. Table II shows the results in the literature, comparing the morbidity-mortality between patients operated by conventional surgery and HALS. From now, these results seem to be comparable even though the HALS results come from preliminary studies. Furthermore, our recent experience in 58 patients treated by HALS shows that 82% were eating at the second postoperative day and 59% were walking the same day [13]. Mean postoperative hospital stay was 5.7 days and decreased from 7 days at the beginning of our series to 4.5 days for the last patients. In a prospective study, Kolvenbach et al. compared the results in 41 patients treated by means of HALS (29 obstructive disease, 12 AAA) and 20 patients treated by conventional surgery, and found a significant shorter intensive care stay (0.41 versus 1.50 days, p = 0.02) and hospital stay (4.3 versus 9.3 days, p = 0.01) [8].

Table I	MODIFICATION OF THE CONTRA-INDICATIONS OF HAND-ASSISTED LAPAROSCOPIC AORTIC SURGERY DURING THE EVOLUTION OF OUR EXPERIENCE
Permanent contra-indications	*Initial but abrogated contra-indications*
Emergency aortic surgery	Obesity (body mass index > 30)
ASA IV	Suprarenal aortic clamping
Severe aortic calcifications	Combined repair of renal or inferior mesenteric ostial disease
Hostile abdomen	Retroperitoneal venous anomalies (left retro-aortic renal vein)

Table II	RESULTS OF CONVENTIONAL AND HAND-ASSISTED LAPAROSCOPIC SURGERY IN PATIENTS WITH AORTO-ILIAC OCCLUSIVE DISEASE AND ABDOMINAL AORTIC ANEURYSMS								
1st author [ref.]	Year	Number of patients	Disease	Early complications Mortality %	Morbidity %	Mean postoperative stay - days	Mid-term patency Primary % (months)	Secondary % (months)
Conventional surgery								
Nevelsteen [20]	1991	869	AIOD	4.5	20	-	-	87 (36)
Poulias [21]	1992	1000	AIOD	3.3	19.8	-	90 (24)	-
Williamson [19]	2001	154	AAA	4	13	10.7	-	-
Carpenter [18]	2002	163	AAA	4.4	9.8	-	-	-
Hand-assisted laparoscopic surgery								
Fabiani [4]	1997	9	AIOD	0	11	5.5	-	-
Kline [6]	1998	20	AAA	0	5	5.8	-	-
Kolvenbach [22]	2001	29	AIOD	0	3.4	4.3	-	-
Alimi [12]	2003	24	AAA	4.2	20.8	5.3	100 (17)	100 (17)
Alimi [13]		58	AIOD	3.4	8.6	5.7	89.3 (26)	91 (26)

AAA: abdominal aortic aneurysm
AIOD: aorto-iliac occlusive disease

12
123

Equivalent midterm graft patency. In order to assess the quality of the reconstructions by means of HALS we have evaluated the patency rate of our first procedures. After a mean follow-up of 17.1 months (range 3 to 38 months), no re-interventions were necessary in the first 24 patients treated for AAA [12]. Concerning the first 58 patients treated for occlusive lesions, 5 re-interventions (9%) were required during a mean follow-up of 26.7 months (range 1 to 66 months). Four of these were performed for graft-limb occlusion due to myo-intimal hyperplasia occurring between 13 and 15 months after the initial intervention. Primary and secondary patency rates were 89.3% and 91%, respectively [13].

ADVANTAGES OF HALS COMPARED TO TOTAL LAPAROSCOPIC SURGERY

A more secure surgical procedure. A mini-laparotomy and intra-abdominal introduction of a hand comprises two important advantages. Keeping tactile perception allows assessment of the degree of aortic calcification, evaluation of the preferred location of clamp position, and easy passage of the prosthetic limbs. Furthermore, this mini-incision enables classic aorto-prosthetic suturing, under direct vision, with standard surgical instruments. Table III summarizes the duration of the procedure and aortic clamp times for both techniques, showing an obvious difference with longer times in total laparoscopic surgery, despite highly skilled surgical teams.

A shorter learning curve. During the training sessions of the *European Institute of Telesurgery* (IRCAD, Strasbourg, France) we observe that the majority of vascular surgeons are able to perform a laparoscopic dissection of the abdominal aorta within three days of training. However, few are able to perform a watertight, non-stenotic aorto-prosthetic anastomosis, which can be explained by the difficult adaptation of instruments and the necessity of a prolonged training of several months at the "pelvic trainer".

The reduced number of patients undergoing surgical repair due to endovascular developments does not encourage surgeons to learn these techniques.

Table III		RESULTS OF TOTAL LAPAROSCOPIC AND HAND-ASSISTED LAPAROSCOPIC SURGERY IN PATIENTS WITH AORTO-ILIAC OCCLUSIVE DISEASE AND ABDOMINAL AORTIC ANEURYSMS				
1st author [ref.]	*Year*	*Number of patients*	*Disease*	*Mean time (min)* Operation	Clamp time	*Mean hospital stay - days*
Total laparoscopic surgery						
Barbera [3]	1998	24	AIOD	276	70	10
Edoga [5]	1998	22	AAA	438	160	4.5
Coggia [9]	2002	14	AIOD	269	57	7.25
Dion [10]	2002	49	AIOD (46) AAA (3)	311	101	6
Hand-assisted laparoscopic surgery						
Kline [6]	1998	20	AAA	245	-	5.8
Kolvenbach [22]	2000	12	AAA	198	43	5
		29	AIOD	148	36	4.3
Castronuovo [7]	2000	60	AAA	462	112	6.3
Alimi [12]	2003	24	AAA	238	76	5.3
[13]		58	AIOD	238	54	5.7

AAA: abdominal aortic aneurysm
AIOD: aorto-iliac occlusive disease

On the other hand, the rapidly expanding laparoscopic techniques in the majority of surgical specialties will allow vascular surgeons in training to familiarize themselves with these techniques.

WHAT IS THE FUTURE OF HALS?

During the last decade, medical attitude has focused on the importance of quality of life. One of the targets of the innovative techniques is to reduce the stay in intensive care and in the hospital, leading to an earlier and more comfortable return to the pre-operative status. The endovascular techniques constitute a simple, fast, and minimally invasive treatment for certain aorto-iliac diseases. However, several indications for surgical treatment remain. *The TransAtlantic Intersociety Consensus* recommends that the most severe obstructive lesions (class TASC C) should preferably or class D exclusively be treated by conventional surgery [1]. In other respects, the complications of aortic endografts such as endoleak, migration, and rupture as illustrated by the EUROSTAR registry have directed the French authorities to reserve endovascular AAA repair only for patients at increased surgical risks [2].

These experiences emphasize the importance of developing less invasive surgical techniques, decreasing surgical trauma, and maintaining high-quality long-term results. The preliminary results of HALS have demonstrated that these procedures can be performed in a large number of patients, including obese people, patients requiring supra-renal clamping, and patients with a hostile abdomen because of the possibilities of video-assisted thoracofemoral grafting.

The duration of surgery and aortic clamp times are close to conventional surgery. Midterm patency rates are also comparable. However, the results do not show a beneficial effect on early morbidity-mortality (Table II). This might be explained by the prolonged aortic clamping, especially in patients with cardiac failure.

Technical progress during the last years has allowed for efficient and reliable laparoscopic dissection of the abdominal aorta. Other technological innovations will improve the procedure and make aorto-prosthetic anastomoses easier [22]. These developments represent important steps toward total laparoscopic interventions.

Conclusion

Following important experimental studies, the preliminary clinical results have demonstrated the feasibility of hand-assisted laparoscopic aortic surgery. Reduced surgical trauma has reduced the time of hospitalization with a more rapid return to a normal physical activity. Besides conventional and endovascular surgery, hand-assisted laparoscopic aortic surgery represents a third solution in the surgical armamentarium to respond to the wishes of modern treatments.

REFERENCES

1 Management of peripheral arterial disease (PAD). TASC Working Group. TransAtlantic Inter-Society Consensus (TASC). *J Vasc Surg* 2000; 31: S1-296.

2 Dattilo JB, Brewster DC, Fan CM, et al. Clinical failures of endovascular abdominal aortic aneurysm repair: incidence, causes, and management. *J Vasc Surg* 2002; 35: 1137-1144.

3 Barbera L, Mumme A, Metin S, et al. Operative results and outcome of twenty-four totally laparoscopic vascular procedures for aortoiliac occlusive disease. *J Vasc Surg* 1998; 28: 136-142.

4 Fabiani JN, Mercier F, Carpentier A, et al. Video-assisted aortofemoral bypass: results in seven cases. *Ann Vasc Surg* 1997; 11: 273-277.

5 Edoga JK, Asgarian K, Singh D, et al. Laparoscopic surgery for abdominal aortic aneurysms. Technical elements of the procedure and a preliminary report of the first 22 patients. *Surg Endosc* 1998; 12: 1064-1072.

6 Kline RG, D'Angelo AJ, Chen MH, et al. Laparoscopically assisted abdominal aortic aneurysm repair: first 20 cases. *J Vasc Surg* 1998; 27: 81-88.

7 Castronuovo JJ Jr, James KV, Resnikoff M, et al. Laparoscopic-assisted abdominal aortic aneurysmectomy. *J Vasc Surg* 2000; 32: 224-233.

8 Kolvenbach R, Ceshire N, Pinter L, et al. Laparoscopy-assisted aneurysm resection as a minimal invasive alternative in patients unsuitable for endovascular surgery. *J Vasc Surg* 2001; 34: 216-221.

9 Coggia M, Bourriez A, Javeliat I, Goëau-Brissonière O. Totally laparoscopic aortobifemoral bypass: a technical note. In: Juhan C, Alimi YS (eds). *New instruments in laparoscopic aortoliac surgery*. Marseille, Angio-techniques 2002: pp 134-141.

10 Dion YM, Gracia CR, Douville Y, Estakhri M. The "Apron technique": mid-term results. In: Juhan C, Alimi Y (eds). *New instruments in laparoscopic aortoliac surgery*. Marseille, Angio-techniques 2002: pp 168-183.

11 Da Silva L, Kolvenbach R, Pinter L. The feasibility of hand-assisted laparoscopic aortic bypass using a low transverse incision. *Surg Endosc* 2002; 16: 173-176.

12 Alimi YS, Di Molfetta L, Hartung O, et al. Laparoscopy-assisted abdominal aortic aneurysm endoaneurysmorraphy: early and mid term results. *J Vasc Surg* 2003; 37: 744-749.

13 Alimi YS, De Caridi G, Hartung O, et al. Laparoscopy-assisted reconstructions for severe aortoiliac occlusive disease: early and mid-term results. *J Vasc Surg* (in press).

14 Alimi YS, Hartung O, Cavalero C, et al. Intestinal retractor for transperitoneal laparoscopic aortoiliac reconstruction: experimental study on human cadavers and initial clinical experience. *Surg Endosc* 2000; 14: 915-917.

15 Alimi YS, Hartung O, Lonjon T, et al. Laparoscopic transperitoneal replacement of abdominal aorta with left renal artery reimplantation: experimental study on pigs. *J Mal Vasc* 2002; 27: 199-204.

16 Kolvenbach R, Deling O, Schwierz E, et al. Reducing the operative trauma in aortoiliac reconstructions. A prospective study to evaluate the role of video-assisted vascular surgery. *Eur J Vasc Endovasc Surg* 1998; 15: 483-488.

17 Cerveira JJ, Halpern VJ, Faust G, Cohen JR. Minimal incision abdominal aortic aneurysm repair. *J Vasc Surg* 1999; 30: 977-984.

18 Carpenter JP, Baum RA, Barker CF, et al. Durability of benefits of endovascular versus conventional abdominal aortic aneurysm repair. *J Vasc Surg* 2002; 35: 222-228.

19 Williamson WK, Nicoloff AD, Taylor LM Jr, et al. Functional outcome after open repair of abdominal aortic aneurysm. *J Vasc Surg* 2001; 33: 913-920.

20 Nevelsteen A, Wouters L, Suy R. Aortofemoral dacron reconstruction for aorto-iliac occlusive disease: a 25-year survey. *Eur J Vasc Surg* 1991; 5: 179-186.

21 Poulias GE, Doundoulakis N, Prombonas E, et al. Aorto-femoral bypass and determinants of early success and late favourable outcome. Experience with 1000 consecutive cases. *J Cardiovasc Surg* 1992; 33: 664-678.

22 Kolvenbach R, Da Silva L, Deling O, Schwierz E. Video-assisted aortic surgery. *J Am Coll Surg* 2000; 190: 451-457.

23 Garitey V, Rieu R, Alimi YS. Prostheto-prosthetic and aortoprosthetic anastomosis using stents, threads, clips and staples: in vitro comparative study. *J Mal Vasc* 2003; 28: 173-177.

13

ROBOT-ASSISTED LAPAROSCOPIC SURGERY OF THE INFRARENAL AORTA

WILLEM WISSELINK, MIGUEL CUESTA, CARLOS GRACIA
JELLE RUURDA, IVO BROEDERS, JAN RAUWERDA

Laparoscopic aortic surgical techniques [1-5], despite admirable efforts of a small number of pioneers, have not been widely embraced in the vascular surgical community. The technical difficulty of performing a vascular anastomosis with laparo-endoscopic instruments has been the main drawback and has led to development of hybrid *procedures whereby laparoscopic dissection is followed by hand-sewn anastomosis via a small incision or, alternatively, hand-assisted laparoscopic surgery. The real benefit of laparo-endoscopic surgery, however, is avoidance of an incision altogether, and robotic technology may represent the missing link that can bring this ideal to common practice.*

To evaluate this presumption, we have compared the efficacy of robot-assisted videoscopic aortic replacement to a standard videoscopic approach in a porcine model. Subsequently, we report on five patients with disabling intermittent claudication who have been treated with robot-assisted, totally laparoscopic aortobifemoral bypass grafting.

Introduction to currently available robotic surgical systems

Recently, two US companies have obtained European Union clearance for clinical use of their robotic telemanipulation devices: *Computer Motion,* *Goleta, CA, USA* (the Zeus® system), and *Intuitive Surgical, Sunnyvale, CA, USA* (the Da Vinci® system) (Figs. 1,2).

In the summer of 2003, the two companies merged. Detailed descriptions of the two systems may be found elsewhere [6]. In short, each system consists of a console containing a viewing system and manipulating devices from which multi-joined

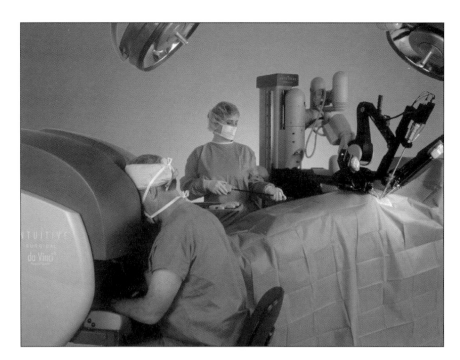

FIG. 1 The *Da Vinci®* system. Surgeon control unit, on the left.

FIG. 2 Three-dimensional screen and control panel of the *Zeus®* surgical system. Two telemanipulator arms control two surgical instruments; the camera arm is voice controlled.

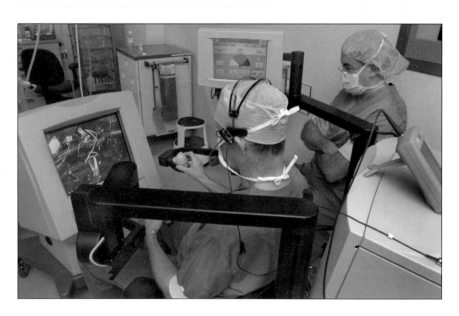

robotic arms can be controlled. These arms may be mounted on the operating table (Zeus®) or on a separate mobile surgical cart (Da Vinci®). Special laparoscopic surgical instruments with "wrists" providing six or more degrees of freedom of movement are brought into the body cavity and connected to the robotic arms. Potential advantages over conventional endoscopic surgery are the improved ergonomics and increased dexterity enabling "regular" surgeons to perform complex surgical tasks such as performing vascular anastomoses with relatively short learning curves. Despite tremendous interest in the subject displayed at vascular meetings, a MEDLINE search produces very little information on the use of robotic technology in the field of vascular surgery. Clinical vascular experience with robotics has been limited to an incidental case report [7] (see below), whereas other fields such as cardiac, pediatric, urologic, and gastro-intestinal surgery [8] have produced an abundance of literature, which is beyond the scope of this chapter.

Experimental work

The aim of our experimental study was to assess the safety and efficacy of robot-assisted laparoscopic interposition grafting of the abdominal aorta in a porcine model and to compare this to the standard laparoscopic approach [9].

Toward this goal, 20 laparoscopic aortic tube interposition prostheses were sutured in an end-to-end fashion through a retroperitoneal approach: 10 using the Da Vinci® robot system and 10 using laparoscopic suture techniques (control). Operating room time divided into separate time frames, blood loss, and complications, were registered. Blood loss after clamp removal was scored separately. Efficacy of the anastomoses was evaluated by measuring flow after the procedure by inspection of the distal aorta and palpation of the femoral artery and by measuring passage, circumference, and number of stitches.

Total operating time (skin-to-skin) was 164 minutes (range 116-225) in the robot-assisted group versus 205 minutes in controls (range 162-244) (Table). Proximal anastomosis time was 22 minutes (range 15-37, robot) versus 40 minutes (range 31-75, con-

trols), distal anastomosis time was 22 minutes (range 14-40, robot) versus 41 minutes (range 28-46, controls). No intra-operative complications occurred in the robot-assisted group. In the control group, the vena cava was injured in one case and subsequently tamponated before the procedure was continued. At autopsy, all robot-assisted anastomoses were macroscopically adequate. In the control group, a large distance (greater than 0.3 mm) between two stitches was measured in 10 cases. This study demonstrated the efficacy and safety of robot-assisted laparoscopic aortic graft interposition. The procedure could be performed faster, with fewer complications and less blood loss with robotic assistance than through a standard laparoscopic approach.

Clinical experience

Following ample clinical experience with laparoscopy-assisted aortofemoral bypass, in which laparoscopic retroperitoneal dissection of the infrarenal aorta was followed by hand-sewn aortic anastomosis via a small incision, we have embarked on total laparoscopic procedures whereby the anastomosis was constructed with the help of a robotic system (Fig. 2).

Between February 2002 and February 2003, five men, 54±4 year old, presented with disabling intermittent claudication due to extensive aorto-iliac occlusive disease [10]. Previous attempts at endovascular recanalization had failed in four patients. Following extensive laboratory practice sessions with a robotic surgical system (Zeus®), approval of our hospital Investigational Review Board, and patient informed consent, all underwent robot-assisted laparoscopic aortobifemoral bypass grafting.

SURGICAL TECHNIQUE

Details of the surgical technique have been described elsewhere [1,7]. In short, under general anesthesia, the patient is positioned supinely with a pillow under the left flank. Three robotic positioner arms are connected to the operating table rails and prepared into the sterile field: one for a 30-degree endoscope *(Aesop Endoscope Positioner, Computer Motion)* on the right, and two instrument arms on the left side of the patient. Care is taken to position the arms in such a fashion that interference between instruments and abdominal wall is avoided. The arms are then simply rotated away to allow

13

Table	Differences between robotic (N=10) and laparoscopic (N=10) aortic tube interposition in a porcine model		
		Robot	Laparoscopy
Total operating time (minutes)		164	205
Proximal anastomosis (minutes)		22	40
Distal anastomosis (minutes)		22	41
Intraoperative complications (N)		0	1

aortic dissection with conventional laparoscopic techniques. Via small groin incisions, the common femoral arteries are dissected free bilaterally. Laparoscopic retroperitoneal dissection of the aorta is performed following the creation of a peritoneal "apron" that is being suspended to the anterior abdominal wall. This technique, using six 10 millimeter trocars, has been described in detail by one of the authors (CG). Trocar positions are depicted in Figure 3. Once the infrarenal aorta and bifurcation have been dissected free, lumbar arteries at the proposed site of aortic clamping are ligated with clips and the inferior mesenteric artery is temporarily occluded. Two retroperitoneal tunnels are made from the groin incision towards the aorta by means of passing a blunt clamp, visualizing the intra-abdominal part with the videoscope. Full heparinization is instituted, the aorta is clamped just distal to the renal arteries and below the inferior mesenteric artery and an aortotomy is made. A bifurcated polytetrafluoroethylene (PTFE) prosthesis (diameter 16 x 8 millimeters or 14 x 7 millimeters, depending on the anatomy) is anastomosed end-to-side by means of robotically steered instruments consisting of a needle driver on the right and a grasper on the left, as well as a voice-controlled robotically positioned endoscope, (Micro Joint Heavy Needle Driver, *Micro Joint DeBakey Grasper,* and Aesop Robotic Endoscope Positioner, *Computer Motion*), (Fig. 4).

The robotic positioner arms are controlled from a separate control console. Following completion of the aortic anastomosis, the two graft limbs are tunneled to the groins where a conventional end-to-side anastomosis is performed to the common femoral artery.

RESULTS

There were no operative complications. Operating times were 220 to 360 minutes (mean 250), respectively, with aortic clamp times of 35 to 110 minutes (mean 47). The long clamp time in one patient was due to technical problems with the camera system. Time to set up the robotic positioner arms and connect the robotic instruments was 17 (±5) minutes. Blood loss was less than 200 mL in all cases. A normal diet was resumed on the second postoperative day and four of five patients were discharged home between postoperative days 4 and 7. One patient died on postoperative day 3 due to a massive myocardial infarction. At autopsy, pinpoint coronary stenoses were found that had been missed during pre-operative cardiac work-up. The aortic anastomosis was found to be intact.

Discussion

In a continued search to reduce operative trauma, minimally invasive procedures such as laparoscopy-assisted and hand-assisted laparoscopic aortofemoral bypass have been developed whereby the entire aortic dissection is performed laparoscopically except for the aortic anastomosis, requiring an abdominal incision of 7 centimeters or more. Indeed, creation of an aortic anastomosis with conventional laparoscopic techniques is demanding, in particular when laparoscopic experience is limited. The addition of robotic technology, however, provides an ergonomic and natural interface between the surgeon's hands and the instrument tips, as well as increased freedom of motion due to wrist action of the robotic instruments. In the patients described, the aortic anastomosis was performed successfully by a vascular surgeon (WW) with limited laparoscopic training and experience, under supervision and assistance, however, of two surgeons with ample laparoscopic (MAC

13

130

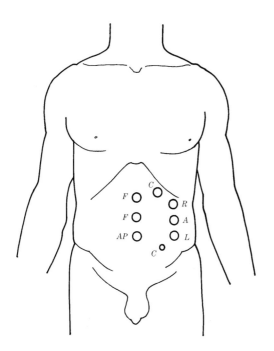

FIG. 3 Trocar positions: A: surgical endoscope positioner *(Aesop)*. AP: assistants' port. C: aortic clamps. F: fan retractors. L: left robotic arm. R: right robotic arm.

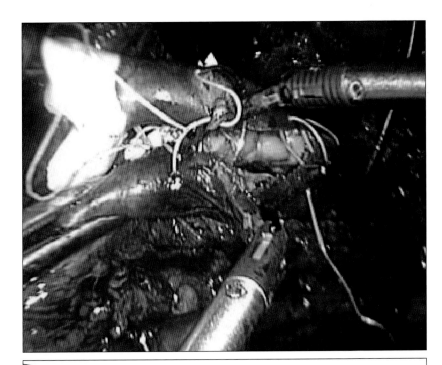

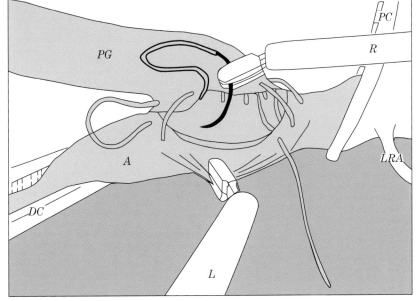

FIG. 4 Robot-assisted end-to-side aortic anastomosis. A: aorta. L: left arm. LRA: left renal artery. PC, DC: proximal and distal aortic clamps. PG: prosthetic graft. R: right arm.

and CG) and robotic (CG) skills. Clearly, considering the limitations of this small report, nothing more than feasibility of the procedure has been demonstrated. However, the early conclusion that robotic technology holds a significant potential in pushing the envelope of minimally invasive vascular surgery seems justified.

Conclusions and future prospects

Whereas for "occlusive" aorto-iliac disease, surgical bypass grafting has been largely replaced by endovascular techniques, "aneurysmal" disease still poses considerable challenges to the endovascular therapist. Long-term results of endovascular abdominal aortic aneurysm repair, especially, have been disappointing, leaving opportunities for conventional surgical techniques. Moreover, if with the development of videoscopic and robotic technology invasiveness and complication rates of surgical aortic replacement can be reduced, a comeback of surgical replacement, especially in younger patients, may be anticipated. Also, in conjunction with endovascular graft placement, robot-assisted videoscopic suturing techniques may prove invaluable in graft fixation and aortic branch management at both thoracic and abdominal levels [9]. Celiac, mesenteric, and renal revascularization procedures, if unsuitable for endovascular repair, will be greatly facilitated by robotic techniques. One of the drawbacks of robotic technology is the complete lack of tactile feedback. The forces of the surgical instruments are therefore rather uncontrollable and may potentially damage the arterial tissue. Furthermore, pulling the stitches, performing the anastomosis,

and making the knots are hampered by this lack of tactile feedback. The latest robotic set-up contains a fourth robotic arm, which can be used as a retractor but also as an active working arm. The surgeon, however, must be aware of the arms in "play" to avoid damaging or tearing aortic and/or arterial tissue. Currently, major research is focused on the development of tactile feedback. In summary, we have demonstrated that robotic technology offers significant benefit over conventional laparo-endoscopic techniques in the surgical treatment of infrarenal aorto-iliac occlusive disease. Whether similar advantages exist for treatment of aorto-iliac "aneurysmal" disease remains to be seen. However, with the expected further technical advancement and availibility of robotically aided videoscopic techniques, it seems important for vascular surgeons to gain or maintain at least basic laparoscopic skills in anticipation. Prospective studies must be performed to assess the beneficial effects, also related to the additional costs of the robotic equipment.

REFERENCES

1 Dion YM, Gracia CR, Ben El Kadi HH. Totally laparoscopic aortic abdominal aortic aneurysm repair. *J Vasc Surg* 2001; 33: 181-185.

2 Kolvenbach R, Ceshire N, Pinter L, et al. Laparoscopy-assisted aneurysm resection as a minimal invasive alternative in patients unsuitable for endovascular surgery. *J Vasc Surg* 2001; 34: 216-221.

3 Ahn SS, Hiyama DT, Rudkin GH, et al. Laparoscopic aortobifemoral bypass. *J Vasc Surg* 1997; 26: 128-132.

4 Alimi YS, Hartung O, Orsoni P, Juhan C. Abdominal aortic laparoscopic surgery: retroperitoneal or transperitoneal approach? *Eur J Vasc Endovasc Surg* 2000; 19: 21-26.

5 Coggia M, Bourriez A, Javerliat I, Goeau-Brissonniere O. Totally laparoscopic aortobifemoral bypass: a new and simplified approach. *Eur J Vasc Endovasc Surg* 2002; 24: 274-275.

6 Rockall TA, Darzi AW. Tele-manipulator robots in surgery. *Br J Surg* 2003; 90: 641-643.

7 Wisselink W, Cuesta MA, Gracia C, Rauwerda JA. Robot-assisted laparoscopic aortobifemoral bypass for aortoiliac occlusive disease: a report of two cases. *J Vasc Surg* 2002; 36: 1079-1082.

8 Ruurda JP, Broeders IA, Simmermacher RP, et al. Feasibility of robot-assisted laparoscopic surgery: an evaluation of 35 robot-assisted laparoscopic cholecystectomies. *Surg Laparosc Endosc Percutan Tech* 2002; 12: 41-45.

9 Ruurda JP, Wisselink W, Cuesta MA, et al. Robot assisted versus standard videoscopic aortic replacement in an experimental model. *Eur J Vasc Endovasc Surg* (In press).

10 Wisselink W, Cuesta MA, Berends FJ, et al. Retroperitoneal endoscopic ligation of lumbar and inferior mesenteric arteries as a treatment of persistent endoleak following endoluminal aortic aneurysm repair. *J Vasc Surg* 2000; 31: 1240-1244.

14

ENDOVASCULAR AORTIC RECONSTRUCTION COMBINED WITH ELECTIVE OPEN SURGERY

JEAN-PIERRE BECQUEMIN, LAURENCE DESTRIEUX-GARNIER
PASCAL DESGRANGES, ERIC ALLAIRE, HISCHAM KOBEITER

Treatment of abdominal aortic aneurysm (AAA) by means of stent-grafts can be considered in patients with favorable anatomical features of the aorta such as adequate landing zones and vascular access. The most common exclusion criterion for stent-graft concerns the proximal neck morphology [1,2] when it is too short, too angulated, or contains thrombus. Iliac artery configurations may also preclude the use of stent-grafts. Heavily calcified aortic neck, severe tortuosity, aneurysms involving the iliac bifurcation, small sized or severely diseased external iliac or common femoral arteries are additional limitations [1,2].

The continuous improvement of stent-graft technology allows more patients to be treated. Larger main body grafts and tapered limb grafts overcome the limitations due to a large proximal and distal neck. Smaller and more flexible introducer sheaths facilitate vascular access. However, there is still a subset of patients in whom stent-graft alone cannot be used safely. In those cases endovascular aortic reconstruction combined with elective open surgery can be an option.

In this chapter we will present the various combinations of open and endovascular techniques that can be associated with AAA stent-grafting in order to deal with difficult anatomy.

Indications and techniques

VISCERAL ARTERY RELOCATIONS.
INDICATIONS

Relocation of the visceral arteries is indicated if the proximal neck is too short, conically shaped, severely angulated (in frontal or lateral direction), and/or contains thrombus. These kinds of neck are associated with an unacceptably high number of failures and complications [3,4], including proximal endoleak, migration, and kidney infarcts. When the portion of the aorta above the renal arteries is healthy, relocation of the renal arteries and, if needed, the superior mesenteric artery increases the length of the proximal landing zone. As a result, the fixation of the stent-graft is proper and the sealing better achieved.

Optimally, the relocations and reconstructions are performed prior to stent-graft deployment; however, it may happen that these procedures must be done urgently when the graft is not properly delivered, occluding one or both renal arteries. In the latter situation, if the aneurysm is excluded by the stent-graft, we strongly believe that visceral artery relocation is a much better option than the surgical conversion requiring celiac clamping, stent-graft removal, and placement of an aortic graft. Association of warm ischemia of the kidneys, hemodynamic variations due to clamping and unclamping of the aorta, and blood loss can be fatal, especially in patients with major associated risk factors [5].

Atheromatous lesions of the renal arteries and/or of the superior mesenteric artery are also good indications for visceral artery reconstruction. In most cases these arteries can be dilated by means of percutaneous transluminal angioplasty. However, some lesions are not accessible for percutaneous transluminal angioplasty, and bypasses must be performed. The latter is applicable to renal artery stenoses that develop months or years after stent-graft placement. The struts of the proximal bare stents may cross the ostium of the renal artery while their remaining parts are healed and fixed within the adjacent aortic wall: this situation does not allow full balloon expansion.

VISCERAL ARTERY RELOCATION.
TECHNIQUES

Iliac to renal artery bypass. Through a retroperitoneal approach the common iliac artery is easily dissected free. Next, the proximal part of the renal artery is also dissected leaving the left kidney in place (anterior route) or mobilized anteriorly (posterior route). These approaches can be followed using the left or right side, however, usually only the ipsilateral renal artery can be revascularized. When both renal arteries must be bypassed, a bilateral retroperitoneal approach or a median laparotomy is required. Polyester or polytetrafluoroethylene (PTFE) grafts can be used. The iliac anastomosis is performed first in an end-to-side fashion. Great care must be taken with the limb of the stent-graft, which must not compromise the renal bypass flow if the stent-graft is placed afterward, and not clamped if already in the iliac artery. Following, the renal anastomosis is performed in an end-to-end fashion [6]. Despite a relatively long length and an extra-anatomical route, long-term patency rates of these iliorenal grafts are good [7] (Fig. 1).

Hepato-renal and spleno-renal bypass. Prior to these procedures, a selective arteriogram with antero-posterior and lateral views of the celiac trunk and superior mesenteric artery is mandatory. It is necessary to confirm that the diameter is adequate and that there is no stenosis at the ostium

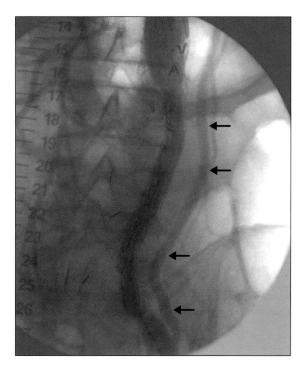

FIG. 1 Post-operative angiography of iliac-renal bypass *(arrows)*, combined with aortic endograft after unintentional covering of renal ostium.

of the donor artery. The right renal artery can be revascularized using the hepatic or the gastroduo- denal artery (Figs. 2, 3). The surgical approach is usually via median laparotomy or a subcostal inci-

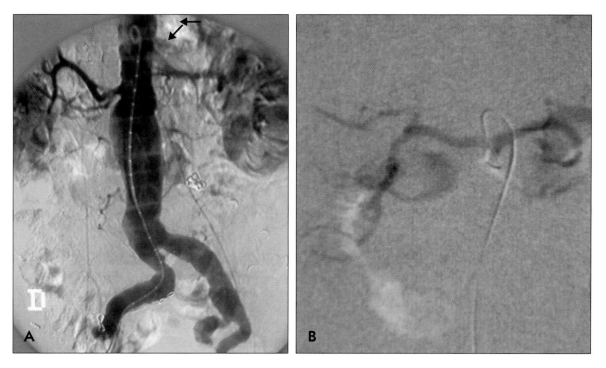

FIG. 2 A - Pre-operative arteriography of AAA with a short neck. Note the differences in level of renal orifices; the left *(arrows)* being some two centimeters higher. B - Postoperative angiography showing the right hepato-renal anastomosis.

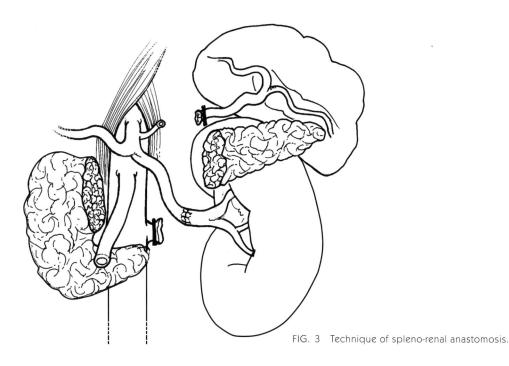

FIG. 3 Technique of spleno-renal anastomosis.

sion. The renal artery is dissected free behind the vena cava. The hepatic and gastroduodenal arteries are freed in front of the pancreas. Before dividing the arteries, one must verify that the anastomosis can be performed without tension or twist. Otherwise, a short graft (preferably saphenous vein) is interposed between the two arteries.

The left renal artery is revascularized with a spleno-renal bypass. The splenic artery is dissected above the tail of the pancreas, then divided and anastomosed in an end-to-end fashion to the proximal part of the left renal artery. Finally, if both renal arteries must be spared, both procedures can be performed simultaneously.

Superior mesenteric bypass. Contrary to the situation of a thoraco-abdominal aneurysm [8,9], superior mesenteric artery bypasses are very rarely required in the context of an infrarenal aneurysm. The exceptions are patients in whom the ostium of the superior mesenteric artery is close to the renal arteries or patients with renal insufficiency and dialysis in whom the proximal tip of the stent-graft will cross the ostia of the visceral arteries. Similarly, the iliac artery is used as a donor site. The superior mesenteric artery is divided anteriorly of the pancreas and anastomosed end-to-end to the tube graft. The main problem is the route of the graft, which should be wide enough to prevent kinking of the graft. A large loop in front of the left kidney is generally appropriate. In our opinion, polyester grafts are more flexible than PTFE grafts for these reconstructions.

INTERNAL ILIAC RELOCATION. INDICATIONS

The internal iliac artery can intentionally be crossed by the limb of a stent-graft, or this might be an inadvertent act. When the internal iliac artery is patent and the graft not fully applied against the arterial wall, as commonly seen in case of associated aneurysm of the common iliac artery, a large type II distal endoleak is almost inevitable. This finding has led to the practice of internal iliac artery coil embolization. There remains controversy about the potential danger of this internal artery exclusion. Most authors have reported uneventful outcomes [10,11], however, severe adverse events have been published including paraplegia, colonic and pelvic ischemia. These complications were favored by multiple micro-embolizations and were more frequent in the setting of bilateral internal iliac occlusions [12-14]. More benign and generally transient are buttock claudication and sciatic neu-

ropathy, occurring in almost 30% of internal iliac exclusion [11,15,16]. Internal iliac relocation of at least of one of these arteries is indicated when the graft crosses two patent internal iliac arteries (Fig. 4). Obviously, severe calcification and aneurysms of the internal iliac artery contraindicate relocation.

INTERNAL ILIAC ARTERY RELOCATION. TECHNIQUES

The surgical approach is relatively simple. A short oblique abdominal incision allows access to the retroperitoneal space. The external iliac artery is dissected up to the iliac bifurcation and the internal iliac artery. The dissection can be difficult when the common iliac artery is affected by aneurysmal disease. Several techniques to perform the revascularization are available [11,15,16]. If the external iliac artery is curved and long enough, a direct end-to-side suture can be performed between the two arteries. However, in most cases, the direct anastomosis is not easy and graft interposition offers a much safer and more convenient solution. The proximal anastomosis is performed on the external iliac or the common femoral artery [17,18]. Again, great attention must be given to the route of the graft in order to avoid any kink or twist.

With aorto-uni-iliac grafts and femorofemoral bypasses, the contralateral internal iliac artery can

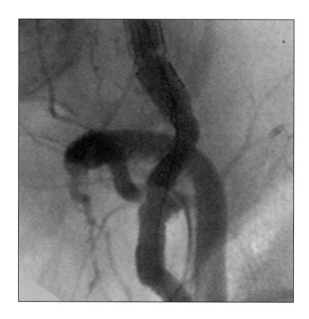

FIG. 4 Bypass from the common femoral artery to the internal iliac artery.

be directly sutured end-to-end to the origin of the external iliac artery [19].

LOWER LIMB REVASCULARIZATION. INDICATIONS AND TECHNIQUES

These procedures are mainly indicated if aorto-uni-iliac grafts are implanted or when thrombosis occurs during or after stent-graft placement [20-24]. Furthermore, in some patients with severe atherosclerosis, the common femoral and/or the superficial femoral artery have to be repaired.

Femorofemoral crossover bypasses can be performed before or after graft deployment. The donor site can be the common femoral artery or the external iliac artery (Fig. 5). We found that in obese patient the external iliac site allowed a more harmonious route with less risk of graft compression or kink. The graft is tunneled either subcutaneously or in the prevesical space.

Common femoral endarterectomy, femorofemoral bypass, and femoropopliteal bypass may be necessary in patients with severely diseased femoral arteries or when the introducer sheath has damaged

the common femoral artery. Combined repair before or after stent-graft placement aims for preserving flow in the limb.

Axillary bifemoral grafts are indicated in case of aortic stent-graft thrombosis. The endograft is left in place to treat the aneurysm.

VASCULAR ACCESS FOR STENT-GRAFTS

Frequently, the current stent-grafts cannot be advanced through small or severely diseased external iliac arteries, often in women [25-27]. Therefore, various endovascular and open techniques must be used to facilitate the access. In some cases, angioplasty with or without stent placement is sufficient. However, the endovascular procedure may fail or the external iliac artery ruptures, requiring open vascular surgery.

Several techniques to obtain improved vascular access are available, such as common femoral or external iliac endarterectomy through the groin. These procedures might be difficult and should not be recommended, except for limited flaps at the level of the introducer sheath.

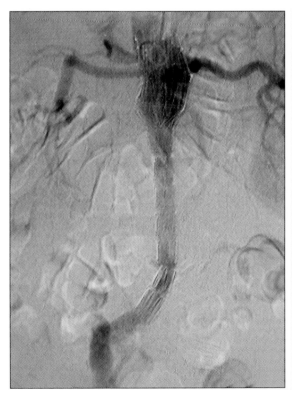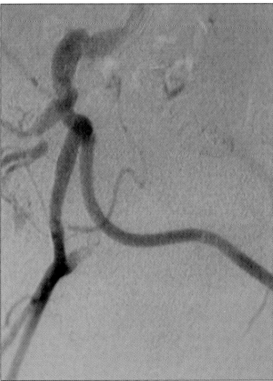

FIG. 5   Right aorto-uni-iliac endoprosthesis with a femoro-femoral cross-over bypass.

An iliofemoral bypass graft is constructed via a retroperitoneal incision with the proximal anastomosis on the common iliac artery. The stent-graft is then passed through the graft. After stent-graft placement, the iliac graft can be removed or used as a conduit to the ipsilateral limb or the contralateral limb instead of a femorofemoral bypass.

MANAGEMENT OF SEALING ZONES

Failure of adequate sealing may occur in case of an unfavorable proximal or distal neck, including conically shaped, severely angulated, or enlarging segments. In many cases endovascular solutions can be found. The most commonly employed strategy comprises placement of a cuff or a new stent-graft. However, in some occasions, endovascular solutions are not feasible and banding of the sealing zone is an alternative solution [28,29].

The proximal infrarenal neck of the iliac artery is dissected through a retroperitoneal access or by means of a laparoscopic approach. A teflon mesh is placed around the aorta and tied by polypropylene sutures. In order to appropriately secure the banding, placement of an inflatable balloon in the lumen of the artery is recommended while the mesh is tied up.

ANEURYSM SAC MANAGEMENT

Following stent-grafting and during follow-up, aneurysm with or without endoleaks may continue to enlarge. Remodeling of the sac and closure of the endoleak can be achieved through a retroperitoneal incision or by laparoscopic means. These techniques can be attempted in fragile patients in order to avoid the risk of a surgical conversion. However, it is necessary to confirm that the stent-graft is firmly attached to the landing zones with perfect integrity of the fabric [28].

The first step is to place a large balloon in the aorta above the stent-graft. Following this, the aorta is approached via a retroperitoneal incision or by a laparoscopic technique. Lumbar arteries can be clipped from outside the sac (Fig. 6). However, the inflammatory reaction and the volume of the sac make this technique demanding. Lumbar arteries at the right side of the aorta are almost impossible to reach. In our experience, the most appropriate way to manage this problem is to open the sac, remove the clots, and suture the lumbar arteries from inside the aneurysm. Back-bleeding can be stopped by inflating the balloon. The sac can be resected and tightly sutured over the graft.

Results and comments

The combination of endovascular aortic reconstruction and elective open surgery comprises a hybrid strategy to overcome limitations of the past and current stent-grafts and to deal with vascular complications during stent-grafting. The rate of associated procedures varies between 1.5% and 22% depending on the time of the reports, the grafts used, and the choice of the physicians. Table I

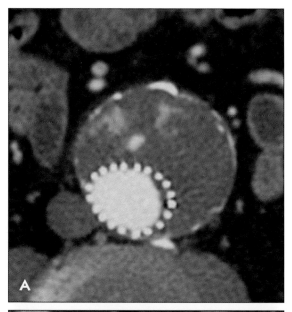

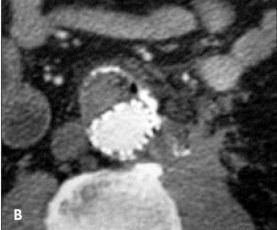

FIG. 6 A - Postoperative CT scan showing type II endoleak. B - CT scan after laparoscopic ligation of lumbar arteries and resection of the sac: absence of endoleak and reduction of sac volume.

shows the rate and distribution of these procedures in several series reported in the literature.

We were able to find 11 series that specifically addressed the issue of combined open and endovascular procedures for AAA treatment (Table II).

Lee et al. [38] reported on 38 combined retroperitoneal iliac procedures in 32 patients to facilitate endovascular AAA repair. The procedures consisted of 8 temporary iliac conduits, 14 common iliac to femoral bypass grafts, and 16 internal iliac reconstructions. The patients' outcomes were compared to those of a group of 132 patients treated without adjunct open procedures. Table III summarizes the findings of Lee et al. and compares them with a series [20] of sole endovascular grafting.

The experience of Lee et al. shows that adjunctive retroperitoneal surgical procedures extended the number of patients amenable for endovascular aneurysm repair. However, these results were obtained at the cost of increased complication rates and longer hospital stays. Their study, however, provides the answer to the fundamental question of whether patients in whom a combined procedure was necessary benefit from this strategy as compared to a similar group of patient treated by open surgery alone.

Since reports are scarce, long-term results of combined procedures are rarely assessed. There are no studies reporting on long-term results of visceral artery relocation. Femorofemoral bypass patency in this setting has been reported by Clouse et al. [20] and Hinchliffe et al. [21]. The 2-year primary patency was 93% and 97.8%, respectively. The infection rate was 2.6% and 4%, respectively. No long-term data are reported with internal iliac relocation.

For the purpose of this presentation we reviewed our experience with combined open and endovascular procedures in our institution. From June 1995 to November 2003, 338 patients underwent endovascular AAA repair. Among them, 40 patients (11%) had 53 elective open surgery combined with a stent-graft placement. Table IV shows the distribution of the open procedures, intra-operative data, length of stay, mortality, and complications.

In our current series the causes of death were colonic necrosis (n = 1), septicemia (n = 1), and myo-

Table I	RATE OF COMBINED OPEN PROCEDURES IN SERIES OF ENDOVASCULAR GRAFTING OF INFRARENAL AORTIC ANEURYSMS				
1st author [ref.]	Year	Number of endovascular AAA repairs	Number of combined procedures	Rate %	Procedures
Gorich et al. [30]	1999	52	1	1.9	- Iliofemoral crossover
Criado et al. [31]	2001	127	28	22.0	- Femorofermoral crossover
Yano et al. [27]	2001	390	50	12.0	- 35 access management + 15 proximal and distal sealing zone management
Bergamini et al. [19]	2002	222	4	1.8	- Femorofemoral crossover EIA-IIA endograft
Pfammatter et al. [32]	2002	66	1	1.5	- 1 iliac bypass for rupture of iliac artery
Carpenter et al. [33]	2002	174	33	19.0	- Aorto-uni-iliac + crossover
Moore et al. [34]	2003	532	24	4.5	- 13 bifurcated stent-graft + crossover - 11 postoperative crossover

EIA: external iliac artery
IIA: internal iliac artery

Table II	RESULTS OF COMBINED OPEN PROCEDURES AND ENDOVASCULAR GRAFTING OF INFRA RENAL AORTIC ANEURYSMS			
1st author [ref]	*Year*	*Procedures*	*Number*	*Complications*
Chuter et al. [26]	1997	Access iliac reconstruction	1	No
Gough et al. [35]	1998	Laparoscopic occlusion of the IIA + femofemoral crossover	5	1 lower limb ischemia
Urayama et al. [36]	1999	Hypogastric artery exclusion	43	No
Parodi et al. [16]	1999	Relocation of the iliac artery bifurcation	5	1 surgical drainage of a wound hematoma
Faries et al. [37]	2001	External iliac-internal iliac bypass	11	1 intra-operative arterial dissection of the AIE
Bergamini et al. [19]	2002	External iliac-internal iliac	4	No
Rhee et al. [11]	2002	Common femoral artery-to-hypogastric artery bypass	6	No
Hinchliffe et al. [17]	2002	Surgical anastomosis of the endograft to the CIA or to the EIA	7	2 asymptomatic occlusions of the hypogastric artery
Lee et al. [18]	2002	EIA – IIA bypass	1	No
Clouse et al. [20]	2003	Aorto-uni-iliac + femorofemoral crossover	121	8/58 endoleak type II were failure of completely occluded contralateral iliac flow
Lin et al. [6]	2003	Iliorenal bypass	1	No

CIA: common iliac artery
EIA: external iliac artery
IIA: internal iliac artery

cardial infarction (n = 1). The death rate was significantly higher than in the group of patients without associated open procedure (1 in 298). Postoperative complications included groin hematoma (n = 1), wound healing delays (n = 2), pneumonia (n = 2), urethral injury (n = 1) following bladder catheterism, and urinary bladder retention (n = 1).

Conclusion

The combination of elective open surgery and endovascular reconstruction increases the number of patients treatable by stent-graft. Visceral artery reconstructions are justified in high-risk patients who would not benefit from a direct open repair of the aortic aneurysm. The benefit of internal iliac reconstructions is not clear since the sacrifice of internal iliac arteries is not clinically significant in most cases. Crossover grafting is current practice with aorto-uni-iliac grafts and is generally followed by good results. The availability of fenestrated branched stent-grafts [8,39] will probably reduce the need for such combined procedures.

Finally, the most dramatic perspective for the future remains the possibility of modeling the aneurysm sac via laparoscopic approach, which may solve the difficult problem of type II endoleaks and aneurysm growth after endovascular repair.

Table III MORTALITY AND MORBIDITY OF COMBINED OPEN PROCEDURES AND ENDOVASCULAR GRAFTING [38], AND ENDOVASCULAR GRAFTING ALONE [20]

	Endovascular grafting		Endovascular grafting alone	
	Number	%	Number	%
Mortality	1 *	3	2 **	2
Arterial injury	6	19	19	14
Claudication	5	16	9	7
IIA occlusion	3	9	9	7
MI, A, CHF	3	9	3	2
Wound complication	2	6	14	11
Renal insufficiency	2	6	3	2
Ischemic colitis	2	6	1	1
Bleeding	2	6	1	1
Respiratory failure	2	6	0	0
Arterial thrombosis	2	6	0	0
Ileus	2	6	0	0
Patients with complications	**19**	**59**	**43**	**33**

* Myocardial infarction
** 1 colonic infarction, 1 unspecific cardiac event

A: arythmia
IIA: internal iliac artery
MI: myocardial infarction
CHF: chronic heart failure

Table IV PERSONAL EXPERIENCE: COMBINED OPEN AND ENDOVASCULAR SURGICAL PROCEDURES (N = 53) IN 40 PATIENTS

Open procedures	Number	Intervention duration (median, mn)	Operative bleeding (average, mL)	Hospital stay duration (median in days)	Morbidity N (%)	Mortality N (%)
Femorofemoral crossover graft	31	150	261	7	3	2
Femoral endarterectomy	6	145	266	8.5	1	0
Iliofemoral graft	5	180	380	7	1	0
Internal iliac revascularization	5	200	400	7	1	0
Internal iliac ligature	2	160	1300	12	1	0
Axillofemoral bypass graft	1	180	500	13	1	0
Ilio-renal bypass graft	2	240	100	2	0	1
Hepato-renal reconstruction	1	120	0	9	0	0
Total	**53**	**160**	**277**	**7**	**8 (15)**	**3 (7)**

REFERENCES

1 Carpenter JP, Baum RA, Barker CF, et al. Impact of exclusion criteria on patient selection for endovascular abdominal aortic aneurysm repair. *J Vasc Surg* 2001; 34: 1050-1054.

2 Wolf YG, Fogarty TJ, Olcott C, et al. Endovascular repair of abdominal aortic aneurysms: eligibility rate and impact on the rate of open repair. *J Vasc Surg* 2000; 32: 519-523.

3 Albertini J, Kalliafas S, Travis S, et al. Anatomical risk factors for proximal perigraft endoleak and graft migration following endovascular repair of abdominal aortic aneurysms. *Eur J Vasc Endovasc Surg* 2000; 19: 308-312.

4 Alric P, Hinchliffe RJ, Wenham PW, et al. Lessons learned from the long-term follow-up of a first-generation aortic stent graft. *J Vasc Surg* 2003; 37: 367-373.

5 Harris PL, Vallabhaneni SR, Desgranges P, et al. Incidence and risk factors of late rupture, conversion, and death after endovascular repair of infrarenal aortic aneurysms: the EUROSTAR experience. European collaborators on stent/graft techniques for aortic aneurysm repair. *J Vasc Surg* 2000; 32: 739-749.

6 Lin PH, Madsen K, Bush RL, Lumsden AB. Iliorenal artery bypass grafting to facilitate endovascular abdominal aortic aneurysm repair. *J Vasc Surg* 2003; 38: 183-185.

7 Mingoli A, Sapienza P, di Marzo L, et al. Iliorenal bypass for the treatment of type-3 Takayasu's disease. A case report with 10-year follow-up. *J Cardiovasc Surg* 1999; 40: 49-53.

8 Bleyn J, Schol F, Vanhandenhove I, Vercaeren P. Side-branched modular endograft system for thoracoabdominal aortic aneurysm repair. *J Endovasc Ther* 2002; 9: 838-841.

9 Quinones-Baldrich WJ, Panetta TF, Vescera CL, Kashyap VS. Repair of type IV thoracoabdominal aneurysm with a combined endovascular and surgical approach. *J Vasc Surg* 1999; 30: 555-560.

10 Henretta JP, Karch LA, Hodgson KJ, et al. Special iliac artery considerations during aneurysm endografting. *Am J Surg* 1999; 178: 212-218.

11 Rhee RY, Muluk SC, Tzeng E, et al. Can the internal iliac artery be safely covered during endovascular repair of abdominal aortic and iliac artery aneurysms? *Ann Vasc Surg* 2002; 16: 29-36.

12 Karch LA, Hodgson KJ, Mattos MA, et al. Adverse consequences of internal iliac artery occlusion during endovascular repair of abdominal aortic aneurysms. *J Vasc Surg* 2000; 32: 676-683.

13 Kibria SG, Gough MJ. Ischaemic sciatic neuropathy: a complication of endovascular repair of abdominal aortic aneurysm. *Eur J Vasc Endovasc Surg* 1999; 17: 266-267.

14 Kritpracha B, Pigott JP, Price CI, et al. Distal internal iliac artery embolization: a procedure to avoid. *J Vasc Surg* 2003; 37: 943-948.

15 Criado FJ. Iliac bifurcation relocation: more complex and controversial. *J Endovasc Surg* 1999; 6: 348-349.

16 Parodi JC, Ferreira M. Relocation of the iliac artery bifurcation to facilitate endoluminal treatment of abdominal aortic aneurysms. *J Endovasc Surg* 1999; 6: 342-347.

17 Hinchliffe RJ, Hopkinson BR. A hybrid endovascular procedure to preserve internal iliac artery patency during endovascular repair of aortoiliac aneurysms. *J Endovasc Ther* 2002; 9: 488-492.

18 Lee WA, Berceli SA, Huber TS, Seeger JM. A technique for combined hypogastric artery bypass and endovascular repair of complex aortoiliac aneurysms. *J Vasc Surg* 2002; 35: 1289-1291.

19 Bergamini TM, Rachel ES, Kinney EV, et al. External iliac artery-to-internal iliac artery endograft: a novel approach to preserve pelvic inflow in aortoiliac stent grafting. *J Vasc Surg* 2002; 35: 120-124.

20 Clouse WD, Brewster DC, Marone LK, et al. Durability of aortouniiliac endografting with femorofemoral crossover: 4-year experience in the EVT/Guidant trials. *J Vasc Surg* 2003; 37: 1142-1149.

21 Hinchliffe RJ, Alric P, Wenham PW, Hopkinson BR. Durability of femorofemoral bypass grafting after aortouniiliac endovascular aneurysm repair. *J Vasc Surg* 2003; 38: 498-503.

22 Pereira AH, Sanvitto PC, de Souza GG, et al. Aortomonoiliac stent-grafts for abdominal aortic aneurysm repair: association with iliofemoral crossover grafts. *J Endovasc Ther* 2002; 9: 765-771.

23 Walker SR, Braithwaite B, Tennant WG, et al. Early complications of femorofemoral crossover bypass grafts after aorta uni-iliac endovascular repair of abdominal aortic aneurysm. *J Vasc Surg* 1998; 28: 647-650.

24 Yilmaz LP, Abraham CZ, Reilly LM, et al. Is cross-femoral bypass grafting a disadvantage of aortomonoiliac endovascular aortic aneurysm repair? *J Vasc Surg* 2003; 38: 753-757.

25 Abu-Ghaida AM, Clair DG, Greenberg RK, et al. Broadening the applicability of endovascular aneurysm repair: the use of iliac conduits. *J Vasc Surg* 2002; 36: 111-117.

26 Chuter TA, Reilly LM. Surgical reconstruction of the iliac arteries prior to endovascular aortic aneurysm repair. *J Endovasc Surg* 1997; 4: 307-311.

27 Yano OJ, Faries PL, Morrissey N, et al. Ancillary techniques to facilitate endovascular repair of aortic aneurysms. *J Vasc Surg* 2001; 34: 69-75.

28 Kolvenbach R, Pinter L, Raghunandan M, et al. Laparoscopic remodeling of abdominal aortic aneurysms after endovascular exclusion: a technical description. *J Vasc Surg* 2002; 36: 1267-1270.

29 Puech-Leao P. Banding of the common iliac artery: an expedient in endoluminal correction of aortoiliac aneurysms. *J Vasc Surg* 2000; 32: 1232-1234.

30 Gorich J, Rilinger N, Soldner J, et al. Endovascular repair of aortic aneurysms: treatment of complications. *J Endovasc Surg* 1999; 6: 136-146.

31 Criado FJ, Wilson EP, Fairman RM, et al. Update on the Talent aortic stent-graft: a preliminary report from United States phase I and II trials. *J Vasc Surg* 2001; 33 (2 Suppl): S146-149.

32 Pfammatter T, Lachat ML, Kunzli A, et al. Short-term results of endovascular AAA repair with the Excluder bifurcated stent-graft. *J Endovasc Ther* 2002; 9: 474-480.

33 Carpenter JP, Baum RA, Barker CF, et al. Durability of benefits of endovascular versus conventional abdominal aortic aneurysm repair. *J Vasc Surg* 2002; 35: 222-228.

34 Moore WS, Matsumura JS, Makaroun MS, et al. Five-year interim comparison of the Guidant bifurcated endograft with open repair of abdominal aortic aneurysm. *J Vasc Surg* 2003; 38: 46-55.

35 Gough MJ, MacMahon MJ. A minimally invasive technique allowing ligation of the internal iliac artery during endovascular repair of aortic aneurysms with an aorto-uni-iliac device. *Eur J Vasc Endovasc Surg* 1998; 16: 535-536.

36 Urayama H, Ohtake H, Katada S, et al. Exclusion of internal iliac arterial aneurysm concomitant with abdominal aortic aneurysm repair. *J Cardiovasc Surg* 1999; 40: 243-247.

37 Faries PL, Morrissey N, Burks JA, et al. Internal iliac artery revascularization as an adjunct to endovascular repair of aortoiliac aneurysms. *J Vasc Surg* 2001; 34: 892-899.

38 Lee WA, Berceli SA, Huber TS, et al. Morbidity with retroperitoneal procedures during endovascular abdominal aortic aneurysm repair. *J Vasc Sur.* 2003; 38: 459-465.

39 Stanley BM, Semmens JB, Lawrence-Brown MM, et al. Fenestration in endovascular grafts for aortic aneurysm repair: new horizons for preserving blood flow in branch vessels. *J Endovasc Ther* 2001; 8: 16-24.

15

HYBRID PROCEDURES
AND HOMEMADE DEVICES
FOR AORTIC REPAIR

MARTIN MALINA, BJÖRN SONESSON
BENGT LINDBLAD, KRASSI IVANCEV

The Latin word hybrida *denotes the offspring of two different species. Operations that involve both open and endovascular techniques are usually called hybrid procedures.*

The main trauma in open vascular surgery is caused by exploration of the blood vessels. Endovascular repair is less traumatic because it is performed from a remote, easily accessible site. Commercially available stents, stent-grafts, and catheters, however, cannot be applied in all patients for anatomical reasons. Furthermore, the high cost of catheters, stents, and stent-grafts is the main reason why the required equipment cannot always be on the shelf. Emergency cases therefore tend to be performed with conventional open techniques. Difficult iliac or femoral access is another common reason for open repair. Hybrid procedures, combining the open and endovascular techniques, are seldom fully exploited. The endovascular approach is rejected when a specific part of the operation requires open repair even if the rest of the procedure would have been better performed endovascularly.

Overall, many patients are subjected to unnecessary surgical trauma that can be avoided by hybrid open and endovascular techniques. Customizing an existing endovascular device in the operating room also helps to reduce the number of open procedures.

The need for "homemade" devices and hybrid procedures changes and will hopefully decrease as novel endovascular techniques develop. In this chapter, we summarize some of the procedures that presently seem useful to reduce the surgical trauma in selected patients with complex aorto-iliac disease.

Combining stents and stent-grafts

Each type of stent-graft has its own specific advantages and drawbacks. There are no clinical data suggesting that we should refrain from combining different stent-graft components. The different properties of various stent-grafts need to be fully exploited. A rigid device may not fit tortuous vessels, while a self-expanding stent with limited radial force is unsuitable for tight stenoses or kinks. Multiple stents and stent-grafts need to be combined to achieve a satisfactory result in challenging cases. A strong balloon-expanded stent may assist the flexible self-expanding stent-graft to overcome focal recoil at the site of a calcified stenosis. A self-expanding stent may also straighten out an angulated portion of the artery [1] or flatten out the folds of an oversized prosthesis to improve the sealing of the stent-graft. The more compliant self-expanding device is favorable in frail dissections or long and tortuous lesions.

The homemade devices

Aorto-iliac lesions span over a wide range of anatomical variations. Uncommon stent-graft configurations are frequently needed. A specific stent-graft that is required for a particular patient may not be available in the emergency setting or even commercially on the market.

The easiest way to obtain a stent-graft with uncommon dimensions is by modifying a device that already exists. Lengths, diameters, and shapes can easily be altered in the operating room under sterile conditions with conventional vascular instruments. It may suffice to turn an available stent-graft upside-down (Fig. 1). The stent-graft diameter can be increased by inserting a wedge of dacron (Fig. 2). Tapering is provided by removing a similar wedge of fabric. Elongation can be achieved by anastomosing two devices (Fig. 2). Meticulous care has to be taken to provide a blood-tight and durable anastomosis because sutures cannot be added after deployment. All sutures must be delicate, usually 6/0,

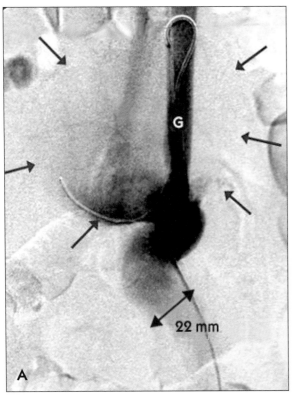
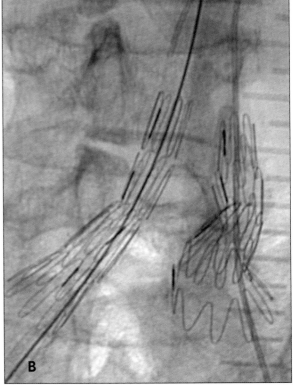

FIG. 1 A - Aorto-bi-iliac bypass graft (G) with bilateral distal anastomotic insufficiency and 22 millimeter wide iliac arteries *(arrows indicate aneurysm)*. B - Two converters turned upside-down bridge the leaks.　　*(To be continued)*

and approximate the graft edges accurately. Too thick sutures and bites of fabric will increase the profile of the stent-graft and make reloading into the sheath difficult. The profile of an end-to-end anastomosis is reduced by cutting both graft ends obliquely. The dacron edges should be cauterized with a sterile heat probe to avoid fabric tears (Fig. 3).

Stent-grafts may also be manufactured de novo by adding stents to conventional vascular grafts. The crimps of dacron grafts are removed by ironing. It is important to appreciate the forces that will act on the stent-graft. The stent needs to be anchored firmly, yet without excessive sutures. Generally, the whole graft should be stented to avoid kinks and

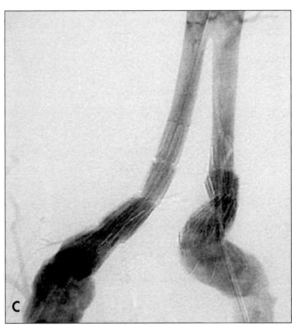

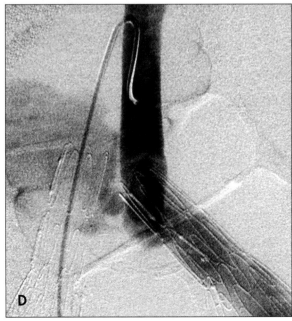

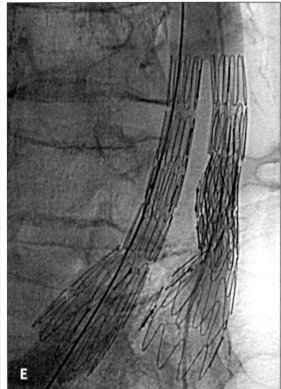

FIG. 1 C - Completion angiography. D - Three years later, the converter has slid out of the graft limb. E - Proximal extension with two additional converters turned upside-down.

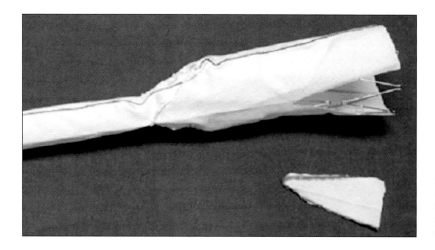

FIG. 2 A stent-graft has been tapered by an oblique, low-profile, end-to-end anastomosis. The proximal end is widened by insertion of a dacron wedge.

FIG. 3 Cauterizing the edges of dacron to avoid tears.

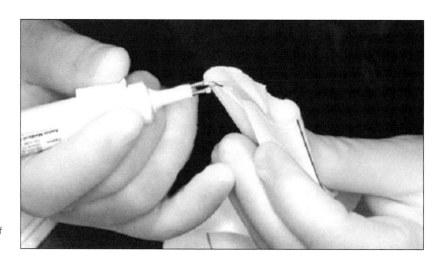

twisting. Whenever orientation of the device is important, radiopaque markers should be added. The gold tip of a readily available "014" wire can be cut at any length and serves as an excellent marker, easy to attach with a fine running suture.

Loading the stent-graft

Reloading a modified stent-graft into the original sheath is not always feasible. Some devices can be partially deployed, modified, and then reloaded. Usually, however, the stent-graft must be entirely unloaded. Large introducers up to 24F should

therefore be kept on the shelf for delivery of modified devices.

It is difficult to push a stent-graft through the valve of a sheath. The stent-graft therefore needs to be preloaded in a cartridge that allows expedient insertion through the valve (Fig. 4). The cartridge itself is prepared from a piece of another sheath. A low-profile catheter (4F) placed within the stent-graft allows insertion of the cartridge over a wire. Loading the stent-graft into the cartridge itself is facilitated by constricting sutures and by a suture to pull the device into the cartridge instead of pushing it. The completed cartridge is passed over a wire into the valve of the delivery sheath. The low-profile catheter is withdrawn and the stent-graft is

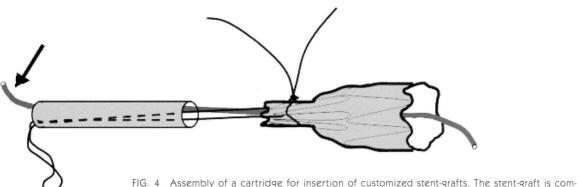

FIG. 4 Assembly of a cartridge for insertion of customized stent-grafts. The stent-graft is compressed by a suture before it is pulled by another into a piece of introducer sheath. The central catheter *(arrow)* allows the cartridge to be passed over a guidewire for final deployment.

pushed out of the cartridge into the sheath. The dilator of the introducer is conveniently used as a pusher after its tip has been cut off.

The modified, reloaded stent-graft is deployed simply by pushing it out of the sheath. The blood stream tends to dislocate the stent-graft distally as it starts deploying, and the accuracy of such placement is limited. Accuracy can be improved by partially deploying the stent-graft above the intended landing site and then slowly pulling it back. A prolene suture inserted into the distal end of the stent-graft holds the stent-graft within the sheath and prevents premature complete deployment during the pullback maneuver. The prolene suture is withdrawn once deployment is completed.

Proximal sutures, holding the tip of the device in place during deployment, are very useful (Fig. 5) but cannot readily be produced in the operating room with an ordinary introducer sheath. Excellent sheaths with proximal safety wires for easy loading and accurate deployment of homemade stent-grafts have been designed but remain, sadly enough, unavailable on the market.

Femoral access: percutaneous, open, or both?

Surgical dissection of the femoral artery is a minor operation. It still deserves attention because it is associated with complications such as hemorrhage, infection, arterial occlusion, pseudoaneurysm, lymphocele, etc. Percutaneous stent-graft insertion is less traumatic and quicker, and does not require the

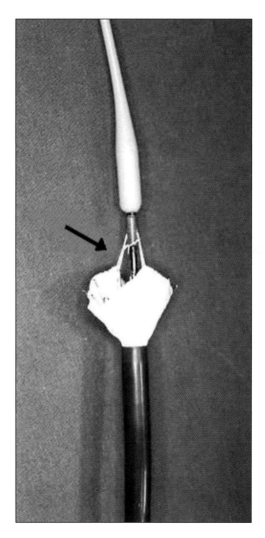

FIG. 5 Sutures holding the proximal end of a stent-graft *(arrow)* prevent distal migration during deployment.

15
147

presence of surgical staff or equipment. Perfusion of the limbs is not interrupted. Narrow and calcified iliac arteries are better negotiated by large sheaths while the artery remains unexposed and supported by surrounding tissues.

Multiple vascular sutures can be applied percutaneously to the femoral artery [2] with a catheter device (Prostar®, *Abbott Laboratories Co., Redwood, CA, USA*). The puncture hole is subsequently dilated to the required diameter: the so-called "pre-close technique." The sutures are tied upon withdrawal of the final large sheath. Large bore introducer sheaths of up to 24F (28F outer diameter) can be inserted percutaneously in this manner.

Bleeding is the major reason why exposure of the femoral artery is still preferred by many surgeons. Hemorrhage does occur upon sheath withdrawal in about 20% of the percutaneous cases with 20F sheaths, due to failure of the closure device. However, a percutaneous transluminal angioplasty (PTA) balloon catheter can be re-inserted into the femoral artery, inflated, and pulled back to obliterate the puncture hole and provide instant hemostasis (Fig. 6). Unrushed open arteriography can then be performed.

The aorto-uni-iliac stent-graft requires a femoro-femoral crossover bypass, and initial cut down therefore seems logical. The alternative is to exclude the aneurysm percutaneously and make the cut down at the end of the procedure, before withdrawing the sheaths. This approach is convenient in urgent repair of ruptured aortic aneurysms when expedient exclusion of the sac must not be delayed by groin dissection. The ruptured aneurysm repair thereby becomes a pure catheter intervention until the sac has been excluded. The operation is initiated under local anesthesia without any delay and without the presence of surgical staff or instruments.

Difficult iliac stenosis: the endo-exo graft

The excessively tortuous or stenotic iliac artery is difficult to handle with a large sheath [3]. An ultra-stiff guidewire is helpful but may not suffice. An iliac bend can often be overcome by external manual manipulation. A "through-and-through," brachial-to-femoral guidewire can be stretched from both ends to straighten out the vessels. Occasionally, the vessels need to be grasped through a retroperitoneal incision.

Whenever resistance to the sheath is encountered, pushing the introducer from below tends to com-

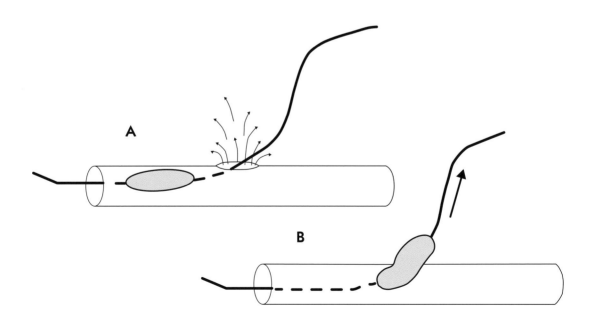

FIG. 6 A - A PTA balloon is inflated in the femoral artery and pulled (B) into the puncture hole to stop hemorrhage after a closure device has failed.

press the sheath and provide little kinks. As Brian Hopkinson clearly phrased: "It is easier to pull a snake through a hole by its tail than pushing it." The device can be towed through the iliac vessels by placing clamps on the wire distal to the sheath and then applying traction from the arm (Fig. 7).

Occasionally, it is impossible to pass the device through the external iliac artery and the sheath may

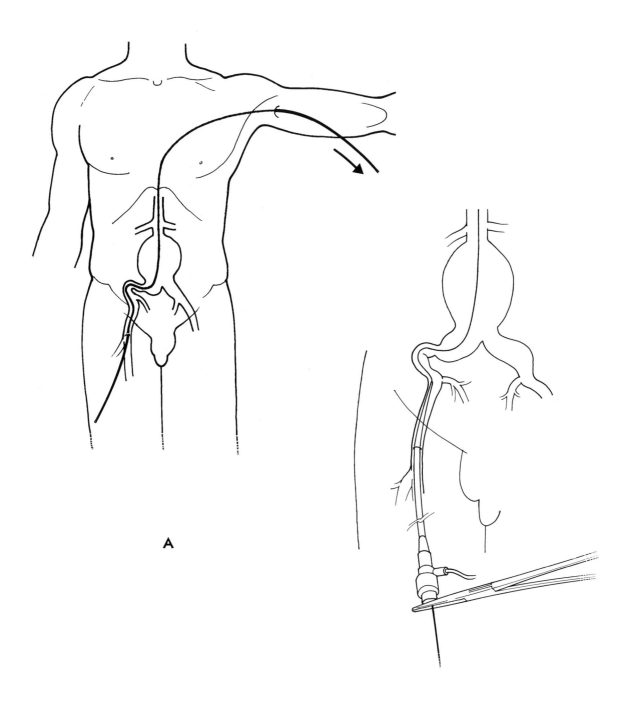

A

B

FIG. 7 Schematic drawing of towing the device through the iliac artery by placing clamps on the wire distal to the sheath and applying traction from the arm.

need to be inserted directly into the common iliac artery via a retroperitoneal surgical access. This approach is perpendicular to the course of the iliac vessel and the large sheath may not readily be inserted at such an angle. A temporary dacron conduit, sutured end to side to the iliac artery for easier sheath insertion, has been proposed. An alternative is to pass the sheath parallel to the external iliac artery from the groin. This provides a more favorable angle for insertion into the common iliac artery and avoids the need for a temporary conduit.

Frequently, it is necessary for the external iliac artery to be bypassed permanently in this type of patient [4]. An excessively long stent-graft can be brought all the way to the common femoral artery where a conventional end-to-side anastomosis is performed. Since the graft passes inside the aorta but exits the common iliac artery to run outside the external iliac artery, the term *endo-exo graft* is handy (Fig. 8).

The iliac aneurysm

Aortic aneurysms frequently extend into the common iliac artery. The established endovascular approach in these cases includes sacrifice of the hypogastric artery by coil embolization and extension of the stent-graft into the external iliac artery. Some patients, however, present bilateral common iliac artery aneurysms. Bilateral sacrifice of the hypogastric artery as well as unilateral sacrifice in patients with compromised colonic perfusion are associated with ischemic complications and should be avoided if possible. There are several options to preserve the hypogastric artery and still avoid open aortic surgery.

Common iliac arteries with a diameter up to 20 to 25 millimeters can be considered for distal landing of the aorto-iliac stent-graft in selected patients. A wide iliac stent-graft can be obtained either by narrowing the proximal end of a 24 to 28 millimeter aortic stent-graft to make it fit the distal orifice of the aorto-iliac main body or by deploying a converter upside-down. A converter is a tapered stent-graft for conversion of an aorto-bi-iliac stent-graft into an aorto-uni-iliac device (Fig. 9). Our own experience of 26 patients with a follow-up of at least one year suggests that this is a durable approach. Particular attention should be paid to extending the stent-graft all the way to the iliac bifurcation.

The distended common iliac artery is likely to dilate further if its distal portion is left unprotected by stent-graft.

Another way to preserve a hypogastric artery in patients with large common iliac arteries is by ligating the common iliac artery and adding a retroperitoneal bypass from the external to the internal iliac artery [5]. Translocation of the internal to the external iliac artery is preferred in selected cases. These procedures can be performed from a limited retroperitoneal incision. Occasionally, the anatomy is favorable enough to pass a flexible stent-graft from the external iliac artery into the hypogastric artery [6].

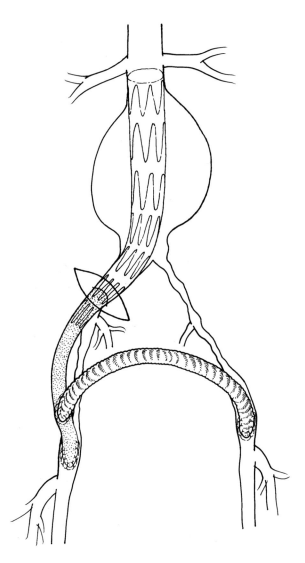

FIG. 8 Schematic drawing of the *endo-exo* graft.

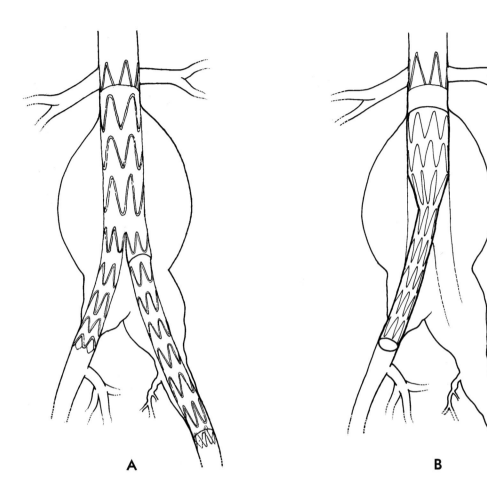

FIG. 9 Schematic drawing of a *converter:* a tapered stent-graft for conversion of bifurcated stent-grafts in to uni-iliac stent-grafts.

The most elegant solution is the branched iliac stent-graft [7]. The common trunk of the hypogastric artery must be long and straight enough to enable safe distal anchoring of the stent-graft. A very short bifurcated stent-graft is needed and can be obtained by shortening a small size aorto-bi-iliac device. The bifurcated stent-graft is deployed into the common iliac artery with the shortest limb pointing toward the hypogastric orifice and the long-er limb extending into the external iliac artery (Fig. 10A). The stent-graft must not protrude above the aortic bifurcation to allow catheterization of the hypogastric artery from the contralateral side. The hypogastric limb is then extended with another stent-graft passed over the bifurcation (Figs. 10B,C). The arteries in patients with large aorto-iliac aneu-rysms provide poor support for the sheath to pass across the aortic bifurcation and the sheath may need to be pulled down from the ipsilateral groin with a "014" wire (Fig. 7). Extension of the stent-graft into the hypogastric artery can also be attempted from the arm but the long distance provides poor torque control and pushability.

Several manufacturers are presently developing branched iliac stent-grafts (e.g., *Cordis Corp., a John-son & Johnson Company, Miami Lakes, FL, USA,* and *William Cook Inc., Bloomington, IN, USA*). The com-mercial product will probably include a more sophisticated mechanism of deployment with a self-expanding branch to be pushed into the hypogas-tric vessel and then released by separate safety wires.

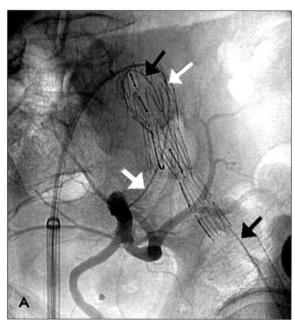

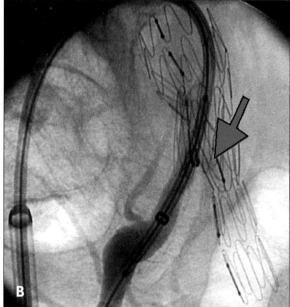

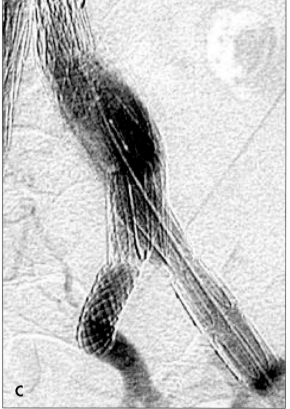

FIG. 10 A - A shortened aorto-bi-iliac stent-graft is deployed in the left common iliac artery. The hypogastric artery is catheterized from the contralateral side *(white arrows)* while the sheath is bent down by traction on a "014" wire *(black arrows).* B - The sheath is advanced into the hypogastric artery to deploy. C - Completion angiography of the branched iliac stent-graft.

The inadequate aortic neck

The most common reason for rejecting a patient from endovascular aneurysm repair is an inadequate proximal neck. The short neck can occasionally be made to suffice for graft anchoring by adding some adjunctive steps. The procedures listed below should be reserved for patients who are at high risk of rupture but are not candidates for open surgery.

Fenestrated stent-grafts are beyond the scope of this presentation and will most likely become commercially available in the near future. It deserves to be mentioned that renal fenestrations can readily be added to a conventional aortic stent-graft [8] in the operating room. It is not always necessary to unload the stent-graft entirely to make a fenestration. The sheath can be retracted partially to uncover the upper portion of the stent-graft (Zenith®, *William Cook*). Fenestrations can then be cut at an appropriate level and the sheath re-advanced to contain the stent-graft. The drawback of homemade fenestrations is that the stent-graft must be fully deployed before catheterization of the renal arteries is attempted. It is therefore impossible to re-adjust the position of the stent-graft. The commercial fenestrated device will provide diameter-reducing sutures that allow partial graft deployment and accurate repositioning for convenient renal catheterization.

Banding of a wide and short neck is another option for patients who require endovascular repair [9]. We have banded the neck of thoracic and abdominal aortic aneurysms, both the proximal and distal neck. Two main problems are encountered. First, it is difficult to make the band sit firmly across the end of the stent-graft in a truly short neck. The adjacent aneurysm tends to push the band and transmural aortic sutures are needed to hold the band and the stent-graft in place. Secondly, an aortic balloon needs to be inflated within the neck to indicate the correct diameter of the band. Combining transabdominal surgery and fluoroscopy is cumbersome and tying the band at the neck is not easily guided by fluoroscopy. The durability of banding is unknown. The strain on the band is high and late erosion of the aortic wall is of concern.

Many patients are not fit for open repair of a suprarenal aneurysm and alternate approaches are required [10]. The branched stent-graft remains too complex to be offered in the routine clinical set-ting [11]. A transabdominal bypass from the iliac artery to the visceral vessels combined with a long aortic stent-graft may be an option for selected patients [12,13]. This procedure does, however, include extensive abdominal dissection with revascularization of vital organs and the mortality rate is significant.

Rescuing failed stent-grafts

Failure of the limb extensions of a stent-graft comprises limb dissociation, migration, kinking, thrombosis, or type III endoleakage. Limb failure is usually treated by additional placement of stents or stent-grafts. Thrombosis of the limbs is more demanding. Thrombolysis is tempting but reperfusion of the sac with rapid aneurysm expansion has occurred [14]. Mechanical thrombectomy may be attempted under fluoroscopy [15,16] but should not be pursued if fixation of the rest of the stent-graft is jeopardized. Spillover of thrombus into the contralateral limb or into renal arteries must be avoided. Re-stenting with additional stent-grafts may open the thrombosed limb surprisingly well and is worth trying. Often, however, the occlusion of one limb is best treated with a crossover bypass and bilateral occlusion may require conversion to open repair or insertion of an axillobifemoral bypass.

Failure of the proximal part of a stent-graft is a critical condition. It is associated with type I endoleakage due to migration of the device or to neck dilation.

Migration must be treated with a proximal extension. Most bifurcated stent-grafts have a high bifurcation and there is little space for a tubular extension within the original device. An overlap of at least five centimeters is recommended between two stent-graft components to avoid continued late dissociation (Fig. 1D). Accurate placement of short aortic stent-grafts is inherently difficult although the aforementioned distal safety suture is helpful. The safest way to achieve a proximal extension with adequate overlap between the stent-graft components is by inserting an aorto-uni-iliac device (Fig. 11). A stent-graft with a bare cross-renal top stent should be selected to reduce the risk of repeat migration. Proximal extension of a stent-graft with a device that is fenestrated for the renal arteries is hazardous. Stent-grafts placed inside each other tend to interlock and accurate positioning of the fenestrations is difficult.

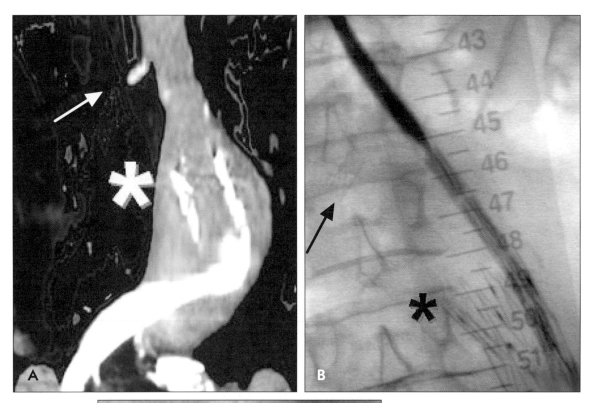

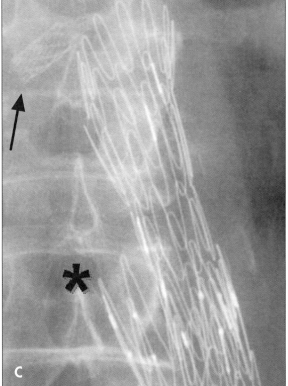

FIG. 11 A - Complete migration of a stent-graft. The stented right renal artery is seen *(arrow)*. B - A novel stent-graft is passed through the failed device to the level of the renal arteries.

Dilation of the neck also leads to a type I endoleak. A proximal and larger stent-graft may be added if the initial device sits a couple of centimeters below the renal arteries. However, if the initial device was correctly placed very near the renal arteries, no reliable endovascular option is presently available to treat neck dilation. Banding the neck or coiling the type I endoleak may be attempted if open repair is not an option.

Total replacement of a stent-graft by open repair is rarely indicated. While replacement of an infrarenal stent-graft is a standard open procedure, stent-grafts with a bare cross-renal stent are more challenging. An occlusion balloon is useful for suprarenal aortic cross-clamping above the top stent. A compliant latex balloon should be selected. Transfemoral insertion over a stiff guidewire is most convenient. The inflated balloon needs to be supported from below by the introducer sheath to prevent sudden intra-operative blowout and hemorrhage. Whenever possible, the bare top stent should be left in-situ and only the graft covered portion of the stent-graft should be replaced. Extraction of the top stent can be carried out after the sac has been incised by compressing the stent manually in order to disengage the aortic wall. Some proximal stents carry barbs and hemorrhage may occur from puncture holes at the suprarenal aorta.

REFERENCES

1 Dias NV, Resch T, Malina M, et al. Intraoperative proximal endoleaks during AAA stent-graft repair: evaluation of risk factors and treatment with Palmaz stents. *J Endovasc Ther* 2001; 8: 268-273.

2 Hahn U, Betsch A, Wiskirchen J, et al. A new device for percutaneous suture-mediated closure of arterial puncture sites using exteriorized needles: initial experience. *J Invasive Cardiol* 2001; 13: 456-459.

3 Lee WA, Berceli SA, Huber TS, et al. Morbidity with retroperitoneal procedures during endovascular abdominal aortic aneurysm repair. *J Vasc Surg* 2003; 38: 459-465.

4 Wain RA, Lyon RT, Veith FJ, et al. Alternative techniques for management of distal anastomoses of aortofemoral and iliofemoral endovascular grafts. *J Vasc Surg* 2000; 32: 307-314.

5 Faries PL, Morrissey N, Burks JA, et al. Internal iliac artery revascularization as an adjunct to endovascular repair of aortoiliac aneurysms. *J Vasc Surg* 2001; 34: 892-899.

6 Bergamini TM, Rachel ES, Kinney EV, et al. External iliac artery-to-internal iliac artery endograft: a novel approach to preserve pelvic inflow in aortoiliac stent grafting. *J Vasc Surg* 2002; 35: 120-124.

7 Abraham CZ, Reilly LM, Schneider DB, et al. A modular multibranched system for endovascular repair of bilateral common iliac artery aneurysms. *J Endovasc Ther* 2003; 10: 203-207.

8 Faruqi RM, Chuter TA, Reilly LM, et al. Endovascular repair of abdominal aortic aneurysm using a pararenal fenestrated stent-graft. *J Endovasc Surg* 1999; 6: 354-358.

9 Tzortzis E, Hinchliffe RJ, Hopkinson BR. Adjunctive procedures for the treatment of proximal type I endoleak: the role of peri-aortic ligatures and Palmaz stenting. *J Endovasc Ther* 2003; 10: 233-239.

10 Lawrence-Brown M, Sieunarine K, van Schie G, et al. Hybrid open-endoluminal technique for repair of thoraco-abdominal aneurysm involving the celiac axis. *J Endovasc Ther* 2000; 7: 513-519.

11 Chuter TA, Gordon RL, Reilly LM, et al. An endovascular system for thoracoabdominal aortic aneurysm repair. *J Endovasc Ther* 2001; 8: 25-33.

12 Rimmer J, Wolfe JH. Type III thoracoabdominal aortic aneurysm repair: a combined surgical and endovascular approach. *Eur J Vasc Endovasc Surg* 2003; 26: 677-679.

13 Macierewicz JA, Jameel MM, Whitaker SC, et al. Endovascular repair of perisplanchnic abdominal aortic aneurysm with visceral vessel transposition. *J Endovasc Ther* 2000; 7: 410-414.

14 Resch T, Lindblad B, Lindh M, et al. Aneurysm expansion and retroperitoneal hematoma after thrombolysis for stent-graft limb occlusion caused by distal endograft migration. *J Endovasc Ther* 2000; 7: 446-450.

15 Ruckert RI, Romaniuk P, Rogalla P, et al. Combined surgical and endovascular removal of thrombus entirely occluding a bifurcated aortic stent-graft. *J Endovasc Surg* 1998; 5: 323-328.

16 Milner R, Golden MA, Velazquez OC, Fairman RM. A new endovascular approach to treatment of acute iliac limb occlusions of bifurcated aortic stent grafts with an exoskeleton. *J Vasc Surg* 2003; 37: 1329-1331.

16

ENDOVASCULAR AORTIC RECONSTRUCTION COMBINED WITH LAPAROSCOPIC SURGERY

JOHN EDOGA

The aim of surgery for abdominal aortic aneurysm (AAA) is to avoid rupture, which is still associated with an overall mortality of approximately 70% to 80% and a postoperative mortality of 40% to 50%. The mortality rate in the case of elective surgery is lower and varies between 3% and 5% in any type of patients and between 6% and 10% in high-risk patients. The increasing incidence of high-risk patients referred to vascular surgeons prompted the search for a less aggressive solution than open surgery in order to decrease the operative risk. Additional goals of this process were to decrease the non-lethal morbidity, to improve the postoperative comfort of the patients, and to shorten the postoperative recovery time. Endovascular aortic repair (EVAR) and laparoscopic surgery were proposed in order to achieve these goals. It quickly became clear that EVAR was associated with substantial problems and/or complications during follow-up, requiring complementary procedures. The laparoscopic approach was proposed in this context to resolve some type II endoleaks. Later, some authors proposed to associate the armamentarium of laparoscopic techniques with the principle of EVAR in order to improve the technical result and to avoid the mid and long-term complications.

The goal of this chapter is to present the current experiences of some pioneering groups and to consider the future endo-aortic procedures performed by this hybrid technology.

Background

The single most important development in the surgical treatment of AAAs was the introduction of endo-aneurysmorrhaphy by Oscar Creech [1] in 1966. His technique has, to this day, remained the gold standard in the management of infrarenal AAAs because it has established an excellent track

record of safety and broad applicability. The durability of the results seen when aortic aneurysms are treated by the Oscar Creech method is directly derived from the very components of that approach:
- evacuation of the laminated thrombus,
- removal of the diseased intimal lining of the aneurysm sac,
- suture ligation of the aortic side branches,
- aortic replacement with a durable conduit permanently fixed to the native aorta and the iliac arteries,
- closure of the endarterectomized aortic wall around the fabric conduit to encourage graft incorporation.

However, the access incision has usually been large and the required dissection extensive. Besides, this technique required aortic cross-clamping, the duration of which was dependent on the surgeon's experience and skill, proficiency of the surgical assistant, and anatomical considerations.

Even as recent developments in mechanical vascular anastomoses and modular grafting promise to reduce the cross-clamp times for the vast majority of cases, and despite advances in anesthesia and critical care, postoperative recovery following the Creech operation is usually arduous and the return to normal activity slow. Yet the Creech operation for AAAs predictably produces durable long-term results, usually without need for re-interventions.

In 1991, an endovascular method for aortic grafting was introduced [2]. Since then, many technical improvements have been made in device construction and deployment mechanics. The basic principles governing endovascular surgery for AAAs have remained the same – *bridging the aneurysm with a watertight prosthetic conduit while avoiding the debilitating incision and invasive dissection associated with the Creech procedure and while virtually eliminating the aortic cross-clamp*. When interruption of aortic blood flow is needed to prevent device movement during deployment of the proximal device fixation, it is extremely brief and produces no measurable changes in cardiac function.

As anticipated, the postoperative recovery following endovascular graft implantation has been less taxing and resumption of normal activity more prompt.

However, conduit attachment is largely only by friction, the laminated thrombus and the diseased intima are left in place, and the "excluded" aneurysm sac continues to be perfused by arterial flow through side branches (endoleak). Persistent side branch flow (type II endoleak) may not be apparent on any of the imaging studies. It is therefore not surprising that a significant percentage of "successful" endovascular aneurysm repairs do go on to fail. Some failures have been reported within days or weeks following the repair while others have occurred several years later. These failures are usually manifested by:
- device migration (caudad or cephalad) [3],
- prosthetic fabric and/or stent fatigue,
- continued aneurysm growth,
- aneurysm repressurization, with or without demonstrable endoleak [4],
- aneurysm rupture, frequently fatal, which has been seen in a disturbingly high number of "treated" cases [5].

Laparoscopic surgery for AAAs became a reality also in the early 1990s, soon after Yves-Marie Dion demonstrated the feasibility of aorto-iliac reconstruction using laparoscopic techniques and instrumentation [6]. Other centers soon followed and a number of approaches and variations were developed to achieve the same goal. The procedures were soon adapted to resect AAAs [7-9]. As a group, patients who have undergone AAA resection by purely laparoscopic or laparoscopic-assisted techniques have consistently shown the same benefits seen following laparoscopic operations for other conditions: quicker postoperative recovery, shorter hospital lengths of stay (Fig. 1), earlier resumption of nor-

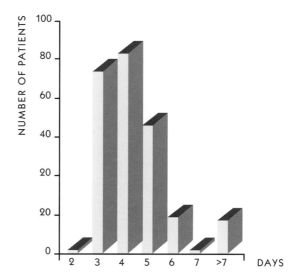

FIG. 1 Bar graph showing the hospital length of stay for patients in our series of laparoscopic and laparoscopy-assisted aortic aneurysm resections.

mal activity, and improved cosmetic results (Figs. 2 and 3). These advantages have been achieved without any increase in mortality or complications attributed solely to the laparoscopic approach. In addition, the mid-term observations and reports following laparoscopic abdominal aneurysm repair portend a durability of the results similar to that seen following the Creech procedure.

Wide acceptance of laparoscopic abdominal vascular surgery has, however, been impeded directly by the steep learning curve encountered in the acquisition of the necessary skills, especially laparoscopic vascular suturing and indirectly by the widening separation of vascular surgery as a specialty from general abdominal surgery. General surgeons who are very skilled in laparoscopy currently have little or no incentive to learn vascular applications of laparoscopy. Established vascular surgeons have very little opportunity to acquire the level of expertise in laparoscopy that is required to perform laparoscopic aortic surgery. Earlier weaning of future vascular surgeons from the general surgical training

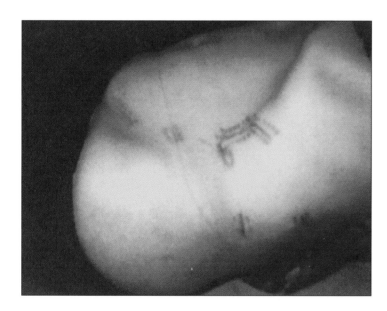

FIG. 2 Cosmetic result 6 weeks following laparoscopy-assisted AAA resection. *(Two adjacent trocar sites had been connected to create a trap door incision to facilitate performance of the proximal anastomosis.)* The introduction of vascular stapling is expected to make this incision unnecessary.

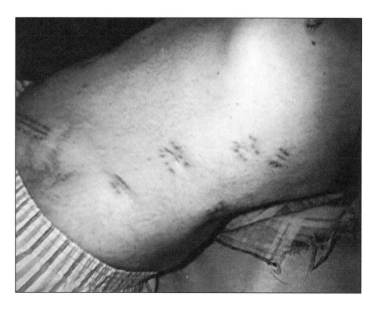

FIG. 3 Cosmetic result 3 months following a totally laparoscopic aortic aneurysm resection.

pathway [10], a concept being proposed by some opinion leaders in the field of vascular surgery, would reduce this opportunity even further.

It is clear that whenever equivalent surgical results have been achieved using minimally invasive techniques, those approaches have quickly gained preference among physicians and patients. It is also evident that EVAR, despite the seductive appeal of the underlying concept, is rarely, if ever, equivalent to the Creech repair. The changing trends in the utilization of EVAR [11] are indicative of the sobering effects that the mid-term results of this venture have had on both physicians and patients.

Laparoscopic technique associated with EVAR

Since 1998 we have used laparoscopic techniques to salvage failing endovascular grafts. We have, however, noted a very severe inflammatory peri-aortic tissue reaction in patients in whom these interven-tions have had to be carried out several months following the initial EVAR. This inflammatory reaction, which obliterates most of the tissue planes, makes an already challenging task even more difficult. For that reason we had, up till now, limited the application of these procedures to situations in which the threat of imminent aneurysm rupture was clearly present. However, other surgeons have described the preemptive use of laparoscopic techniques to treat persistent type II endoleaks by ligation of lumbar and inferior mesenteric arteries [12].

At least two investigators have, in addition, begun to proactively combine laparoscopy and video-assisted minimally invasive surgical approaches with endovascular techniques for the primary treatment of AAAs. Kolvenbach et al. [13] have reported on a series of 8 patients in whom laparoscopic suture fixation of the aortic prosthesis, ligation of the aortic side branches with evacuation, and remodeling of the AAA sac were carried out immediately after implantation of an endovascular graft (Fig. 4). Piquet and his group have developed a hybrid procedure that combines a video-assisted left retroperitoneal

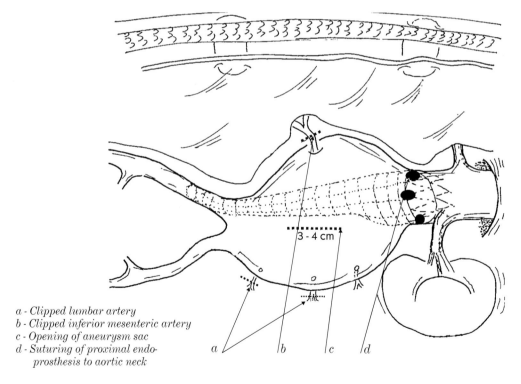

a - Clipped lumbar artery
b - Clipped inferior mesenteric artery
c - Opening of aneurysm sac
d - Suturing of proximal endo-
  prosthesis to aortic neck

FIG. 4 The hybrid procedure proposed and performed by R. Kolvenbach. An endovascular graft, in this case an aorto-uni-iliac endograft, is secured to the aortic neck by laparoscopically placed sutures. The lumbar and inferior mesenteric arteries have been ligated. The aneurysm sac is incised, evacuated, and surgically remodeled.

aortic exposure and repair utilizing a standard bifurcated aortic graft. In this approach, the proximal aortic anastomosis is performed using standard suture technique between the divided aortic neck and the vascular graft, while the distal fixation of the graft limbs is accomplished by deployment of self-expanding stents with hooks. This is an extension of their published treatise on video-assisted mini-invasive retroperitoneal approach for treatment of infrarenal aortic diseases [14]. Pre-operative computed tomography scanning is used to evaluate the iliac artery landing sites, and fluoroscopy is not routinely employed at the time of surgery. The anticipated introduction of mechanical vascular anastomotic devices and graft connectors is expected to facilitate this approach.

Personal technique

Our plan for the combination of laparoscopic and endovascular surgical techniques for the treatment of AAAs calls for the use of laparoscopically applied bands to secure specially designed EVAR prostheses (Fig. 5 A and B) at the proximal and distal landing sites with the addition of barbs to augment the proximal fixation (Fig. 6). We believe that fixation of the prostheses at the banding sites combined with reduction of the band widths will reduce the possibility of ischemic deterioration of the aortic wall due to compression, while providing a better configuration for engagement of the barbs. Similar to the procedure described by Kolvenbach, we advocate ligation of the aortic side branches to

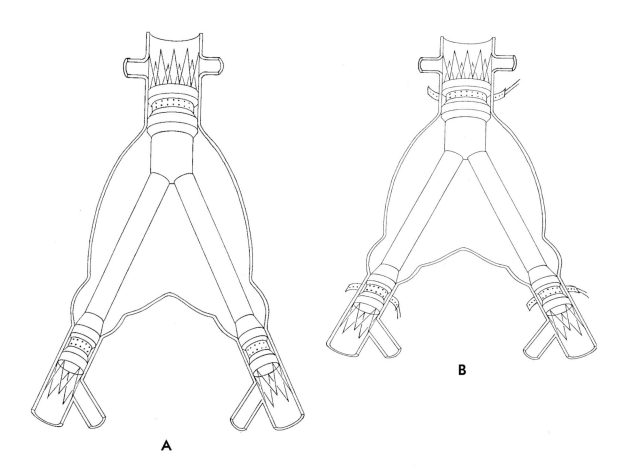

A

B

FIG. 5   A - A specialized endograft designed for combined procedures. The banding at the proximal and distal fixation points provides for better, safer fixation and a tighter seal. The banding segment bears radiopaque markings.
B - Narrow laparobands with radiopaque markings designed to fit into the banding segments of the endograft reduce the compressive forces on the aortic wall. We believe that long-term ischemic degeneration of the aortic wall is less likely using this approach.

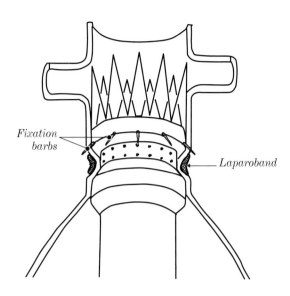

Fixation barbs

Laparoband

FIG. 6 Augmentation of proximal endograft fixation with barbs, which may be deployed once the laparobands have been closed.

isolate the aneurysm sac. Once the EVAR device has been deployed and secured, we believe the aneurysm sac should be opened to remove the laminated thrombus and diseased intima. Surgical remodeling of the sac to tightly fit around the endovascular prosthesis will probably prove to be a useful adjunctive maneuver, as it would encourage *healing* around the aortic graft.

Other concepts being considered include the use of laparoscopy to facilitate the deployment of endovascular tackers, T-fasteners, and staples designed to secure the endoprostheses to the aortic neck and prevent migration.

Rationale for the development of combined procedures

Aortic cross-clamping is one of the major contributors to the morbidity associated with traditional aortic replacement surgery. The deleterious effects of aortic clamping and declamping have been widely documented [15,16]. The need for and the duration of interruption of aortic blood flow even at the infrarenal level is probably the single most important factor in determining which patients, particularly those with cardiac comorbidities, are likely

to survive conventional aortic surgery. The sudden increase in impedance to ventricular ejection and the resultant fall in cardiac output have been found to be more pronounced in patients undergoing aortic surgery for aneurysms than in similar patients operated on for occlusive disease [17].

EVAR results in virtual elimination of aortic cross-clamping. This probably explains why even the most cardiac-impaired high-risk patients are able to tolerate this method of conduit placement within the aneurysmal abdominal aorta.

Questions, however, abound regarding the efficacy of this therapy. Device-related failures due to device migration, device breakdown due to stent fracture, fabric rupture, kinking, separation of device segments, and aorta-related failures due to continuing growth and/or morphologic alterations most significantly at the "landing sites" have re-inforced the doubts expressed by those who have been skeptical all along about the ability of endovascular surgery to survive as a stand-alone operation for aortic aneurysms. Sudden aneurysm enlargement and rupture are frequently reported, even among patients in whom EVAR initially met all the radiologic criteria for successful aneurysm exclusion [18]. The cost has not decreased appreciably and the expense of mandatory follow-up studies and needed re-interventions keeps growing as more patients are treated with an increasing number of available endovascular devices.

It has therefore become necessary, may be even mandatory, for supplemental measures to be added to the endovascular technique to broaden its applicability, ensure its efficacy, and increase its durability while preserving its known advantages. Any of the laparoscopic approaches that have been described and used for the treatment of AAAs can be adapted to provide the features of the Creech procedure not currently addressed by the endovascular operation. Adjustments will have to be made in the design of endografts and their delivery systems in order to take full advantage of these developing techniques at an affordable cost.

It is possible that in the near future, nearly all aneurysms can be treated with an endovascularly inserted fabric conduit that is actively fixed to the aorta by means of laparoscopically aided banding, stapling, or suturing devices. It has already been demonstrated that laparoscopic techniques can be used to ligate all the pertinent aortic side branches, evacuate the laminated thrombus, remove the diseased intima, and surgically remodel the aneurysm sac around the vascular conduit. When endovascular aortic reconstruction is combined with laparoscopic surgery, all of the above objectives can be achieved while remaining minimally invasive and eliminating the need for aortic cross-clamping.

Conclusion

The most formidable obstacle to this approach is the cost and logistics involved in the combination of the needed skills sets, especially at a time when the repositories of the necessary know-how are being further separated by the perceived need for subspecialization. In addition, the introduction of surgical devices and systems for the performance of large and small vascular anastomoses and for coupling of prosthetic grafts is imminent. The clinical application of these systems is expected to produce marked reductions in aortic cross-clamp times and is more likely to make minimally invasive or purely laparoscopic resections the preferred treatment for AAAs.

REFERENCES

1 Creech O Jr. Endo-aneurysmorrhaphy and treatment of aortic aneurysm. *Ann Surg* 1966; 164: 935-946.

2 Parodi JC, Palmaz JC Barone HD. Transfemoral intraluminal graft implantation for abdominal aortic aneurysms. *Ann Vasc Surg* 1991; 5: 491-499.

3 Harris PL, Vallabhaneni SR, Desgranges P, et al. Incidence and risk factors of late rupture, conversion, and death after endovascular repair of infrarenal aortic aneurysms: the EUROSTAR experience. European collaborators on stent-graft techniques for aortic aneurysm repair. *J Vasc Surg* 2000; 32: 739-749.

4 Terramani TT, Najibi S, BrinkmanWT, Chaikof EL. Complications associated with endovascular repair of abdominal aortic aneurysms. *Adv Vasc Surg* 2002; 10: 109-116.

5 Zarins CK, White RA, Fogarty TJ. Aneurysm rupture after endovascular repair using the AneuRx stent graft. *J Vasc Surg* 2000; 31: 960-970.

6 Dion YM, Katkhouda N, Rouleau C, Aucoin A. Laparoscopy-assisted aortobifemoral bypass. *Surg Laparosc Endosc* 1993; 3: 425-429.

7 Castronuovo JJ Jr., James KV, Resnikoff M, et al. Laparoscopic-assisted abdominal aortic aneurysmectomy. *J Vasc Surg* 2000; 32: 224-233.

8 Dion YM, Gracia CR, Ben El Kadi HH. Totally laparoscopic abdominal aortic aneurysm repair. *J Vasc Surg* 2001; 33: 181-185.

9 Alimi YS, Di Molfetta L, Hartung O, et al. Laparoscopy-assisted abdominal aortic aneurysm endoaneurysmorraphy: early and mid-term results. *J Vasc Surg* 2003; 37: 744-749.

10 Veith FJ. Vascular surgery won a battle but is losing the war: a call to arms for every vascular surgeon. *Ann Vasc Surg* 2003; 17: 229-233.

11 Sternbergh WC, Nordness PJ, York JW, et al. Endo-exuberance to endo-reality: trends in the management of 431 AAA repairs between 1996 and 2002. *J Endovasc Ther* 2003; 10: 418-423.

12 Wisselink W, Cuesta MA, Berends FJ, et al. Retroperitoneal endoscopic ligation of lumbar and inferior mesenteric arteries as a treatment of persistent endoleak after endoluminal aortic aneurysm repair. *J Vasc Surg* 2000; 31: 1240-1244.

13 Kolvenbach R, Pinter L, Raghunandan M, et al. Laparoscopic remodeling of abdominal aortic aneurysms after endovascular exclusion: a technical description. *J Vasc Surg* 2002; 36: 1267-1270.

14 Rollet G, Amabile P, Piquet P. Video-assisted mini-invasive retroperitoneal approach for treatment of infrarenal aortic disease. In: Becquemin JP, Loisance D, Watelet J (eds). *Controversies and update in vascular and cardiovascular surgery.* Torino, Edizioni Minerva Medica 2003: pp 283-289.

15 Carroll RM, Laravuso RB, Schauble JF. Left ventricular function during aortic surgery. *Arch Surg* 1976; 111: 740-743.

16 Lunn JK, Dannemiller FJ, Stanley TH. Cardiovascular responses to clamping of the aorta during epidural and general anesthesia. *Anesth Analg* 1979; 58: 372-376.

17 Dunn E, Prager RL, Fry W, Kirsh MM. The effect of abdominal aortic cross-clamping on myocardial function. *J Surg Res* 1977; 22: 463-468.

18 Fransen GAJ, Vallabhaneni SR, van Marrewijk CJ, et al. Rupture of infra-renal aortic aneurysm after endovascular repair: a series from EUROSTAR registry. *Eur J Vasc Endovasc Surg* 2003; 26: 487-493.

17

HYBRID TECHNIQUES AFTER ENDOVASCULAR ANEURYSM EXCLUSION

RALF KOLVENBACH

Endoleaks, endotension, and graft migration are the major problems of endovascular abdominal aortic aneurysm (AAA) exclusion (EVAR). There is an increasing number of patients with endotension and aneurysms that increase in diameter without any evidence of patent lumbar arteries or a patent inferior mesenteric artery (IMA) [1,2]. Endovascular coiling of patent lumbar arteries or of the IMA is cumbersome and often requires several treatment sessions by experienced radiologists.

Laparoscopically we can offer the following techniques to patients with endografts: clipping of the IMA and of lumbar arteries to treat type II endoleaks, thrombus removal [3], fixation of the endograft to the aortic neck, and banding of the aorta to prevent neck dilatation.

Yet, the major advantage is that we can go much further compared to an interventional procedure: laparoscopically the thrombus can be removed, which permits wrapping of the endograft like in a Creech procedure. Using special suturing techniques, the endoprosthesis can actively be attached to the aortic wall preventing graft migration. This can be combined with a banding procedure to enlarge the landing zone and to prevent neck dilatation.

Operative technique

The operative technique is basically identical to a total laparoscopic aortic aneurysm resection. We prefer a left retrocolic transabdominal approach originally described by Dion [4,5]. The patient is placed on the operating table, which is flexed in the middle, on a suction vacuum bag. When the table is tilted to the right, the patient is positioned almost 70 degrees on the right side (Fig. 1).

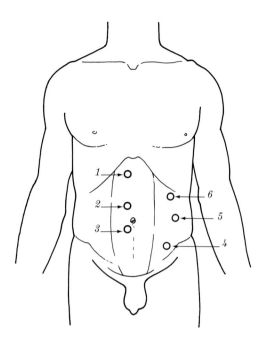

FIG. 1 Placement of trocars.
1 - 1.5 mm instrument port for graspers.
2 - 10 millimeter port for the laparoscopic scissors and for a retractor.
3 - Camera port.
4 - Camera port.
5 and 6 - Instrument ports.

The left hemicolon and the splenic flexure are mobilized medially (Figs. 2A,B). Laparoscopic dissection and suturing is performed with the surgeon standing on the right side of the patient. Laparoscopic retractors can be avoided because of traction sutures placed through the mesentery of the sigmoid colon and the right lateral decubital position of the patient. A similar stay suture is used to prevent the left kidney from taking a medial rotation. Laparoscopic exposure of the aorta is initiated at the level of the neck of the aneurysm. Only limited exposure of the aortic bifurcation is performed to reduce the incidence of nerve damage.

In obese patients access to the right groin, if necessary, can best be obtained by opening the valve of the suction vacuum bag, which permits the patient to fall back in a supine position.

A 5 millimeter suction-irrigation device is connected with a cell saving machine, and a large bore 10 millimeter suction device (*Storz, Tuttlingen, Germany*) is used to evacuate the thrombus material.

When an endograft has been in place for several months there is quite often a dense inflammatory retroperitoneal reaction. In very rare cases, these circumstances force the surgeon to choose a transperitoneal approach.

The origin of the IMA is identified and the artery is divided between clips (Fig. 3A). When clips are too small to safely occlude the IMA, a vascular stapler is used. This facilitates further mobilization of the aorta. The aneurysm and the aortic neck are identified. As many lumbar arteries as accessible are clipped on the left side of the aorta. Since access to the right-sided lumbar arteries is often very difficult because of the inflammatory changes, we now prefer a more direct approach stitching lumbar arteries from inside the aneurysm sac, like in open surgery.

Laparoscopic remodelling of the aorta after EVAR

The principal laparoscopic steps outlined above are performed without clamping the aorta since it would damage the endograft. Instead, under fluoroscopic guidance an aortic balloon occlusion catheter is introduced from the groin through a hemostatic sheath. This balloon is inflated before the sac of the aneurysm is incised to stabilize the graft inside the aorta. Dislodgement of the endograft when taking out the thrombus, is impossible if the balloon is inflated. This is accomplished by gradually monitoring the patient's blood pressure and after systemic heparinization of the patient.

The sac of the aneurysm is incised and opened with laparoscopic scissors in an H-shaped configuration. The graft is inspected using the magnification of the 30-degree endoscope to exclude any damage of the fabric or stents (Fig. 3B). Laparoscopic graspers and a 10 millimeter suction-irrigation device are used to remove the thrombus material [6]. Patent lumbar arteries are stitched with a vicryl suture blocked with a pledget at the end.

With a laparoscopic running suture (2-0 prolene) the sac of the aneurysm is closed, wrapping the aorta tightly around the endograft like in a Creech procedure. In addition to these measures we like to place an aortic band around the neck of the aneurysm to prevent neck dilatation. This requires careful circumferential dissection of the proximal aorta. Using a curved grasping instrument origi-

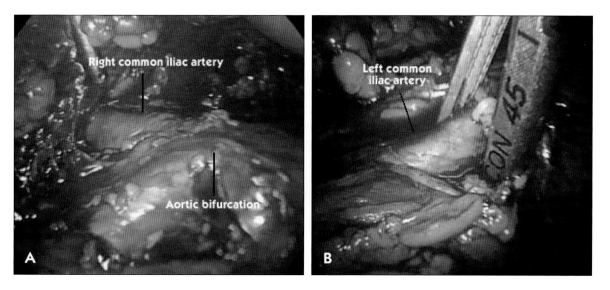

FIG. 2   A - Aortic bifurcation.   B - Stapling of the left common iliac artery after aorto-uni-iliac endograft exclusion.

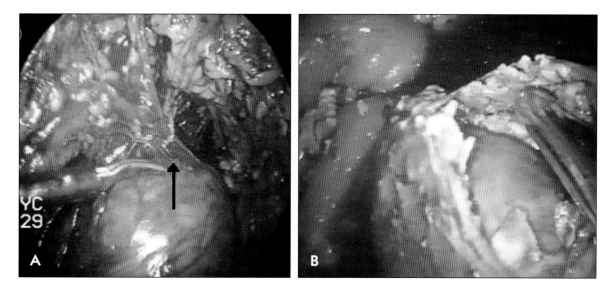

FIG. 3   A - Inferior mesenteric artery.   B - Endograft after incision of the sac of the aneurysm. There is no graft incorporation.

nally designed for laparoscopic fundoplication, a band of polytetrafluoroethylene is wrapped around the aortic neck. The band is put on tension and secured with several interrupted prolene sutures. When this can be accomplished successfully, there is probably no need for placing additional sutures to prevent migration. When sutures cannot be avoided, it is necessary to perform fluoroscopy first

to identify the bare springs and the part of the graft where the interrupted stitches go through the fabric of the endograft's body.

During the study period, in three patients the lumbar arteries were stitched with the help of a master-slave robot (Zeus®, *Computer Motion, Santa Barbara, CA, USA*) after incision of the sac of the aneurysm. Because of the five degrees of freedom of the robotic arms, stitching of the lumbar arteries was significantly easier as compared to with the laparoscopic needle holders. The surgical team was again standing on the right side of the patient (Figs. 4A, B).

A system engineer was present in the operating room during all robotic procedures, helping with the set-up.

Results

In a prospective feasibility study, the technique described was used in 12 patients. The mean age of all patients was 74.5 years. In 4 cases laparoscopy was performed after a mean period of 20.2 months ±4.7 following endovascular AAA exclusion for increase in diameter size. In three patients out of this small group, no type II endoleak could be detected pre-operatively (Table I). However, at surgery, we found between one and three patent lumbar arteries, which were clipped extraluminally after incision of the aneurysm sac. During the short mean follow-up period of 11 months after the laparoscopic procedure, we have not yet detected further increase in aneurysm diameter. In all cases, at surgery the grafts were found intact.

In all cases, there was a decrease of the diameter of the AAA after laparoscopic intraluminal thrombus removal.

There were no major complications and no graft dislodgement when incising the sac of the AAA. We did not have to cross-clamp the infrarenal aorta in either case.

Discussion

The smaller number of lumbar arteries clipped on the right side was due to the significant technical difficulties encountered when we tried to elevate the aorta to clip lumbar arteries on the right side of the aorta from underneath [7,8]. Thrombus is not an inert substance. Macrophages generating oxygen free radicals in the cannaliculi of the intraluminal thrombus can cause further degeneration of the aortic wall by enhancing tissue hypoxia [3]. Thrombus transmits pressure, which can further complicate a differentiation between type II endoleaks and endotension [9]. Theoretically, there is a fear that removal of thrombus can weaken the outer shell of the aneurysm. Yet we hope that partial wrapping of the endograft will accelerate incorporation of the graft and prevent device migration.

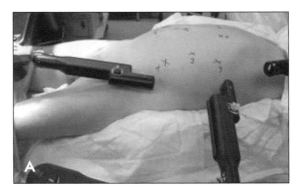

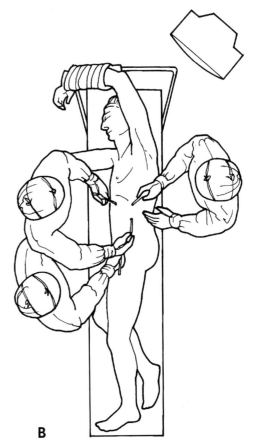

FIG. 4 A - Set-up of the robotic arms. B - Typical position of the surgeon and assistant on the right side of the operating table that we use in all aortic laparoscopic procedures. The laparoscopic camera is placed in the left upper abdomen.

Table	INTRA-OPERATIVE DATA AND LAPAROSCOPIC FINDINGS	
Pre-operative diameter of the aneurysm (cm)		6.30 ± 0.97
Postoperative diameter of the aneurysm (cm)		2.95 ± 0.43
Mean number of lumbar arteries detected during laparoscopy on either the left or the right side		1.66 ± 0.65 2.66 ± 0.77
Time required for laparoscopy (minutes)		91.75 ± 7.13
Postoperative hospital stay (days)		4.41 ± 1.37

The indication for treating type II endoleaks is still under debate [8,9]. The intra-operative injection of contrast dye into the sac of the aneurysm after graft deployment ("saccogram") as well as a delayed contrast computed tomography or modern pressure sensor technology could be part of an algorithm defining a suitable candidate for laparoscopic postinterventional exploration. This could also prevent an overtreatment in many cases. Based on the above information, it appears a logical step to try to attach the stent graft directly to the aortic wall using laparoscopic techniques [2]. Improved techniques using radiopaque suture material combined with intravascular ultrasound will probably permit a more exact placement of a fixation device.

There will be an increasing role for these hybrid techniques in the near future. Hybrid procedures can be used to facilitate total laparoscopic aneurysm surgery.

Total laparoscopic aneurysm resection can be offered to patients who are suitable for conventional surgery as a minimally invasive alternative to endovascular aneurysm exclusion. Through a combination of laparoscopic and endovascular techniques, the procedure can be standardized and offered to the majority of patients. A new surgical technique can only be successful when all essential steps are simple and reproducible in a large number of patients.

Hybrid techniques in total laparoscopic aneurysm resection consist of the following steps: occlusion of both common iliac arteries with an occluder device. Subsequently, the aorta is clamped and the sac of the AAA is opened. The proximal anastomosis is performed totally laparoscopically with two running sutures. The right limb of the bifurcated graft is anastomosed to the right external iliac artery using a three centimeter access above the inguinal ligament. The right limb is anastomosed after laparoscopic exposure with the right iliac bifurcation, again through an extraperitoneal mini-incision. Finally, the thrombus is removed and, if necessary, lumbar arteries are clipped. Using this hybrid technique, cross-clamp time can be reduced to less than 60 minutes in most of our cases. This technique can also be used in patients with severe calcifications of the iliac arteries where clamping or stapling can be quite a challenge or even impossible. Completion angiography shows direct perfusion of the hypogastric arteries in these cases.

This feasibility study showed that we currently have the operative technique we need to improve long-term performance of endografts or to salvage failing grafts, reducing the need for conversion to open surgery [10-15].

17

169

R E F E R E N C E S

1 White GH, Yu W, May J, et al. Endoleak as a complication of endoluminal grafting of abdominal aortic aneurysms: classification, incidence, diagnosis and management. *J Endovasc Surg* 1997; 4: 152-168.

2 Cao P, Verzini F, Zannetti S, et al. Device migration after endoluminal abdominal aortic aneurysm repair: analysis of 113 cases with a minimum follow-up period of 2 years. *J Vasc Surg* 2002; 35: 229-235.

3 Adolph R, Vorp DA, Steed DL, et al. Cellular content and permeability of intraluminal thrombus in abdominal aortic aneurysm. *J Vasc Surg* 1997; 25: 916-926.

4 Dion YM, Gracia CR. A new technique for laparoscopic aorto-bifemoral grafting in occlusive aortoiliac disease. *J Vasc Surg* 1997; 26: 685-692.

5 Dion YM, Gracia CR, Ben El Kadi HH. Totally laparoscopic abdominal aortic aneurysm repair. *J Vasc Surg* 2001; 33: 181-185.

6 Kolvenbach R, Ceshire N, Pinter L, Da Silva L. Laparoscopy-assisted aneurysm resection as a minimal invasive alternative in patients unsuitable for endovascular surgery. *J Vasc Surg* 2001; 34: 216-221.

7 Edoga JK, Asgarian K, Singh D, James KV. Laparoscopic surgery for abdominal aortic aneurysm. Technical elements of the procedure and a preliminary report of the first 22 patients. *Surg Endosc* 1998; 12: 1064-1072.

8 Baum R, Carpenter J, Golden MA, et al. Treatment of type II endoleaks after endovascular repair of abdominal aortic aneurysms: comparison of transarterial and translumbar techniques. *J Vasc Surg* 2002; 35: 23-29.

9 Veith F, Baum RA, Ohki T, et al. Nature and significance of endoleaks and endotension: summary of opinions expressed at an international conference. *J Vasc Surg* 2002; 35: 1029-1035.

10 Wisselink W, Cuesta MA, Berends FJ, et al. Retroperitoneal endoscopic ligation of lumbar and inferior mesenteric arteries as a treatment of persistent endoleak after endoluminal aortic aneurysm repair. *J Vasc Surg* 2000; 31: 1240-1244.

11 Kolvenbach R, Schwierz E. Combined endovascular/laparoscopic approach to aortic pseudoaneurysm repair. *J Endovasc Surg* 1998; 5: 191-193.

12 Kolvenbach R, Da Silva L, Deling O, Schwierz E. Video-assisted aortic surgery. *J Am Coll Surg* 2000; 190: 451-457.

13 Kolvenbach R, Deling O, Schwierz E, Landers B. Reducing the operative trauma in aortoiliac reconstructions. A prospective study to evaluate the role of video-assisted vascular surgery. *Eur J Vasc Endovasc Surg* 1998; 15: 483-488.

14 Da Silva L, Kolvenbach R, Pinter L. The feasibility of hand-assisted laparoscopic bypass using a low transverse incision. *Surg Endosc* 2002; 16: 173-176.

15 Kolvenbach R, Schwierz E. Totally laparoscopic aneurysm resection as a routine procedure. *J Vasc Surg* 2004 (in press).

18

EMBOLIZATION OR REVASCULARIZATION OF HYPOGASTRIC ARTERIES DURING ENDOVASCULAR AORTIC ANEURYSM REPAIR

FABIO VERZINI, GIANBATTISTA PARLANI
AGOSTINO MASELLI, PIERGIORGIO CAO

Iliac artery anatomy represents a central factor in endoluminal treatment of aorto-iliac aneurysms. Since as many as 20% of aneurysms involve the common iliac artery, it may be necessary to exclude the hypogastric artery (HA) with the aorto-iliac endograft to achieve a hemostatic seal. HA occlusion may not be innocuous, especially in the case of bilateral interruption or ipsilateral collateral flow deficit. Serious adverse events such as infarction of the colon, buttock necrosis, and spinal cord ischemia as well as buttock claudication and sexual impotence have been reported after HA interruption during open aneurysm repair, and can obviously also occur after endovascular repair. Review of published series suggests that unilateral HA interruption is a relatively safe procedure, however, the issue of bilateral occlusion remains controversial. Recently, HA re-implantation into the external iliac artery has been introduced as a valuable adjunctive procedure to reduce the incidence of ischemic complications. This option should be considered in all cases requiring bilateral HA occlusion during endovascular abdominal aortic aneurysm (AAA) treatment in patients at high risk for open repair.

Importance of HA

Endoluminal AAA repair is becoming a valid alternative to open surgical repair. However, because of anatomical limitations, not all patients are suitable for endografting, because of either unfavorable proximal aortic neck anatomy or iliac contra-indications. Approximately 20% of patients have an extension of the aneurysmal disease into the distal common iliac and/or internal iliac arteries, as shown by a prospective evaluation of computed tomography (CT) studies in patients with AAA [1]. In these cases the endovascular option is still possible but only with HA ostial coverage.

Although studies in gynecology [2], urology [3], and trauma [4] suggest that HA occlusion is generally well tolerated, complications have been reported, particularly after bilateral interruption or in conjunction with aorto-iliac surgery [5-9]. Endovascular aortic repair may be particularly prone to ischemic complications due to the concomitant routine occlusion of the inferior mesenteric artery.

HA interruption has been reported to be associated with significant morbidity including severe lower extremity neurological deficits, ischemic colitis, buttock necrosis, impotence, and gluteal claudication. Moreover, HA circulation can represent a critical point in developing a reflux into the aneurysmal sac after endografting (type II endoleak), eventually leading to aneurysmal sac expansion and, rarely, AAA rupture.

To avoid complications secondary to HA exclusion, two different options should be considered when planning endovascular AAA repair: HA exclusion with eventual embolization to prevent refilling, or HA surgical revascularization (Fig. 1). A third option, already under clinical investigation, will hopefully be available in the near future when industry will provide branched endografts to revascularize both external and internal iliacs with the bifurcated endograft segment.

Anatomical considerations

The HA and its branches are characterized by a network of anastomotic connections with arteries both cephalad and caudal to the pelvis. The visceral branches receive collateral flow primarily from the inferior mesenteric artery via its superior rectal branch. HA parietal branches anastomose with lumbar and midsacral arteries proximally and the circumflex branches of the external iliac, common, and profunda femoral arteries distally. This lumbar-hypogastric-circumflex arterial axis acts as a crucial substitutive pathway in patients with chronic occlusive disease of the iliac arteries. It not only perfuses the pelvis but also relays blood flow to the lower extremity forming what some authors have metaphorically called "a real arterial turntable" [10]. Although the HA collateral system has the potential for enlargement under conditions of chronic ischemia, it may have limited functional reserve in the acute setting.

It is well known that one open HA can provide sufficient collateral flow to the pelvis and prevent ischemic complications if the contralateral artery is

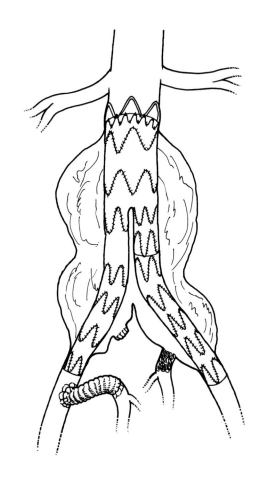

FIG. 1 Fig. 1. Schematic drawing of an AAA extending bilaterally to the common iliac bifurcations. An aorto-bi-iliac endograft with right external-HA bypass and left HA embolization in the main trunk of the artery are displayed.

ligated or oversewn during aorto-iliac reconstructions. Moreover, it has been demonstrated that ipsilateral external iliac and femoral arteries provide a more significant collateral flow than the contralateral HA, and therefore it is of great importance to preserve iliac and femoral circumflex arteries when isolating the common femoral artery for device introduction.

Embolization technique

HA embolization can be performed before or at the same stage of aortic endografting. It is usually advisable to embolize the HA in a staged fashion in cases of scheduled pre-operative angiograms and when bilateral occlusions must be performed. This approach can reduce operation time and total amount of contrast medium administered during aortic endografting, and can enhance development of collateral circulation, hence reducing the ischemic risks. The second procedure, usually performed after at least one week, permits the evaluation of the effectiveness of primary HA embolization, the development of collateral pathways, and the need for adjunctive procedures.

In our experience the HA is usually selectively cannulated with a 5F curved catheter, similar to a *cobra* or a *vertebral* catheter usually from a contralateral approach. In case of a simultaneous procedure, the catheter is left in place during aortic endograft deployment. Coils are positioned at the end of the procedure when the endograft has been fully deployed and the inflow in the native artery stopped, to reduce the risk of distal migration of the coils. To save the collateral flow it is important to coil the main trunk of the HA as close as possible to the ostium; in the case of large HA aneurysm, the coil embolization should be performed in the ostia of the collateral vessels distal to the aneurysm (Fig. 2).

Stainless steel Gianturco® coils with adherent fibers of polyester material *(William Cook, Bjaeverskov, Denmark)* or platinum coils *(Balt, Montmorency, France)* with a spire diameter ranging from 5 to 12 millimeters and from 5 to 10 centimeters in length, are usually preferred for embolization. The number of coils needed depends on HA anatomy. In the case of a non-aneurysmal artery, an average of three coils are usually sufficient to achieve thrombosis of the vessel.

Revascularization technique

HA revascularization is usually accomplished at the same stage of the endovascular procedure using a retroperitoneal approach with an 8 centimeter oblique incision in the lower-lateral abdominal quadrant. After division of the external oblique fascia and splitting the muscles, careful isolation of the common iliac bifurcation and the proximal HA together with both the anterior and posterior branches is performed. When a large common iliac aneurysm is involved, this maneuver can be rather difficult because of the posterior origin of the HA and its relative stiffness.

When needed, the retroperitoneal incision can be used to manipulate the external and common iliac arteries facilitating endograft advancement inside a calcified arterial wall. Moreover, in severely stenotic vessels not amenable to angioplasty, a conduit can be sutured to the common iliac bifurcation and used for endograft access. In this particular case a

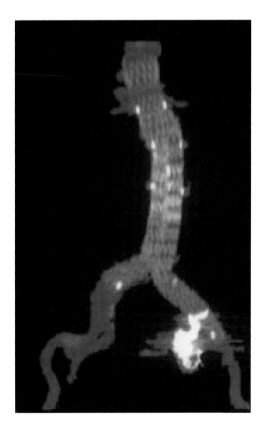

FIG. 2 Postoperative CT reconsturction after aortic endografting with left HA embolization.

branched conduit can be pre-prepared, with a side branch ready to be anastomosed to the HA. Once the artery has been prepared, revascularization is usually postponed after deployment of the aortic endograft in order to ensure that there is a valid inflow segment on the external iliac artery, distal to the endograft landing zone. After clamping and dividing the HA, the proximal stump of the artery is generally oversewn with a running suture, or with a calcified artery, with the aid of pledgets and buttress sutures. The distal portion of the HA is anastomosed end-to-end to a 7 or 8 millimeter dacron graft whereafter the graft is sutured to the external iliac artery in an end-to-side fashion (Fig. 3).

With redundant arteries, direct HA re-implantation on the external iliac artery can be done with an end-to-side anastomosis. Alternatively, a different technique described by Parodi and Ferreira can be applied: the redundant external iliac artery can be divided, the proximal end sutured end-to-end to the HA, and the distal stump anastomosed end-to-side to the proximal external iliac artery [11]. Those different techniques are described in Figure 4.

In cases of difficult anatomies, as with obese patients, and when the scheduled endografting procedure is expected to be time consuming, staged HA re-implantation before AAA repair should be considered.

Review of the literature

Several reports have suggested that acute HA interruption during open AAA repair can result in a number of complications such as buttock necrosis, spinal cord ischemia, and ischemic colitis, with an associated mortality rate greater than 70% [12,13]. More recent studies have been published in which one or both HAs have been sacrificed to facilitate endovascular AAA repair (Table I). A relatively lower incidence of serious adverse events has been reported in these series (Table II).

Buttock claudication occurs most often after HA interruption and AAA endografting, and can be disabling. In the study by Karch et al., of the 22 patients with HA occlusion, 7 (32%) complained of hip and buttock claudication, 2 of them after bilateral occlusion. By 6 months, 4 of these 7 patients still complained of buttock pain but were able to continue walking and did not complain of a limited lifestyle [16]. Bilateral occlusion seems to result in regression of symptoms in a similar manner to unilateral occlusion. In the series of Mehta et al. the incidence of intermittent claudication reduced from 36% at one month to 12% at one year in patients with unilateral HA occlusion; in patients with bilateral interruption, claudication was reported in 40% of the cases at one month and 11% at one year [22]. Coil embolizations can increase the incidence of buttock claudication if deployed in the distal HA. In a study by Cynamon et al. 12 of 22 patients (55%) with coil embolization in the HA bifurcation experienced claudication whereas only 1 of 10 (10%) claudicated after coil placement in the proximal HA [23].

Buttock necrosis is very seldom reported. Non-healing sacral decubitus in a debilitated patient and scrotal skin sloughing have been described and can be considered major pelvic ischemic complications as well [14].

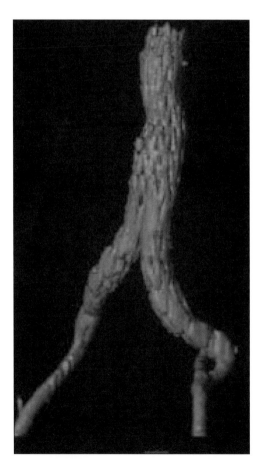

FIG. 3 Postoperative CT reconstruction after aortic endografting showing bilateral HA ostial coverage and revascularization of left HA (external-internal iliac bypass).

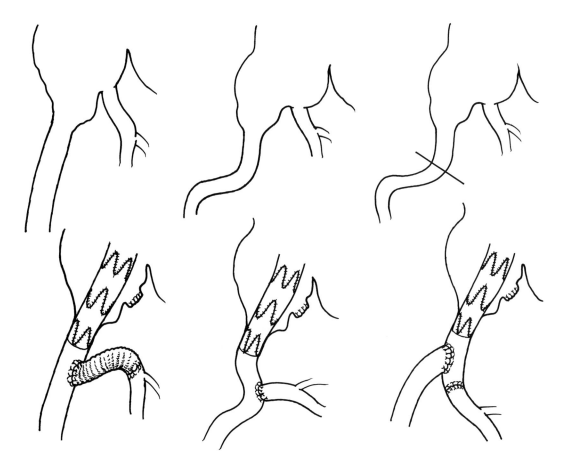

FIG. 4 Schematic representation of internal iliac artery surgical reconstruction during endovascular AAA-repair.

18
175

Colon ischemia is one of the most feared complications of HA interruption. Interestingly, in the series of Karch et al. the incidence of symptomatic colon ischemia was 5% (1/20) for unilateral HA interruption and 100% (2/2) for bilateral occlusion. Various degrees of ischemia have been reported, most being a mild degree of mucosal ischemia [16].

Sexual dysfunction was reported in a high percentage of patients after HA occlusion in a study by Lin et al. In unilateral occlusion, the incidence was 43% (3/7) and 50% (2/4) after bilateral interruption. Only one patient reported moderate improvement of erectile capacity with time [14]. Such a high incidence of impotence was not reported in most other series, but the true incidence of the disease may be underestimated because of difficulties in data retrieval with retrospective evaluations, the relatively small sample size of the studies published to date, or difficulties in sexual function evaluation in the elderly population.

Neurologic deficit occurs very rarely. To our knowledge, only one series focusing on endovascular aortic repair with HA sacrifice reported two minor symptoms (one drop foot, one minor bilateral lower extremity weakness) [22]. A single case of delayed (after 48 hours) lower extremity paraparesis secondary to HA unintentional occlusion due to atheroembolism has been reported, which fortunately improved after treatment [24].

All these complications can hopefully be avoided with HA revascularization especially when bilateral HA ostial coverage is needed. Faries et al. have published a promising series of 11 revascularizations in 10 patients. After the procedure no gluteal claudication, erectile dysfunction, colon and perineal ischemia, and mortality occurred, and all of the

Table I	INCIDENCE OF HA INTERRUPTION AND EMBOLIZATION IN PATIENTS WITH ENDOLUMINAL TREATMENT FOR AAA						
1st author [ref.]	*Year*	*Total patients*	*Patients with HA occlusion (%)*		*Bilateral HA occlusion*	*HA coil embolization*
Lin et al. [14]	2002	NA	12		4	12
Wolpert et al. [15]	2001	65	18	(28)	7	18
Karch et al. [16]	2000	96	22	(23)	2	15
Criado et al. [17]	2000	156	39	(25)	11	39
Lee et al. [18]	2001	157	23	(15)	NA	NA
Schoder et al. [19]	2001	147	55	(37)	10	55
Razavi et al. [20]	2000	71	32	(45)	5	32
Lee et al. [21]	2000	94	28	(30)	3	13
Mehta et al. [22]	2001	NA	107		8	103
Personal experience		530	77	(15)	9	14

AAA: abdominal aortic aneurysm
NA: not available

Table II	INCIDENCE OF ISCHEMIC COMPLICATIONS AFTER HA INTERRUPTION IN PATIENTS WITH ENDOLUMINAL TREATMENT FOR AAA					
1st author [ref.]	*Year*	*Buttock claudication %*	*Colon ischemia %*	*Sexual dysfunction %*	*Buttock necrosis %*	*Neurological deficit %*
Lin et al. [14]	2002	50	0	45	17	-
Wolpert et al. [15]	2001	50	0	7	NA	NA
Karch et al. [16]	2000	32	12.5	NA	0	0
Criado et al. [17]	2000	13	0	3	0	0
Lee et al. [18]	2001	39	NA	NA	0	0
Schoder et al. [19]	2001	45	0	25	NA	0
Razavi et al. [20]	2000	28	0	12	0	0
Lee et al. [21]	2000	18	0	8	8	NA
Mehta et al. [22]	2001	16	2	6	0	2
Personal experience		23	0	10	0	0

AAA: abdominal aortic aneurysm
NA: not available

revascularizations remained patent at a mean follow-up of 10 months [25].

Personal experience

Between April 1997 and October 2003, 530 consecutive patients underwent endovascular repair for AAA at *Struttura Complessa di Chirurgia Vascolare, Policlinico Monteluce, Perugia, Italy*. Pre-operative, operative, and follow-up data of patients were entered in a prospective database. A total of 77 patients (14.5%) underwent HA occlusion: 46 (8.7%) intentionally and 31 (5.8%) unintentionally. In 9 patients (1.7%) both HA had been occluded; unilateral HA revascularization was carried out in 7 patients, with external iliac-internal iliac bypass in 6 patients, and internal iliac re-implantation in one patient. In 2 patients with bilateral HA occlusion, no revascularization was performed: one patient was scheduled for elective colonic resection for cancer the following day, and the other patient presented with heavily calcified common and internal iliac arteries at surgical exploration; none experienced colon infarction in the postoperative course.

HA embolization was performed in 14 cases, all of them at the time of the main procedure: in 6 cases from ipsilateral femoral approach and in the remaining 8 cases from a contralateral approach; in 3 cases the embolization procedure was unsuccessful because cannulation of the hypogastric ostium did not succeed. Direct HA interruption was performed in 5 cases: in 2 cases after a failed attempt at embolization, and in 3 cases after the advancement of the endograft with retroperitoneal approach. In 18 cases HA embolization was not performed either because the graft itself occluded the ostium or because the pre-operative angiogram showed poor hypogastric outflow (Figs. 5,6).

Operative and fluoroscopic times to complete the endografting procedure in HA occlusion were significantly increased compared to patients without HA interruption (160 minutes vs. 124 minutes, p = 0.0001, and 29 minutes vs. 21 minutes, p = 0.0001, respectively); 175 ml mean contrast medium was used in patients with HA occlusion vs. 147 ml in patients with patent HA (p: n.s.). Postoperative hospital stay was longer (5.3 vs. 3.1 days, p = 0.003). There was no peri-operative mortality, colon infarction, or neurological deficit in patients undergoing HA interruption or revascularization. Buttock claudication was the complaint of 23% of the patients with HA interruption (18 patients), which tended to improve but not to disappear over time. New onset of sexual dysfunction after the procedure was recorded in 10% of the males. Only one patient experienced mild colon mucosal ischemia, which

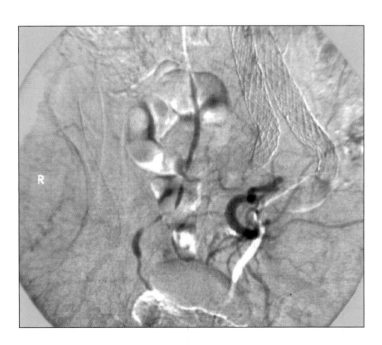

FIG. 5 Completion angiography after aortic endografting showing exclusion of left HA without embolization (early phase).

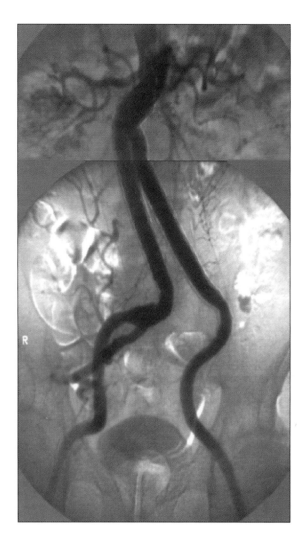

FIG. 6 Completion angiography in the same patient showing refilling in left HA from collateral pathways without aneurysmal sac endoleak (late phase).

was successfully treated with bowel rest and wide-spectrum antibiotic therapy.

Late results at mean follow-up of 26 months showed a mean decrease in AAA diameter of 5 millimeters, similar to patients without HA interruption, and an incidence of type II endoleak of 7.7%; only one endoleak (1.3%) originated from the embolized HA. Three patients (3.9%) experienced an increase of 5 millimeters or more in AAA diameter during follow-up; one was treated with a proximal extension cuff for graft migration, while the second patient was treated with aneurysmal sac embolization for type II endoleak. Both events were not related to HA occlusion. The last patient died from cardiac failure while waiting for further evaluation of AAA enlargement in absence of visible endoleak.

Conclusion

Unilateral HA interruption during endovascular repair of AAA is a relatively safe procedure, particularly with preservation of the collateral flow from the external iliacs, the contralateral internal iliac, and femoral arteries. In bilateral HA involvement, we strongly advocate the preservation of at least one HA in patients with suitable anatomy. HA revascularization represents an useful and effective adjunctive procedure to expand endovascular indications especially in patients at high surgical risk for open repair.

REFERENCES

1 Armon MP, Wenham PW, Whitaker SC, et al. Common iliac artery aneurysms in patients with abdominal aortic aneurysms. *Eur J Vasc Endovasc Surg* 1998; 15: 255-257.

2 Clark SL, Phelan JP, Yeh SY, et al. Hypogastric artery ligation for obstetric hemorrhage. *Obstet Gynecol* 1985; 66: 353-356.

3 Bao ZM. Ligation of the internal iliac arteries in 110 cases as a hemostatic procedure during suprapubic prostatectomy. *J Urology* 1980; 124: 578.

4 Agolini SF, Shah K, Jaffe J, et al. Arterial embolization is a rapid and effective technique for controlling pelvic fracture hemorrhage. *J Trauma* 1997; 43: 395-399.

5 Andriole GL, Sugarbaker PH. Perineal and bladder necrosis following bilateral internal iliac ligation. Report of a case. *Dis Colon Rectum* 1985; 28: 183-184.

6 Senapati A, Browse NL. Gluteal necrosis and paraplegia following postoperative bilateral internal iliac artery occlusion. *J Cardiovasc Surg* 1990; 31: 194-196.

7 Gloviczki P, Cross SA, Stanson AW, et al. Ischemic injury to the spinal cord or lumbosacral plexus after aorto-iliac reconstruction. *Am J Surg* 1991; 162: 131-136.

8 Cikrit DF, O'Donnell DM, Dalsing MC, et al. Clinical implications of combined hypogastric and profunda femoral artery occlusion. *Am J Surg* 1991; 162: 137-141.

9 Paty PK, Shah DM, Chang BB, et al. Pelvic ischemia following aortoiliac reconstruction. *Ann Vasc Surg* 1994; 8: 204-206.

10 Hassen-Khodja R, Batt M, Michetti C, Le Bas P. Radiologic anatomy of the anastomotic systems of the internal iliac artery. *Surg Radiol Anat* 1987; 9: 135-140.

11 Parodi JC, Ferreira M. Relocation of the iliac artery bifurcation to facilitate endoluminal treatment of abdominal aortic aneurysms. *J Endovasc Surg* 1999; 6: 342-347.

12 Picone AL, Green RM, Ricotta JR, et al. Spinal cord ischemia following operation on the abdominal aorta. *J Vasc Surg* 1986; 3: 94-103.

13 Iliopoulos JI, Howanitz PE, Pierce GE, et al. The critical hypogastric circulation. *Am J Surg* 1987; 154: 671-675.

14 Lin PH, Bush RL, Chaikof EL, et al. A prospective evaluation of hypogastric artery embolization in endovascular aortoiliac aneurysm repair. *J Vasc Surg* 2002; 36: 500-506.

15 Wolpert LM, Dittrich KP, Hallisey MJ, et al. Hypogastric artery embolization in endovascular abdominal aortic aneurysm repair. *J Vasc Surg* 2001; 33: 1193-1198.

16 Karch LA, Hodgson KJ, Mattos MA, et al. Adverse consequences of internal iliac artery occlusion during endovascular repair of abdominal aortic aneurysms. *J Vasc Surg* 2000; 32: 676-683.

17 Criado FJ, Wilson EP, Velazquez OC, et al. Safety of coil embolization of the internal iliac artery in endovascular grafting of abdominal aortic aneurysm. *J Vasc Surg* 2000; 32: 684-688.

18 Lee WA, O,Dorisio J, Wolf YG, et al. Outcome after unilateral hypogastric artery occlusion during endovascular aneurysm repair. *J Vasc Surg* 2001; 33: 921-926.

19 Schoder M, Zaunbauer L, Holzenbein T, et al. Internal iliac artery embolization before endovascular repair of abdominal aortic aneurysms. *AJR Am J Roentgenol* 2001; 177: 599-605.

20 Razavi MK, DeGroot M, Olcott C 3rd, et al. Internal iliac artery embolization in the stent-graft treatment of aortoiliac aneurysms: analysis of outcomes and complications *J Vasc Interv Radiol* 2000; 11: 561-566.

21 Lee CW, Kaufman JA, Fan CM, et al. Clinical outcome of internal iliac artery occlusions during endovascular treatment of aortoiliac aneurysmal diseases. *J Vasc Interv Radiol* 2000; 11: 567-571.

22 Mehta M, Veith FJ, Ohki T, et al. Unilateral and bilateral hypogastric artery interruption during aortoiliac aneurysm repair in 154 patients: a relatively innocuous procedure. *J Vasc Surg* 2001; 33: S27-32.

23 Cynamon J, Lerer D, Veith FJ, et al. Hypogastric artery coil embolization prior to endoluminal repair of aneurysms and fistulas: buttock claudication, a recognized but possibly preventable complication. *J Vasc Interv Radiol* 2000; 11: 573-577.

24 Bhama JK, Lin PH, Voloyiannis T, et al. Delayed neurologic deficit after endovascular abdominal aortic aneurysm repair. *J Vasc Surg* 2003; 37: 690-692.

25 Faries PL, Morrissey N, Burks JA, et al. Internal iliac artery revascularization as an adjunct to endovascular repair of aortoiliac aneurysms. *J Vasc Surg* 2001; 34: 892-899.

18

179

19

COMBINED AORTO-ILIAC ANGIOPLASTY AND INFRA-INGUINAL REVASCULARIZATION

EUGENIO ROSSET, MATHIEU POIRIER, BRUNO AUBLET-CUVELLIER,
SYLVAIN BEURTHERET, NICOLAS VALERIO, SAMY POUGET
MATHIEU HERMIER, ISSIFOU MOUMOUNI, ALAIN BRANCHEREAU

The combination of obliterating atherosclerotic lesions at the aorto-iliac and infra-inguinal levels illustrates the presence of a generalized and progressive atheromatous disease. Its treatment poses tactical surgical problems [1]. The rise of endoluminal surgical techniques, of which the results in the treatment of occlusive aorto-iliac lesions are most convincing, offers a less aggressive alternative to a two-stage bypass procedure to treat such lesions. At present, the vascular surgeon is familiar with endovascular surgical procedures, which are practiced routinely in a well-equipped operating room. This has led us to perform more and more combined procedures, comprising iliac transluminal angioplasty together with an ipsilateral infra-inguinal surgical revascularization in patients with two-level lesions.

Description of the problem

The presence of a tandem lesion that is considered significant frequently confronts the surgeon with a therapeutic dilemma, which is never solved completely. Which of these lesions is the most significant? This does not mean the one that is anatomically the most severe, but rather the one that has the most important hemodynamic consequences. Should one or both lesions be corrected? If so, should the treatment be performed simultaneously or in two sessions? And finally, in which order should these two revascularizations be realized if this option is chosen?

Severe ischemia pleads for a two-level revascularization. Particularly when trophic disturbances are present, a considerable increase in arterial blood pressure is required at the ankle if one aims at wound healing within a reasonable period of time. In case of intermittent claudication, revascularization at a single level always leads to an improvement, but some residual claudication may remain. Hemodynamic evaluation of the lesions by means of duplex ultrasound may be predictive of the results, as it may guide the choice of which lesion to treat. The reliability of this method, however, has not been clearly shown.

Hence, one should be more inclined to perform a two-level revascularization when the claudication is severe, when both lesions appear hemodynamically significant, and when the functional demand is high. Two-level lesions also imply tactical surgical problems. Performing a distal revascularization while ignoring a proximal lesion may cause early or midterm postoperative failure. The classic approach, consisting of a proximal reconstruction while ignoring the distal lesion, has two drawbacks. First, this may be insufficiently effective, as described before. Second, because of a high outflow resistance, the reconstruction may deteriorate rapidly and eventually lead to thrombosis.

The standard surgical technique at the aorto-iliac level is an aortofemoral or bifemoral bypass. This technique has long proven its efficacy and excellent patency results. In contrast, it represents a certain surgical trauma, with a peri-operative mortality of 3.3%, as shown by a recent questionnaire among 483 hospitals in the USA [3]. The trauma related to this type of surgery, augmented by a possible infra-inguinal revascularization, should not be regarded as negligible. The possibility of performing an endovascular technique to repair an aorto-iliac lesion is an attractive solution for all these problems. The advantages are obvious. Endovascular treatment avoids the aggressive character of proximal surgery and, because of its simplicity, may easily be combined with an infra-inguinal reconstruction during the same session. However, some questions remain concerning the mortality and morbidity of these combined procedures, their hemodynamic efficacy, and their results in the long term.

The aim of this chapter is to present the technical problems of these two techniques, whether or not simultaneous, as well as the results from our group.

Technical aspects

The patient is positioned on a radiolucent table, which allows for both transluminal angioplasty and arteriographic check of the surgical revascularization. The patients are treated in the operating room on the radiolucent table. The use of a contrast injector that is permanently available when needed is rarely necessary. The radiological images are obtained by means of a mobile device, which enables numbered subtraction images and road mapping. The operating field should include all regions involved in the endovascular and surgical procedure, which allows for surgical conversion in case of failure of the proximal endoluminal procedure.

In the majority of cases the infra-inguinal procedure is performed in the first tempo, followed by a subsequent proximal percutaneous transluminal angioplasty (PTA). This order makes it possible to perform a per-operative angiogram of the distal revascularization. Another advantage is that the common femoral artery does not have to be clamped distal to the iliac artery that has just undergone a PTA and is therefore prone to thrombosis. Post-PTA clamping must be avoided if the angioplasty was performed in an occlusive lesion of the external iliac artery. In case of PTA of the common iliac artery, the flow through the hypogastric artery, if patent, may avoid the risk of thrombosis due to a proper blood flow through the angioplastied area. Inversely, a PTA of an iliac artery should not delay the distal surgical revascularization. It is therefore preferable to place the introducer in a perfused artery. The puncture should be done proximal or distal to the anastomosis or at the level of the femoral anastomosis (Fig. 1). The prerequisite is to choose an area as smooth as possible in order to avoid hemostatic problems, or thrombo-embolic complications due to the occurrence of a post-puncture dissection. In case the arteries are very calcified, we prefer to perform the puncture in a freshly desobstructed arterial segment, or rather in a freshly implanted patch or bypass. Despite the obvious fragility of a freshly desobstructed artery, hemostasis at the puncture site can easily be obtained by means of a superficial suture with a 6 x 0 monofil. Up until now we have not seen any late complication due to this puncture. A technical maneuver is to place the introducer via the arterial suture before finishing it completely. The final sutures are put in place and the two ends are not

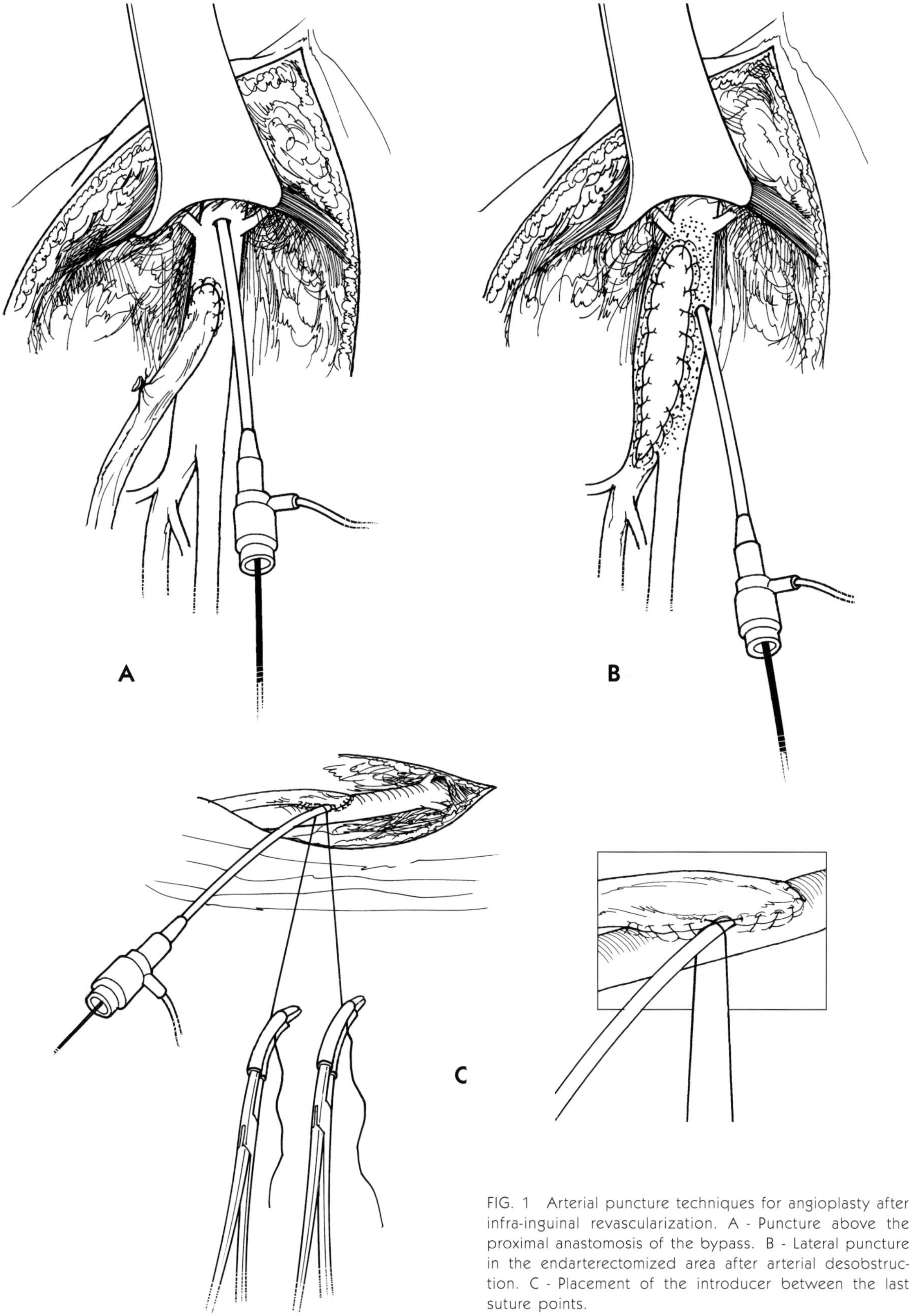

FIG. 1 Arterial puncture techniques for angioplasty after infra-inguinal revascularization. A - Puncture above the proximal anastomosis of the bypass. B - Lateral puncture in the endarterectomized area after arterial desobstruction. C - Placement of the introducer between the last suture points.

tied, but are kept under tension through traction by a clamp. Once the introducer is placed, the arteries are declamped and hemostasis is obtained by "crossing" the sutures over the introducer. This maneuver allows easy retraction of the introducer with direct hemostasis due to the ligation of the two suture ends.

If there is doubt about the success of the PTA, it is preferable to perform the surgical revascularization afterward. In this case we perform the arterial puncture in a smooth area, usually the anticipated site for the bypass anastomosis or arterial desobstruction. After removal of the guidewire and introducer the arteries are clamped and the arteriotomy is performed starting from the opening of the puncture. The intervention is then performed according to the standard procedure.

Study material

We report a retrospective series of 92 consecutive patients, operated from January 1997 to September 2003 in two centers for vascular surgery *(Gabriel Montpied Hospital, Clermont-Ferrand,* and the *Timone Hospital, Marseille)*. All these patients presented with lesions at two levels: the proximal lesion was located at the aorto-iliac level and the distal one infra-inguinally. They were all treated with a combination of an endovascular technique for the proximal lesion and a surgical procedure for the infra-inguinal lesion. Our study reports on 96 interventions (57 on the left, and 39 on the right side), four patients of whom underwent bilateral treatment in two sessions using this technique. They comprised 14 females (15%) and 78 males (85%). Their mean age was 68 years, ranging from 44 to 88 years. Their comorbidity was illustrative of the severity and spread of the atheromatous disease in these patients (Table I). Six patients were treated for acute ischemia (6% of the cases); 11 patients presented with pain at rest (11.5%); 33 with trophic disturbances (34.5%); and 46 with intermittent claudication (48%): 15 patients had a walking distance below 100 meters and 31 patients above 100 meters.

Table II details the proximal lesions treated during these procedures. We have treated 113 lesions in 96 limbs, comprising 17 cases with two-level iliac lesions. This table also shows the associated contralateral and internal iliac lesions. Only significant lesions are mentioned, i.e., a stenosis equal to or above 70% or arterial occlusion. At the infra-in-

guinal level, 46 patients had lesions mainly at the femoral triangle, whereas the other 50 patients showed extended occlusive lesions of the superficial femoral or femoropopliteal arteries.

Table III shows the endovascular techniques used to restore the 113 iliac lesions. During the 96 endovascular procedures 56 stents were placed. In 9 cases the hypogastric artery was occluded. In 5 cases two stents were needed. The surgical revascularizations associated with the endovascular procedures were limited to the femoral arteries in 46 cases: in 35 of these it concerned a reconstruction of the femoral bifurcation using prosthetic material for a bypass or patch, and in 11 cases an endarterectomy of the femoral bifurcation with direct closure or using a venous patch. In the remaining 50 cases a bypass was performed, comprising 20 above-knee femoropopliteal bypass grafts (8 saphenous veins and 12 prostheses), 18 below-knee femoropopliteal bypass grafts (11 saphenous veins, 3 composite grafts and 4 prostheses), and 12 femorocrural bypass grafts (11 saphenous veins, 1 composite) (Table IV).

Additional procedures were performed in 12 cases: one iliac thrombectomy to treat a recent iliac thrombosis before angioplasty and placement of a stent; one endoprosthesis placed to exclude an aneurysm of the common iliac artery; one profound femorofemoral dacron prosthesis together with a below-knee femoropopliteal bypass; 7 PTAs of the superficial femoral artery distal to a revascularization of the femoral bifurcation; one venous bypass from the popliteal to the posterior tibial ar-

Table I	RISK FACTORS		
Risk		*Patients N = 92*	*%*
Hypertension		59	64
Diabetes		27	29
Dyslipidemia		33	36
Smoking		69	75
Renal insufficiency		11	12
Respiratory insufficiency		11	12
Cardiac failure		8	9
Coronary artery bypass graft		13	14
Medically treated coronary disease		27	29

tery distal to a prosthetic above-knee femoropopliteal bypass; and one crural artery dilatation distal to

a prosthetic above-knee femoropopliteal bypass. The contralateral lesions were treated simultaneously in 8 cases: 4 PTAs of the common iliac artery using the kissing-balloon technique; 3 PTAs of the external iliac artery; and one surgical revascularization of the femoral bifurcation. All patients were evaluated in November 2003. The survival, patency, and limb salvage rates were calculated using the Kaplan-Meier method. Comparisons were made using the chi-square test.

Results

EARLY RESULTS

Mean hospitalization duration was 14±10 days, ranging from 2 to 60 days. Three patients died in the first 30 postoperative days or before leaving the hospital, which yields a mortality rate of 3.3%. One patient died 45 days postoperatively due to multiorgan failure. This concerned a 71-year-old patient

Table II	DISTRIBUTION OF ILIAC LESIONS		
Site		Limbs N = 96	%
Occlusion of common iliac artery		2	2
Stenosis of common iliac artery		56	58
Occlusion of external iliac artery		2	2
Stenosis of external iliac artery		53	55
Associated lesions			
Ipsilateral hypogastric artery occlusion		12	13
Contralateral aorto-iliac lesion		54	56

Table III	PROXIMAL ENDOVASCULAR REVASCULARIZATIONS				
Site			Angioplasty	Primary stent	Angioplasty and stent on demand
Occlusion of common iliac artery	2		0	1	1
Stenosis of common iliac artery	56		26	8	22
Occlusion of external iliac artery	2		0	0	2
Stenosis of external iliac artery	53		31	4	18
Total	**113 ***		**57**	**13**	**43**

* 17 limbs required two endovascular revascularizations for two-level iliac lesions

Table IV	INFRA-INGUINAL SURGICAL RECONSTRUCTIONS			
Materials		Autogenous	Composite	Prosthetic or allograft
Revascularization of femoral bifurcation		11	0	35
Above-knee femoropopliteal bypass		8	0	12
Below-knee femoropopliteal bypass		11	3	4
Femorocrural bypass		11	1	0

with hypertension and diabetes, who smoked and suffered from respiratory, renal, and cardiac insufficiency and presented with trophic disturbances, treated with a PTA of the common iliac artery and a femorocrural bypass using an inversed saphenous vein. One patient died 22 days postoperatively due to acute ischemia of the contralateral leg. This concerned an 81-year-old woman with diabetes and renal insufficiency, who presented with trophic disturbances of the foot, and was treated with a stent in the common iliac artery and a femorocrural bypass using an inversed saphenous vein. The third death was two days after surgery due to a myocardial infarction in an 86-year-old hypertensive patient who had undergone an amputation of the contralateral limb and presented with trophic disturbances, and was treated with a PTA of the common iliac artery and a femorocrural bypass using an inversed saphenous vein. The primary postoperative patency of endovascular revascularizations was 95.8%. Four early events were observed: one rupture of the right common iliac artery, several hours after an angioplasty using a kissing balloon, with revascularization of the femoral bifurcation below, which was treated with an emergency aortobifemoral bypass procedure. There was one occlusion three days postoperatively of an external iliac lesion, treated with angioplasty and stent combined with a femorocrural bypass, which was treated by means of an emergency femorofemoral crossover bypass. On the fifth postoperative day, a lesion of the common iliac artery, treated with angioplasty and stent, occluded. The additional femorocrural bypass that the patient had received was occluded three days postoperatively and remained occluded despite a redo bypass procedure. The extensive occlusion of the two revascularizations was resolved with an amputation. An early restenosis of the external iliac artery with revascularization of the femoral bifurcation below was treated with a new angioplasty with two stents on the fourth day after the operation.

The primary postoperative patency of surgical infra-inguinal revascularizations was 92.7%. Seven early events were observed: one thrombosis of the femoral revascularization leading to a major amputation; two thromboses of above-knee prosthetic femoropopliteal bypasses, treated by below-knee extension of the bypass using saphenous vein in one case and by major amputation in the other; one thrombosis of the below-knee femoropopliteal saphenous venous bypass, treated with a redo procedure and inversion of the saphenous vein; one thrombosis of the composite femorocrural bypass treated with thrombectomy; two thromboses of a venous femoropopliteal bypass, of which one required a major amputation. In total, four major amputations were performed in the first postoperative month. The limb salvage rate was 95.8%. Five patients presented general complications (8.7%). These comprised one cerebrovascular event, one acute pulmonary edema, one unstable angina, one phlebitis, and one deregulated diabetes in a patient who had become insulin dependent. Fourteen patients (15.2%) suffered from surgical complications. We observed 6 delayed wound closures, of which one needed a re-intervention; 3 hematomas, of which 2 required surgical correction; 2 lymph fistulae; 2 infections, of which one needed surgical intervention; and one arteriovenous fistula in an in-situ saphenous venous bypass, requiring early embolization using coils. In total, 10 patients (9%) underwent an early re-intervention, 6 times for a redo arterial reconstruction and 4 times for local complications not related to the arterial reconstruction.

LATE RESULTS

The mean survival time was 31 months, ranging from one to 82 months. One patient was lost to follow-up after one month and was excluded while "living and patent" at the time of the last follow-up moment. During follow-up 19 patients died (20.6%). The mortality causes were cardiac in 6 cases and vascular in the other 6 cases; 7 patients died from various reasons. The survival rate was 88±3.4% after 1 year and 66.5±7.3% after 5 years (Fig. 2). The overall primary patency, comprising the two revascularizations, was 72±5% after 1 year and 62.2±6.6% after 5 years (Fig. 3). The overall secondary patency was 75.8±4.7% after 1 year and 74.4±4.9% after 5 years (Fig. 4). The primary and secondary patencies of the endovascular techniques and the infra-inguinal revascularizations are shown separately in Figures 5 and 6. During follow-up, 13 major amputations were performed: the limb salvage rate was 88±3.6% at 1 year and 86.6±3.8% at 5 years (Fig. 7). The overall primary patency after 5 years in case of additional above-knee surgery was higher than of below-knee surgery: 66.2±8.2% versus 54±10% (Fig. 8).

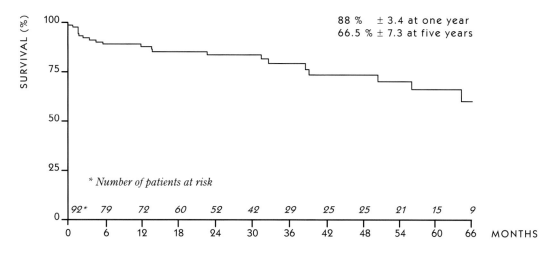

FIG. 2   Survival curve of our patients after combined endovascular and surgical treatment.

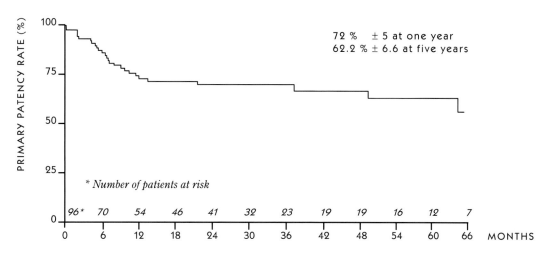

FIG. 3   Overall primary patency rate (both reconstructions patent).

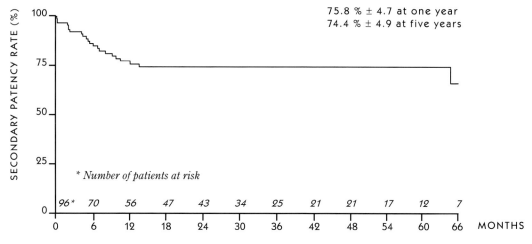

FIG. 4   Overall secondary patency rate (both reconstructions patent).

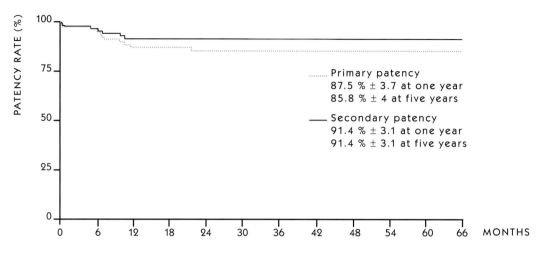

FIG. 5   Primary and secondary patency rates of aorto-iliac angioplasties.

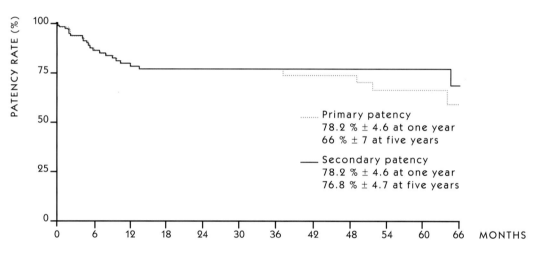

FIG. 6   Primary and secondary patency rates of infra-inguinal reconstructions.

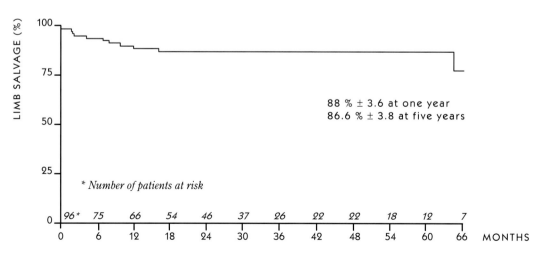

FIG. 7   Limb salvage rate during follow-up in our experience.

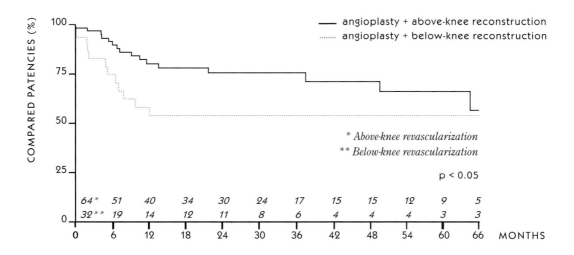

FIG. 8 Overall primary patency (both reconstructions) as compared with angioplasties combined with above-knee and below-knee surgical reconstructions.

Discussion

Many authors have demonstrated the feasibility of treating arterial insufficiency of the lower limbs by means of a combination of surgical and endovascular procedures in a single vascular surgical operation session [4,5]. Thanks to the availability of adequate radiological material and radiolucent operating tables, combined vascular and endovascular surgery has now been realized as a routine procedure by virtually all centers for vascular surgery [6].

The mortality in our experience was 3.3%. This might seem rather high when compared with the mortality of elective aortobifemoral surgery for occlusive lesions. The latter mortality was found to be 3.3% in a 1997 questionnaire comprising 3073 patients [3], and ranged from 0.85% to 5.3% in a study on retrospective series performed since the end of the 1950s up to 2001 (see Table II in reference 7) [7]. The results are difficult to compare for various reasons: half of the patients in the study we present here were treated for critical ischemia, whereas in all series reporting the results of aortic surgery, critical ischemia never comprised more than 20% of the total. For the same reasons it is likely that the severity of the atherosclerotic disease and the number of associated risk factors are higher in our population. Finally, it concerned a two-level revascularization in all cases, which is rarely the case in the series published on aortobifemoral bypass procedures.

The mean hospitalization duration was 14 days, which is an acceptable delay in patients, half of whom presented with critical ischemia when admitted to the hospital. The overall secondary patency was 74.4±4.9% after 5 years. These results are comparable to those observed in the literature, which show a mortality rate ranging between 0% and 4.5% and an overall 5-year primary patency rate above 65%, with a 5-year limb salvage rate close to 90% in most of the series (Tables V, VI). The 5-year secondary patency of the endovascular procedure was 91.4±3.1%, which is comparable to the patency rate after single endovascular reconstruction of the iliac tracts. Some authors have advocated the systematic use of a stent in angioplasty procedures [14]. In our experience we save the indication for a stent for iliac recanalizations (Fig. 9), or in case of a residual stenosis or persistent arterial dissection after prolonged repeated inflation [16]. Timaran et al. have ascribed the improvement of the long-term patency of iliac angioplasties to the improvement of the outflow, obtained by the accompanying infra-inguinal revascularization [15]. However, no series in the literature on these hybrid procedures evaluates the results using the intention-to-treat principle. They all use only those procedures with an initially technically successful angioplasty for the calculations of the patency rate, which flatters the published results [4]. Thus, in our experience, a patient with a secondary iliac rupture eventually benefited from a two-level

Table V MORTALITY OF COMBINED PROXIMAL ENDOVASCULAR AND INFRA-INGUINAL SURGICAL PROCEDURES

1st author [ref.]	*Year of publication*	*Number of patients*	*Number of procedures*	*Number of simultaneous procedures*		*Clinique stage %*			*Mortality %*
				Number	*%*	*II*	*III*	*IV*	
Brewster [4]	1989	75	79	3	4	22	42	36	0
Peterkin [5]	1990	46	46	16	35	11	52	37	0
Wilson [8]	1990	18	18	0	0	30	70	0	0
Van der Vliet [9]	1992	17	17	17	100	100	0	0	0
Bull [10]	1993	46	46	46	100	NA	NA	NA	4.3
Siskin [11]	1999	87	93	0	0	36	22	42	4.5
Sinci [12]	2000	41	41	0	0	NA	NA	NA	0
Faries [13]	2001	126	126	0	0	0	22	78	1
Nelson [14]	2002	34	34	34	100	41	29	30	0
Timaran [15]	2003	31	31	25	80	59	12	29	3.2
Personal experience	2004	92	96	96	100	48	17	35	3.3

NA: not available

Table VI OVERALL PATENCY AND LIMB SALVAGE AFTER COMBINED PROXIMAL ENDOVASCULAR AND INFRA-INGUINAL SURGICAL PROCEDURES

1st author [ref.]	*Year of publication*	*Overall patency*				*Limb salvage rate*	
		Primary		*Secondary*		*%*	*Follow-up year*
		%	*Follow-up - year*	*%*	*Follow-up - year*		
Brewster [4]	1989	76	5	88	5	90	5
Peterkin [5]	1990	72	5	91	5	93	5
Wilson [8]	1990	76	2	NA	NA	NA	NA
Van der Vliet [9]	1992	67	5	NA	NA	NA	NA
Bull [10]	1993	61	5	76	5	93	5
Siskin [11]	1999	63	4	71	4	94	4
Sinci [12]	2000	78	4	NA	NA	NA	NA
Faries [13]	2001	71	3	71	3	85	3
Nelson [14]	2002	84	1	97	1	91	2
Timaran [15]	2003	NA	NA	NA	NA	88	5
Personal experience	2004	72	5	74	5	87	5

NA: not available

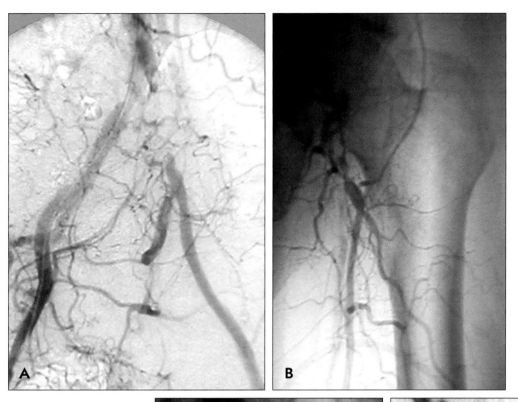

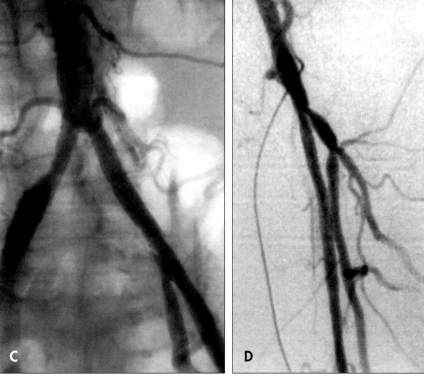

FIG. 9 Examples of severe stenoses at two levels causing critical ischemia and ulceration. A - Angiography showing left common iliac artery occlusion. B - Angiography showing a severe stenosis at the femoral bifurcation. Note that the superficial femoral artery is patent but poorly depicted. C - Completion angiography after recanalization of the common iliac artery with primary stenting. D -Completion angiography following endarterectomy and patch angioplasty of the femoral bifurcation.

surgical procedure and was obviously excluded from the patency calculations.

The secondary patency of surgical revascularizations was 76.8±4.7%. It is difficult to compare these results with surgery only, because of the diversity of the procedures performed. However, in our experience we never observed a postoperative occlusion that could have been caused by the angioplasty performed during the same session. In patients presenting with critical ischemia or disabling intermittent claudication, the necessity of a two-level reconstruction is generally accepted [1,17,18]. This approach is corroborated when at two levels significant lesions are present, which explains their substantial clinical effect (Fig. 10). In contrast, when the functional symptoms are less severe, the question remains regarding the choice of which lesion to treat; classically, the most proximal lesion is treated first [1,17]. This approach is even more preferable when significant proximal lesions exist. The choice may be more difficult when a moderate iliac stenosis exists together with an extensive infra-inguinal lesion that is not compensated by collaterals (Fig. 11). In this case, a single proximal reconstruction may lead to an insufficient functional or even totally ineffective result. Likewise, a single bypass performed distal to a stenosis, albeit moderate, may fail shortly after or, in most cases, later, when the untreated proximal lesion progresses.

An aortobifemoral bypass procedure is the treatment of choice for proximal lesions [19]. Nevertheless, in case of an additional infra-inguinal surgical procedure, the cumulative mortality/morbidity of the two surgical reconstructions may be considerable [11]. A PTA may offer a suitable alternative, because of its speed, lower mortality/morbidity, and acceptable long-term results in particular [2].

Some authors prefer to perform a sequential treatment, in which the iliac angioplasty is performed a few days before the surgical revascularization [4,11,13]. In this case the angioplasty may be performed in the radiology department with more sophisticated equipment, which enables better imaging and, according to these groups, a greater choice of endovascular materials. The interval between the two procedures allows for evaluation of the endovascular procedure and, in case of a dissatisfying result,

modification of the anticipated surgical strategy. On the other hand, an ipsilateral femoral puncture on the desired access side shortly after may increase the infection risk, particularly when the use of prosthetic material is planned. Furthermore, performing two separate procedures implies that the patient has to undergo two operations and prolongs the duration of hospitalization.

In contrast, the advantages of a combined treatment in one session are many: apart from a reduction in hospitalization duration, it is more comfortable for the patient to avoid two successive interventions. The puncture of an already surgically exposed artery avoids the risks of a percutaneous puncture: catheterization of the arterial lumen is easier and the hemostasis of the puncture site is simple. The occurrence of a hematoma, a false aneurysm, or a dissection at the puncture site is avoided. The angioplasty procedure can be performed easily and quickly while the imaging quality in the operating room is largely sufficient to adequately perform angioplasties of the aorto-iliac segment. The presence of an introducer at the level of the common femoral artery in turn allows performing an iliac angioplasty and checking simultaneously the PTA as well as the infra-inguinal surgical reconstruction. Hence, we generally prefer to perform the infra-inguinal revascularization in the same session. Once the revascularization is done, the arterial puncture is performed and an introducer inserted. The puncture is preferably made in an area where the artery is smooth, while avoiding as much as possible puncturing close to a suture or in a recently implanted prosthetic graft (Fig. 1).

Conclusion

Hybrid procedures, combining a proximal angioplasty with an infra-inguinal surgical procedure, nowadays represent the most adequate solution to treat two-level arterial lesions. The mortality varies between 0% and 4.5%, which is mainly related to the medical condition of the patients, half of whom are operated for critical ischemia. The patency, limb salvage rate, and strength of the results appear to be excellent.

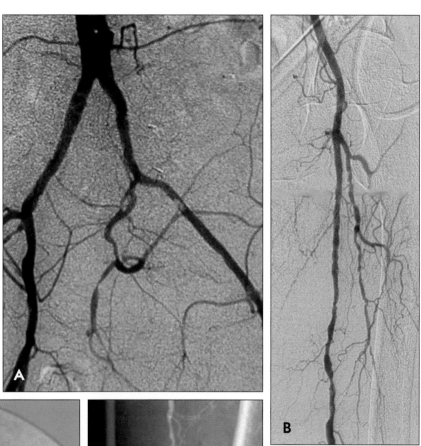

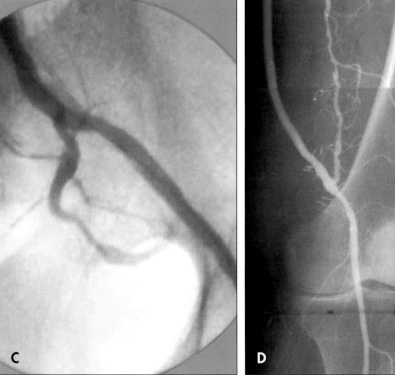

FIG. 10 Examples of tight lesions at two levels causing severe intermittent claudication. Treatment of only one lesion, either the iliac or superficial femoral artery stenosis, will probably not relief the disabling claudication. A - Angiography showing severe external iliac artery stenosis. B - Multiple lesions in the superficial femoral artery. Note the stenoses in the profound femoral artery. Treatment of the iliac lesion alone will probably not resolve the symptoms. C - Completion angiography after balloon dilatation of the iliac artery. D - Completion angiography of the venous femoropopliteal bypass.

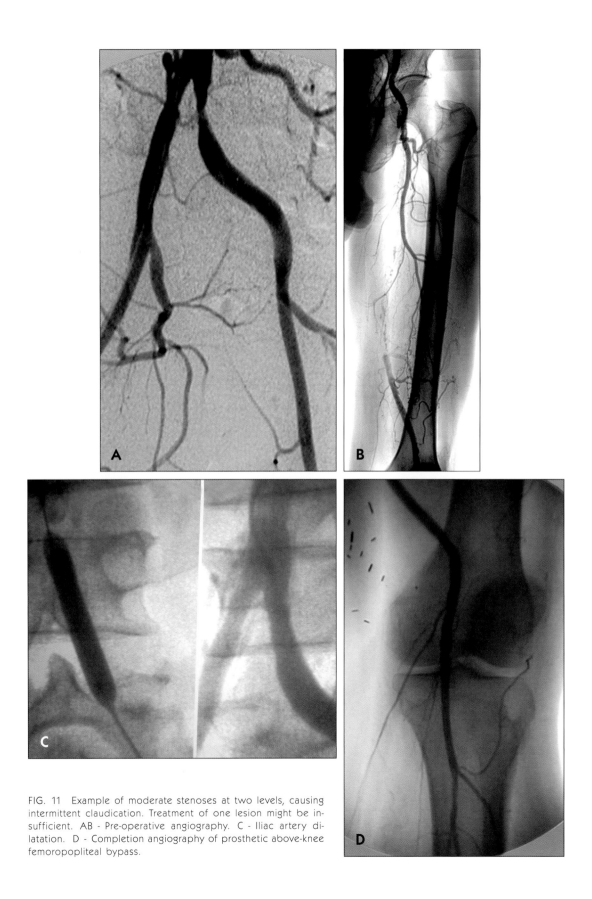

FIG. 11 Example of moderate stenoses at two levels, causing intermittent claudication. Treatment of one lesion might be insufficient. AB - Pre-operative angiography. C - Iliac artery dilatation. D - Completion angiography of prosthetic above-knee femoropopliteal bypass.

REFERENCES

1 Branchereau A, Rosset E, Di Mauro P. Restauration combinée aorto-iliaque et fémorale superficielle. In Branchereau A, Jausseran JM, eds. *Traitement des lésions obstructives de l'artère fémorale superficielle.* Marseille, CVN, 1992, pp 157-170.

2 Johnston KW, Rae M, Hogg-Johnston SA, et al. Five-year results of a prospective study of percutaneous transluminal angioplasty. *Ann Surg* 1987; 206: 403-413.

3 Dimick JB, Cowan JA, Henke PK, et al. Hospital volume. Related differences in aorto-bifemoral bypass operative mortality in the United States. *J Vasc Surg* 2003; 37: 970-975.

4 Brewster DC, Cambria RP, Darling RC, et al. Long-term results of combined iliac balloon angioplasty and distal surgical revascularization. *Ann Surg* 1989; 210: 324-330.

5 Peterkin GA, Belkin M, Cantelmo NL, et al. Combined transluminal angioplasty and infrainguinal reconstruction in multilevel atherosclerotic disease. *Am J Surg* 1990; 160: 277-279.

6 Ricco JB, Camiade C, Mangiacotti N, et al. Angioplastie transluminale associée à une revascularisation chirurgicale dans l'ischémie des membres inférieurs. In Branchereau A, Jacobs M, (eds). *Ischémie critique des membres inférieurs.* Armonk, Futura, 1999, pp 129-144.

7 Branchereau A, Jullian H, Ayari R, Ede B. Complications post-opératoires précoces après chirurgie restauratrice de l'aorte sous-rénale. In: Branchereau A, Jacobs M (eds). *Complications de la chirurgie vasculaire et endovasculaire, 2e partie.* Armonk, Futura publishing Company 2002, pp 33-51.

8 Wilson SE, White GH, Wolf G, et al. Proximal percutaneous balloon angioplasty and distal bypass for multilevel arterial occlusion. *Ann Vasc Surg* 1990; 4: 351-355.

9 Van der Vliet JA, Mulling FJ, Heijstraten FMJ, et al. Femoropopliteal arterial reconstruction with intraoperative iliac transluminal angioplasty for disabling claudication: results of a combined approach. *Eur J Vasc Surg* 1992; 6: 607-609.

10 Bull PG, Schlegl A, Mendel H. Combined iliac transluminal angioplasty and femoropopliteal reconstruction for multilevel arterial occlusive disease. *Int Surg* 1993; 78: 332-337.

11 Siskin G, Darling RC 3rd, Stainken, et al. Combined use of iliac artery angioplasty and infrainguinal revascularization for treatment of multilevel atherosclerotic disease. *Ann Vasc Surg* 1999; 13: 45-51.

12 Sinci V, Kalaycioglu S, Halit V, et al. Long-term effects of combined iliac dilatation and distal arterial surgery. *Int Surg* 2000; 85: 13-17.

13 Faries PL, Brophy D, LoGerfo FW, et al. Combined iliac angioplasty and infrainguinal revascularization surgery are effective in diabetic patients with multilevel arterial disease. *Ann Vasc Surg* 2001; 15: 67-72.

14 Nelson PR, Powell RJ, Schermerhorn ML, et al. Early results of external iliac artery stenting combined with common femoral artery endarterectomy. *J Vasc Surg* 2002; 35: 1107-1113.

15 Timaran CH, Ohki T, Gargiulo NJ, et al. Iliac artery stenting in patients with poor distal runoff: influence of concomitant infrainguinal arterial reconstruction. *J Vasc Surg* 2003; 38: 479-485.

16 Rosset E, Malikov S, Magnan PE, et al. Endovascular treatment of occlusive lesions of the distal aorta: mid-term results in a series of 31 consecutive patients. *Ann Vasc Surg* 2001; 15: 140-147.

17 Brewster DC, Perler BA, Robinson JG, Darling RC. Aortofemoral graft for multilevel occlusive disease: predictors of success and need for distal bypass. *Arch Surg* 1982; 117: 1593-1600.

18 Sumner DS, Strandness DE. Aortoiliac reconstruction in patients with combined iliac and superficial femoral arterial occlusion. *Surgery* 1978; 34: 348-355.

19 Nevelsteen A, Lacroix H, Suy R. Résultats des pontages pour pathologie occlusive aorto-iliaque. In Branchereau A, Jacobs M, eds. *Résultats à long terme des reconstructions artérielles.* Armonk, Futura, 1997, pp 95-112.

19

20

RADIOLOGICAL GUIDED ENDARTERECTOMY WITH STENTING FOR FEMOROPOPLITEAL RECONSTRUCTION

LUUK SMEETS, GWAN HO, FRANS MOLL

In 1946 Dos Santos performed the first endarterectomy, which was originally intended to be a thrombectomy. The patient was a 66-year-old male with an ischemic left limb caused by an iliofemoral endarteritis obliterans. The common femoral artery (CFA) was opened with a longitudinal incision, and an ophthalmic spatula and a U-shaped twisted stiletto were blindly advanced into the iliac artery freeing the thrombus and restoring a strong jet of blood. With a second incision at the level of the adductor ring, the same procedure was performed toward the groin and the periphery, thus opening the superficial femoral artery (SFA). After the arteriotomies were sutured, good pulsations were present everywhere. Although the procedure was a success, the patient died after two days as a result of pre-existing renal failure. Histopathological examination revealed that not only the thrombus but also the whole intima and part of the media had been removed. Four months later Dos Santos performed the procedure through three arteriotomies in the subclavian, axillary, and brachial artery in a 35-year-old female with upper right limb ischemia. Twenty-nine years later the artery was still patent [1,2]. This disobliteration was to be called thrombo-endarterectomy and was, technically speaking, a semi-closed technique. Strikingly he reported these findings as "the fall of the myth of the necessity of an intact intima." In 1954, DeBakey introduced the use of a ring stripper, consisting of a metal ring placed at a 90-degree angle at the end of a metal shaft. From then, modifications were established in the design of the ring loop and shaft. Cannon and Barker positioned the ring with sharp edges at a 105-degree angle [3]. In order to minimize the risk of perforation, Barker preferred that the ring had blunt edges. Eventually Vollmar made his modifications in 1967, changing the angle to 135 degrees instead of 90 degrees and using a smooth elliptic ring instead of a circular one (Fig. 1) [4]. Many other methods of developing a cleavage plane between intima and media have been used, such as gas endarterectomy and saline endarterectomy [5,6]. The shape of the ring stripper was also replaced by a spiral dissector [7]. All proved to be inferior to the ring stripper. Thus, semi-closed endarterectomy was applied for iliac and femoral artery occlusive disease for many years but was largely superseded by prosthetic and venous bypass surgery in the 1970s.

Reappraisal of endarterectomy

Based on several reports, semi-closed endarterectomy with a ring stripper was reappraised in the last decade because 5-year patency rates up to 71% were similar to above-knee femoropopliteal (AKFP) bypass graft surgery [8-17] (Table). In the mid 1990s, digital subtraction angiography and fluoroscopy

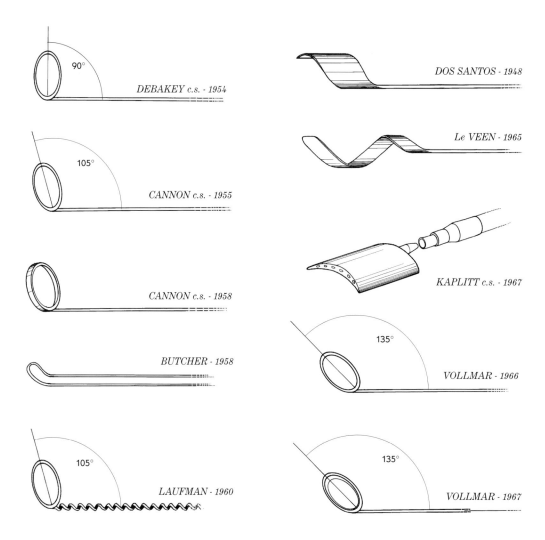

FIG. 1 Evolution of ring strip loops for semiclosed endarterectomy.

Table	PATENCY RATES OF ENDARTERECTOMY, REMOTE ENDARTERECTOMY, AND ABOVE-KNEE FEMOROPOPLITEAL BYPASS				
1st author [ref.]	*Year of publication*	*Technique*	*Three-year follow-up %*	*Five-year follow-up %*
Mukherjee, Inahara [8]	1989	EA	80	70
Vercellio et al. [9]	1986	EA	NA	64
Ouriel et al. [10]	1986	EA	66	NA
Van der Heijden et al [11]	1993	EA	78	71
Rosenthal et al. [12]	2001	REA	61	-
Smeets et al. [13]	2003	REA	64	48
AbuRahma et al. [14]	1999	ASV	-	76
		PTFE	-	68
Green et al. [15]	2000	PTFE	-	45
Johnson, Lee [16]	2000	ASV	-	74
		PTFE	-	39
Klinkert et al. [17]	2003	ASV	-	76
		PTFE	-	52

ASV: autologous saphenous vein bypass
EA: endarterectomy
PTFE: polytetrafluoroethylene bypass
REA: remote endarterectomy
NA: not available

in the operating room for endovascular aneurysm repair were introduced. These radiological techniques in combination with conventional surgical skills led to the development of radiological guided endarterectomy with the use of a new device. This device was a ring strip cutter, and the procedure was called remote endarterectomy (REA) [18]. Remote SFA endarterectomy (RSFAE) and remote iliac artery endarterectomy have been performed and described since by various institutions.

This ring strip cutter (MollRing Cutter®, *Vascular Architects Inc., San Jose, CA, USA)* is additional to and substantially equivalent to the Vollmar ring stripper, except for its remote cutting mechanism. The two rings, with sharpened inner cutting edges, mimic a pair of scissors when the two shafts telescope into each other (Fig. 2). With this device it is possible to perform an endarterectomy through a single, groin incision. The intimal core is transected at a specific endpoint remote from the site of entry.

This, in advantage to the semi-closed endarterectomy, makes a second incision to expose the popliteal artery at the endpoint of the endarterectomized segment unnecessary.

Techniques

CLASSIC SEMI-CLOSED ENDARTERECTOMY

By a vertical groin incision, the CFA, the profunda femoral artery, and the proximal part of the SFA are exposed. A second medial incision is made at the level of the distal part of the SFA or proximal part of the popliteal artery, to expose the endpoint of the endarterectomy. After intravenous administration of a 5000 IU bolus of heparin, the origin of the SFA is encircled with silastic vessel loops instead of clamping. Clamping the artery could make it difficult to obtain an appropriate cleavage plane. A longitudinal arteriotomy (three

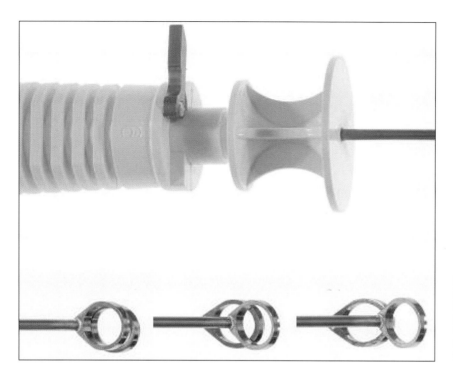

FIG. 2 The ring strip cutter device: two rings with sharpened inner cutting edges mimic a pair of scissors. The remote trigger unlocks the lower ring which is then activated backwards.

centimeters) of the occluded or stenosed SFA permits a meticulous dissection of the intimal core in the right cleavage plane between the lamina elastica interna and the circular fibers of the media or, preferably, between media and the smooth lamina elastica externa of the adventitia (Fig. 3). After transsection of the intimal core in the exposed SFA area, most surgeons prefer blunt dissection of the first two to three centimeters within the closed artery before bringing up a suitably sized ring stripper (Vollmar Dissector®, *Aesculap, South San Francisco, CA, USA*). Ring diameters range from 5 to 10 millimeters. The loop of the ring stripper is advanced distally into the artery with gentle rotating and thrusting movements by one hand while stabilizing the intimal core with the other (Fig. 4). In the event that the ring stripper cannot be passed, different sized strippers can be tried and fluoroscopy can be of great assistance. In some events, a third arteriotomy is necessary. The intimal core is dissected up to the level of the second incision, and an arteriotomy is performed. After transsection of the dissected intimal core, it is removed retrograde together with the ring stripper. The distal transsected intima must be anchored with 6-0 tacking sutures to ensure a smooth distal transition zone to normal intima. After flushing with a solution consisting of

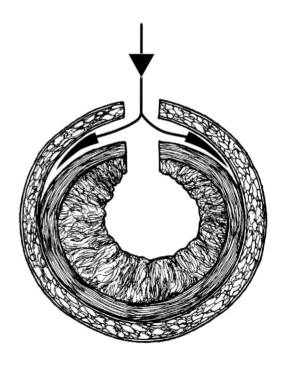

FIG. 3 Cleavage plane for endarterectomy.

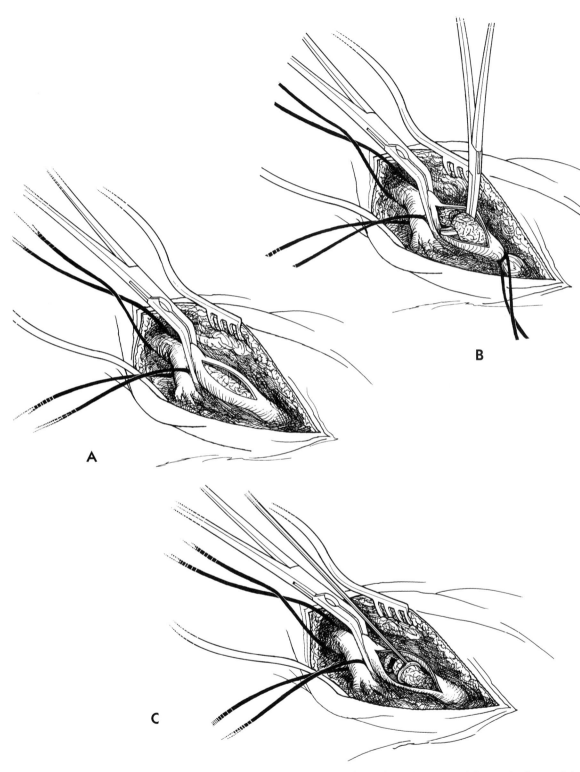

FIG. 4   A - By a vertcal groin incision, the common femoral artery, the profunda femoral artery, and the proximal part of the superficial femoral artery (SFA) are exposed. B - The intimal core is dissected from the SFA arterial wall with the cleavage plane between the lamina elastica interna and the circular fibers of the media or, preferably, between media and the smooth lamina elastica externa of the adventitia. C - A conventional ring stripper is passed over the intimal core and advanced down the SFA beyond the occluded segment.

5000 IU heparin and 1 mg papavarine in 100 cc saline, a completion angiogram is made. Often, re-opened collateral arteries are seen. Additional debris may be removed using a Fogarty graft thrombectomy catheter *(Baxter Health Corporation, Irvine, CA, USA)*. The proximal arteriotomy can be extended to perform an open endarterectomy of the CFA and profunda femoral artery, and both arteriotomies can be closed primarily or with a patch. Patients are prescribed thrombocyte-aggregation inhibitors.

REMOTE ENDARTERECTOMY

The first part of the procedure is the same as described above. Next, the ring stripper is exchanged for a suitable MollRing Cutter, which is passed down along the same cleavage plane until the same level is reached, and under fluoroscopic guidance the intimal core is remotely transsected and removed (Fig. 5). After fluoroscopic examination of the re-opened artery and the distal runoff vessels, the Moll-Ring Cutter can be re-introduced if an additional part of the intimal core must be removed. Also, loose parts can be removed by catching them between the two half closed rings of the device (Fig. 2). To prevent any further distal dissection after restoring blood flow, a short stent (Palmaz®, P204, *Cordis Endovascular, Warren, NJ, USA;* Easy Wallstent®, *Schneider Inc, USA;* diameters 5 to 8 millimeters) is inserted over a guide wire (Terumo®, *Tokyo, Japan;*

Schneider®, *Zurich, Switzerland*) to tack down the distal intimal flap, covering both the endarterectomized surface and proximal part of the artery that is not endarterectomized [19]. Prior to stent placement, the guidewire must be passed across the distal intimal edge. In general this is not a problem and it can be easily achieved under fluoroscopic visualization. If this is not possible, or if the wire causes a further dissection of the distal lumen, the guidewire can be passed in a retrograde fashion via the popliteal artery, also described by Galland et al [20].

Personal experience with REA

From March 1994 to August 2000, 183 RSFAE procedures were scheduled in 164 patients in *the St. Antonius Hospital Nieuwegein, The Netherlands* [21]. Intraoperative technical success was achieved in 161 (88%) procedures, indicating that in 22 procedures an additional procedure was required. A second distal incision was required in four procedures due to a perforation of the distal SFA or popliteal artery, or due to technical difficulties in passing the guidewire across the distal intimal edge. In seven procedures placement of a proximal polytetrafluoroethylene (PTFE) interposition graft (8 millimeter diameter) was required due to poor quality of the CFA. In the remaining 11 cases conversion to bypass surgery was performed due to a perforation of

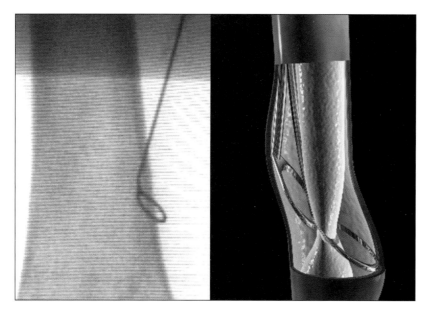

FIG. 5 *Left:* the loop of the ring stripper is advanced distally into the artery with gentle rotating and thrusting movements. *Right:* then the ring stripper is exchanged for a suitable MollRing Cutter which remotely transsects the intima core.

the SFA or the technical inability to perform endarterectomy, e.g., as a result of a too heavily calcified intimal core. The mean length (range) of the endarterectomized segment was 31 centimeters (17-45 centimeters). During the follow-up, 67 of the 183 limbs occluded, but only 1 above-knee and 4 below-knee amputations were required (of which 4 patients were operated for gangrene). The 5-year cumulative primary patency rate as assessed by means of life-table analysis was 38% ± 6.8% (SE) (Fig. 6). To achieve a 5-year primary assisted patency rate of 48% ± 6.3%, percutaneous transluminal balloon (26) and stent (3) angioplasty was performed in 29 patients, and surgical revision of the proximal and distal SFA was performed in 3 patients and 1 patient, respectively. The 5-year secondary patency rate was 49%, after embolectomy (n = 4), fibrinolysis with urokinase (n = 2), and fibrinolysis with surgical revision (n = 8). Females had a statistically significant lower 5-year cumulative primary patency rate (26%) as compared to males (45%), p = 0.01.

Adjacent procedures

ENDOLINING

In order to prevent the high incidence (46%) of early unpredictable but not all symptomatic recurrent stenoses after RSFAE, seen at standard duplex surveillance, new solutions needed to be found [21].

The occurrence of restenosis, which is the net result of both intimal hyperplasia and vascular remodeling, was not related to the site of the stent or adductor hiatus level, but was rather equally distributed throughout the entire SFA. Within stents, both intimal hyperplasia and stent area reduction have been observed to result in restenosis, especially at stent edges and stent junctions [22]. It has been suggested that this myeloproliferative response after plaque treatment may be reduced when the treated segment is covered with an endograft, preventing direct contact of the blood flow with the arterial wall [23,24]. This implies that by placing an endograft, one accepts that the collaterals are also sealed. The concept of endovascular grafting dates back more than a decade, and most experience has been acquired from percutaneous transluminal angioplasty (PTA) and recanalization techniques prior to insertion of an endograft [25,26]. In these procedures the atherosclerotic intimal core was not removed with the conceivability that extensive smooth muscle cell proliferation within the compressed atherosclerotic plaques may indent the endovascular graft and jeopardize the patency. Therefore it seems logical to debulk the arterial lumen first.

RESULTS OF ENDOLINING

An initial study, in which a femoropopliteal endograft was placed after RSFAE, described relative high early failure rates as a result of accidental

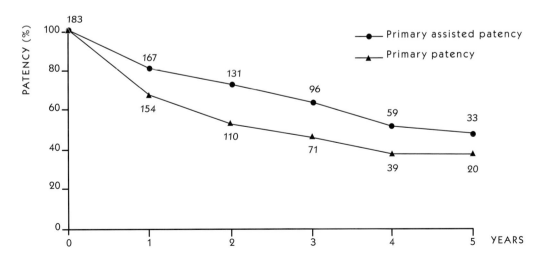

FIG. 6 Primary and primary assisted patency curves, with number of patients at risk (personal experience).

twisting, kinking, and folding of the unsupported grafts [27]. A balloon-expandable PTFE endovascular graft with PTFE rings incorporated (Enduring Vascular Graft, *W.L. Gore & Associates, Inc., Flagstaff, AZ, USA*) (Fig. 7) was then used to provide resistance and to eliminate the need for a distal stent. In the study by Heijmen et al., 41 patients were treated and although 5 (12%) needed intra-operative additional procedures, no conversions to conventional bypass grafting were required [28]. One of the problems was foreshortening of the PTFE while postdilating in small steps from distal to proximal, causing proximal migration of the endograft and subsequent exposure of a segment of the endarterectomized SFA and distal intimal flap. Another problem was a stenosis at the proximal anastomosis seen in 8 patients (28%) with control angiography and duplex scanning during early follow-up. In the first 29 procedures the proximal anastomosis was made through an end-to-side patchplasty. Because of this disproportionate rate of restenosis, in the remaining 12 patients (29%) the endograft was proximally anastomosed in an end-to-end fashion in order to obtain a more rheologically sound transition. However, no significant difference in patency was seen between these two groups.

In a multicenter study including 89 patients [29], overall primary and secondary patency rates were 42% and 56%, respectively, at 18 months' follow-up, and 30% and 44% at 36 months' follow-up. No recurrent stenoses were detected in the central part of the graft, suggesting adequate resistance to compressive forces. Intravascular ultrasound studies have shown that endograft recoil and plaque growth were not encountered at two years' follow-up [30]. Furthermore, at the anastomotic segments adjacent to the endograft, an unexplained local vasodilatory response was observed at 6 months' follow-up, which tended to stabilize at 2 years' follow-up. These positive findings were jeopardized by the occurrence of acute early and late occlusions of the endograft, concluding that endografting cannot be considered an improved treatment modality.

ASPIRE®

The concept of complete endografting was abandoned and a new stent concept was developed that is not characterized by thrombogenicity, compromising collaterals, or forming anastomotic problems. This new stent (aSpire®, *Vascular Architects Inc., San Jose, CA, USA*) combines the advantages of covered and open stents. In contrast with tubular stents, it is designed to better withstand the four major forces: extension/contraction, torsion, compression, and flexion. The specific indication therefore addresses arterial segments prone to flexion and extension such as the external iliac, the distal superficial femoral and proximal popliteal artery. The stent is

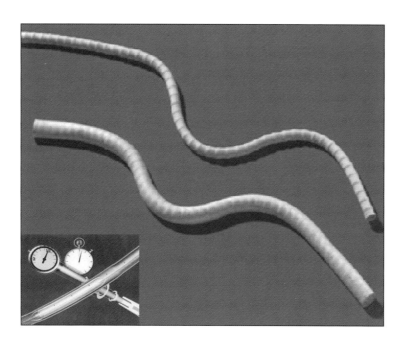

FIG. 7 Samples of a balloon-expandable polytetrafluoroethylene (ePTFE) endovascular graft with ePTFE rings incorporated. The lower is completely dilated.

made from nickel titanium (nitinol), manufactured in a double spiral configuration and covered with a thin sleeve of expanded PTFE (ePTFE) (Fig. 8). It is very flexible with a high radial force, and crush-and-kink resistance. The specific shape and the delivery device with separate proximal and distal releases of the stent add the benefit of not compromising the collaterals, and it can therefore be placed in a longer arterial segment. The early results of a European multicenter trial and a study under clearance of the US Food and Drug Administration, in which patients with occlusive disease of the SFA or iliac artery were treated with an aSpire® stent after PTA or REA, are promising. The aSpire® can be positioned accurately and deployed with ease, preserving side branches in the stented arterial segment. Obviously, long-term follow-up and a randomized controlled study are required to determine its advantage over other stents.

A further improvement might be expected from the drug-eluting stent. Stents are coated or impregnated with an agent such as Sacrolimus, Taxol, or Nitroprusside (nitric oxide donor), in order to inhibit intimal hyperplasia. This might give the aSpire® stent its final advantage because its ePTFE covering can be impregnated and, because the collaterals are not compromised, it is possible to treat the entire endarterectomized segment. In-vitro and animal studies are promising and the first patient will be treated with the nitric oxide drug-eluting stent (Med-aSpire®) in short time.

Determining treatment strategy

The prevalence of intermittent claudication in the general population aged 55 to 74 years is about 5%, that caused by SFA occlusive disease is 49% to 57% [31,32]. Only 30% to 50% of cases of intermittent claudication in these patients are known to their general practitioners [33]. Progression of atherosclerotic disease, seen in 50% of patients after an average follow-up of two years and a half, does not always result in worsening of symptoms [34]. The requirement of arterial reconstruction because of symptomatic progression ranges from 9% to 21% per year [35-37]. Critical leg ischemia affects approximately 1 in 2.500 of the population [38]. One year after developing critical leg ischemia, only 56% of patients will be alive with two legs. Furthermore, approximately 20% will have had an amputation and 10% to 20% will have died from concomitant coronary or cerebrovascular disease [39].

Therefore, it is important to stratify the patient into the group of disabling intermittent claudication or critical ischemia, i.e., rest pain or gangrene. In the first group a conservative regimen should be

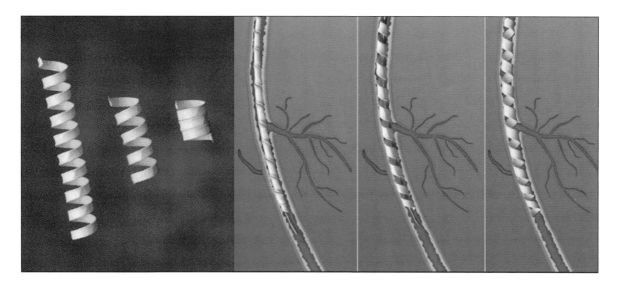

FIG. 8 The *aSpire* stent: a double spiral nickel titanium (nitinol) configuration covered with a thin sleeve of ePTFE. One of the advantages is the possibility of sparing collaterals.

established at first, consisting of cessation of smoking, walking exercise, and antiplatelet medication. If this conservative regimen is unsuccessful after at least six months, more invasive actions are considered. The latter are obviously immediately started in patients with critical ischemia. Further pre-operative evaluation includes a physical examination and ankle-brachial pressure indices measurements. Assessment of the disease is then performed by means of angiography or magnetic resonance angiography to visualize and classify the location, nature (i.e., stenosis or occlusion) and length of the lesion, and distal arterial runoff. Once the decision to intervene is made, a radiological guided endarterectomy is warranted.

Discussion

Current interventional modalities aim for minimal invasiveness. Unfortunately, PTA for long (longer than 10 centimeters) occlusive lesions in the SFA has a disappointing long-term patency or is not possible at all [40]. The use of stents in combination with PTA has not altered these results, despite close surveillance and early re-intervention [41]. These observations leave only a choice between bypass surgery and REA.

AKFP bypass surgery is associated with multiple incisions and the risk of infection and postoperative discomfort. The use of prosthetic material increases this risk of infection. Many additional techniques have been attempted to improve the patency rates, including arteriovenous fistulae, pre-cuffed prosthetic grafts, and the interposition vein cuffs and patches. These techniques may improve patency in below-knee prosthetic bypass grafting but all prove to be of no benefit in AKFP bypass grafting [42]. This actually means that no significant improvement in prosthetic graft technology has been achieved during the last twenty years. With a 5-year patency rate of 47% it offers no advantages over REA [43]. Venous bypass grafting has a significantly better patency rate and no increased risk of infection and should therefore be the first option, even when the vein must be harvested from another extremity. Apart from the question of whether for AKFP grafting it is better to spare the saphenous vein and save it for future cardiovascular surgery, a rising number of patients do not have an adequate saphenous vein

at all. Moreover, we believe that the autologous material is best spared for the event when minimally invasive techniques such as RSFAE have failed.

RSFAE offers a new, safe and effective treatment of long segmental SFA occlusive disease. The only requirements are a patent popliteal artery with at least one crural runoff vessel. It represents a minimally invasive procedure, with less surgical exposure as necessary for semi-closed endarterectomy or any bypass procedure. Operative trauma and postoperative discomfort are reduced, leading to earlier recovery and discharge of the patient as described in other reports. In RSFAE the whole intimal core is removed and a complete disobliteration of the SFA is performed. Complications that can occur during the process of cleaving, transecting, and removing the intimal core are a perforation of the SFA, due to extreme calcification, or a technical failure. In the event of a perforation, a second distal incision is usually enough to solve the problem. If necessary, conversion to a standard above-knee prosthetic bypass can always be performed. A third possibility is a transluminally placed ePTFE endolining. Previous (surgical) interventions in the ipsilateral SFA are not necessarily a contra-indication. When successful, no prosthetic graft material is exposed in the wound without the accompanying risk of infection. The absence of graft anastomoses precludes the risk of both late anastomotic aneurysms and stenoses.

In the event of restenosis, minimally invasive correction is usually possible, as previous studies have shown that PTA with selective stenting of recurrent disease after previous endarterectomy is feasible and safe [44-46]. However, re-intervention is not required in all cases of restenosis. Van der Heijden et al. [11] showed that 48% of failed endarterectomies remained asymptomatic. This is only 9% to 26% following occlusion of a femoropopliteal bypass [47, 48]. In our study the primary patency rate of 38% improved to 48% as a result of minimally invasive re-intervention (PTA with or without stent). The decision for re-intervention should be made on the basis of clinical symptoms or on the time interval between the RSFAE and restenosis. Results of a previous study of our first RSFAE patients showed that revision of early (inferior to one year) recurrent stenoses improves the patency rates but late restenoses developing after one year do not seem to progress to re-occlusion and may be treated conservatively [43].

Conclusion

Radiological guided endarterectomy in the form of RSFAE is an effective, minimal invasive procedure. The long-term patency rates are equal to those of prosthetic above-knee bypass surgery. In case of failure, conventional bypass procedures will still be available. Future developments in RSFAE are focused on drug-eluting stents, pharmaceutical innovations, and improvements.

REFERENCES

1 Dos Santos JC. Sur la désobstruction des thromboses artérielles anciennes. *Mem Acad Chir* 1947; 73: 409-411.

2 Dos Santos JC. Leriche memorial lecture. From embolectomy to endarterectomy or the fall of a myth. *J Cardiovasc Surg* 1976; 17: 113-128.

3 Canon JA, Barker WF. Successful management of obstructive femoral arteriosclerosis by endarterectomy. Experience with a semiclosed technique in selected cases. *Surgery* 1955; 38: 48-59.

4 Vollmar J. Rekonstruktive chirurgie der arterien. Stuttgart, *Thieme Verlag* 1967: p 416.

5 Sobel S, Kaplitt MJ, Reingold M, et al. Gas endarterectomy. *Surgery* 1966; 59: 517-521.

6 Blaisdell FW, Hall AD, Thomas AN. Surgical treatment of chronic internal carotid artery occlusion by saline endarterectomy. *Ann Surg* 1966; 163: 103-111.

7 Leveen HH. Technical features in endarterectomy. *Surgery* 1965; 57: 22-27.

8 Mukherjee D, Inahara T. Endarterectomy as the procedure of choice for atherosclerotic occlusive lesions of the common femoral artery. *Am J Surg* 1989; 157: 498-500.

9 Vercellio G, Castelli P, Coletti M, et al. Semiclosed thrombendoarterectomy on femoro-popliteal tract revisited after a fourteen years experience on 595 cases. *Int Surg* 1986; 71: 59-61.

10 Ouriel K, Smith CR, DeWeese JA. Endarterectomy for localized lesions of the superficial femoral artery at the adductor canal. *J Vasc Surg* 1986; 3: 531-534.

11 van der Heijden FH, Eikelboom BC, van Reedt Dortland RW, et al. Endarterectomy of the superficial femoral artery: a procedure worth reconsidering. *Eur J Vasc Surg* 1993; 6: 651-658.

12 Rosenthal D, Schubart PJ, Kinney EV, et al. Remote superficial femoral artery endarterectomy: multicenter medium-term results. *J Vasc Surg* 2001; 34: 428-433.

13 Smeets L, Ho GH, Hagenaars T, et al. Remote endarterectomy: first choice in surgical treatment of long segmental SFA occlusive disease? *Eur J Vasc Endovasc Surg* 2003; 25: 583-589.

14 AbuRahma AF, Robinson PA, Holt SM. Prospective controlled study of polytetrafluoroethylene versus saphenous vein in claudicant patients with bilateral above knee femoropopliteal bypasses. *Surgery* 1999; 126: 594-602.

15 Green RM, Abbott WM, Matsumoto T, et al. Prosthetic above-knee femoropopliteal bypass grafting: five-year results of a randomized trial. *J Vasc Surg* 2000; 31: 417-425.

16 Johnson WC, Lee KK. A comparative evaluation of polytetrafluoroethylene, umbilical vein and saphenous vein bypass grafts for femoral-popliteal above-knee revascularization: a prospective randomized department of veterans affairs cooperative study. *J Vasc Surg* 2000; 32: 268-277.

17 Klinkert P, Schepers A, Burger DH, et al. Vein versus polytetrafluoroethylene in above-knee femoropopliteal bypass grafting: five-year results of a randomized controlled trial. *J Vasc Surg* 2003; 37: 149-155.

18 Ho GH, Moll FL, Joosten PP, et al. The Mollring Cutter remote endarterectomy: preliminary experience with a new endovascular technique for treatment of occlusive superficial femoral artery disease. *J Endovasc Surg* 1995; 2: 278-287.

19 LeVeen HH, Diaz C, Christoudias G. The postendarterectomy intimal flap. *Arch Surg* 1973; 107: 664-668.

20 Galland RB, Whiteley MS, Gibson M, et al. Remote superficial femoral artery endarterectomy: medium-term results. *Eur J Vasc Endovasc Surg* 2000; 19: 278-282.

21 Ho GH, van Buren PA, Moll FL, et al. Incidence, time-of-onset, and anatomical distribution of recurrent stenoses after remote endarterectomy in superficial femoral artery occlusive disease. *J Vasc Surg* 1999; 30: 106-113.

22 van Lankeren W, Gussenhoven EJ, Honkoop J, et al. Plaque area increase and vascular remodeling contribute to lumen area change after percutaneous transluminal angioplasty of the femoropopliteal artery: an intravascular ultrasound study. *J Vasc Surg* 1999; 29: 430-441.

23 Bray AE. Superficial femoral endarterectomy with intra-arterial PTFE grafting. *J Endovasc Surg* 1995; 2: 297-301.

24 Morris GE, Ahn SS, Quick CR, et al. Endovascular femoropopliteal bypass: a cadaveric study. *Eur J Vasc Endovasc Surg* 1995; 10: 9-15.

25 Diethrich EB, Papazoglou K. Endoluminal grafting for aneurismal and occlusive disease in the femoropopliteal arteries: early experience. *J Endovasc Surg* 1995; 2: 225-239.

26 Spoelstra H, Casselman F, Lesceu O. Balloon-expendable endobypass for femoropopliteal atherosclerotic occlusive disease. A preliminary evaluation of fifty-five patients. *J Vasc Surg* 1996; 24: 647-654.

27 Ho GH, Moll FL, Tutein Noltenius RP, et al. Endovascular femoropopliteal bypass combined with remote endarterectomy in SFA occlusive disease: initial experience. *Eur J Vasc Endovasc Surg* 2000; 19: 27-34.

28 Heijmen RH, Teijink JA, van den Berg JC, et al. Use of a balloon-expandable, radially reinforced ePTFE endograft after remote SFA endarterectomy: a single-centre experience. *J Endovasc Ther* 2001; 8: 408-416.

29 Hagenaars T, Gussenhoven EJ, Smeets L, et al. Midterm follow-up of balloon-expandable ePTFE endografts in the femoropopliteal segment. *J Endovasc Ther* 2002; 9: 428-435.

30 Hagenaars T, Gussenhoven EJ, Athanassopoulos P, et al. Intravascular ultrasound evidence for stabilisation of compensatory enlargement of the femoropopliteal segment following endograft placement. *J Endovasc Ther* 2001; 8: 308-314.

31 Fowkes FG, Housley E, Cawood EH, et al. Edinburgh Artery Study: prevalence of asymptomatic and symptomatic peripheral arterial disease in the general population. *Int J Epidemiol* 1991; 20: 384-392.

32 Mavor GE. Pattern of occlusion in atheroma of lower limb arteries: correlation of clinical and angiographic findings. *Br J Surg* 1956; 43: 352-364.

33 Stoffers HE, Kaizer V, Knottnerus JA. Prevalence in general practice. In: Fowkes FGR (ed). *Epidemiology of peripheral vascular disease*. London, Springer Verlag 1991: pp109-113.

34 Kuthan F, Burkhalter A, Baitsch R, et al. Development of occlusive arterial disease in lower limbs. Angiographic follow-up of 705 medical patients. *Arch Surg* 1971; 103: 545-547.

35 Wilson SE, Schwartz I, Williams RA, Owens ML. Occlusion of the superficial femoral artery: what happens without operation. *Am J Surg* 1980; 140: 112-118.

36 Imparato AM, Kim GE, Davidson T, Crowley JG. Intermittent claudication: its natural course. *Surgery* 1975; 78: 795-799.

37 Whyman MR. Natural history of femoral atheromatous lesions. In: Fowkes FGR (ed). *Epidemiology of peripheral vascular disease.* London: Springer Verlag 1991: pp 301-313.

38 Anonymous. Critical limb ischaemia: management and outcome. Report of a national survey. The Vascular Surgical Society of Great Britain and Ireland. *Eur J Vasc Endovasc Surg* 1995; 10: 108-113.

39 Smith FC. Non-surgical treatment of critical ischaemia. In: Earnshaw JJ, Murie JA (eds). *The evidence for vascular surgery.* Shropshire, TFM Publishing Limited 1999: pp 73-78.

40 Capek P, McLean GK, Berkowitz HD. Femoropopliteal angioplasty. Factors influencing long term success. *Circulation* 1991; 83(2 suppl): I70-I80.

41 Cheng SW, Ting AC, Wong J. Endovascular stenting of superficial femoral artery stenosis and occlusions: results and risk factor analysis. *Cardiovasc Surg* 2001; 9: 133-140.

42 Hamsho A, Nott D, Harris PL. Prospective randomized trial of distal arteriovenous fistula as an adjunct to femoro-infrapopliteal PTFE bypass. *Eur J Vasc Endovasc Surg* 1999; 17: 197-201.

43 Anonymous. Management of peripheral arterial disease (PAD). TransAtlantic Inter-Society Consensus (TASC). Section D: chronic critical limb ischaemia. *Eur J Vasc Endovasc Surg* 2000; 19 Suppl A: S144-243.

44 Ho GH, van Buren PA, Moll FL, et al. The importance of revision of early restenosis after endovascular remote endarterectomy in SFA occlusive disease. *Eur J Vasc Endovasc Surg* 2000; 19: 35-42.

45 Derom A, Vermassen F, Ongena K. PTA and stenting after previous aortoiliac endarterectomy. *Eur J Vasc Endovasc Surg* 2001; 22: 130-133.

46 Tisnado J, Vines FS, Barnes RW, et al. Percutaneous transluminal angioplasty following endarterectomy. *Radiology* 1984; 152: 361-364.

47 Brewster DC, LaSalle AJ, Robinson JG, et al. Femoropopliteal graft failures. Clinical consequences and success of secondary reconstructions. *Arch Surg* 1983; 118: 1043-1047.

48 Blankensteijn JD, Van Vroonhoven TJ. Consequences of failure of femoro-popliteal grafts for claudication. *Eur J Vasc Surg* 1988; 2: 183-189.

21

DISTAL BYPASS COMBINED WITH FREE VASCULAR GRAFT

MAURI LEPÄNTALO, ERKKI TUKIAINEN
MILLA KALLIO, ALAIN BRANCHEREAU, SERGUEI MALIKOV
KOEN VAN LANDUYT, FRANK VERMASSEN

Combined arterial reconstructions and endovascular procedures are the most common hybrid procedures in vascular surgery. However, interventionalists are not the only colleagues with whom vascular surgeons collaborate. Large, infected tissue defects with exposed tendons and bones do not always heal despite successful bypass grafting, local surgery and wound care. Therefore, a number of patients with ischemic tissue loss are at risk for major amputation, despite successful revascularization of the ischemic tissue. The use of free tissue transfer in the management of major tissue loss secondary to atherothrombotic disease with or without diabetes was introduced in the late 1980s. During the last decade, sporadic observations provoked the gradual spread of this method in institutions devoted to leg salvage. Distal bypass and free graft transfer can be done staged or, nowadays more often, simultaneously as a hybrid operation necessitating both vascular and plastic surgical skills. Teamwork among vascular and plastic surgeons has been developed in a number of European centers. Experience of three European centers is presented.

Leg ischemia with infection and tissue loss

Vascular surgery is getting more and more complicated. Moderate peripheral arterial disease is treated conservatively and local lesions endovascularly. An increasing number of patients do not only have local lesions and mere claudication, but have multisegmental arterial occlusive disease and critical ischemia instead. The patients have many concurrent diseases and the vascular reconstructions are more cumbersome. A number of those patients are treated with hybrid procedures by vascular surgeons with interventional skills or by vascular surgeons and angioradiologists during the same operative procedure in the operating theater (Fig. 1). If the patients have large ischemic tissue lesions, vascularized free muscle transfer may be needed to cover the defect and used as an adjunct to long infra-inguinal reconstructions to prevent major amputation. A prerequisite for this activity is a seamless teamwork among vascular and plastic surgeons. When the vascular reconstruction and the free flap transfer are performed in a same operation synchronously, a more uncommon type of hybrid procedure is made (Fig. 1).

Critical leg ischemia is not only a sign of generalized arteriosclerotic disease but also a serious threat to the independence of the patient. Major amputation decreases the mobility of the old and severely comorbid patient population and only few of them are able to learn to walk with a prosthesis. There is evidence that active lower limb revascularization is worthwhile and can decrease the amputation rate by up to 52% to 60% [1,2]. A Finnish population-based study showed that only those types of revascularizations that directly improved the perfusion of the ischemic area could diminish the need for major amputation [3]. The benefit of long infrapopliteal bypass as a leg salvage procedure is especially noteworthy in elderly patients over 80 years of age [4].

Patients with acute deep infection complicating ischemia present a real challenge for leg salvage. The bypass should be delayed until active spreading of the infection is controlled, most often by intravenous antibiotics, bed rest, and debridement or amputation left wide open. After adequate revascularization, restricted acral gangrene can be treated by local, distal amputations. Likewise, superficial and limited tissue lesions can be debrided and covered by split thickness skin grafting. The outcome is only successful if a functional limb is salvaged. Local minor amputations should be regarded as victories of treatment of ischemic tissue lesions [5].

However, infrapopliteal reconstruction cannot always guarantee healing in case of major ischemic tissue loss. Local wound care with wound excisions and skin grafting may not be enough to treat and cover large, infected tissue defects with exposed tendons, bones, or joints, despite successful bypass grafting [6]. Repeated extensive debridement procedures may not ensure secondary healing, especially if the wound does not granulate, which is often the case in these patients. Even when successful they often

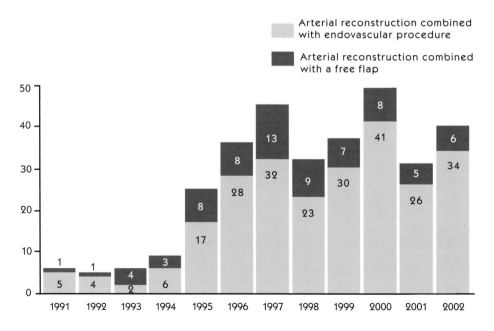

FIG. 1 Hybrid vascular procedures in operating theater: combined vascular and endovascular revascularization vs. combined distal bypass and free vascular graft in Helsinki University Central Hospital.

deform the foot markedly. Local flap coverage is mostly inadequate for wound coverage, as there is only little viable tissue available because of distal anatomical location, infection and fibrosis and, most importantly, their vitality is limited. Therefore, a number of patients with ischemic tissue loss are still at risk for major amputation despite a successful infra-inguinal bypass graft.

A solution to this problem was introduced in the late 1980s, when free tissue transfer was included in the management of major tissue loss secondary to atherothrombotic disease with or without diabetes [6-9]. Vascular anastomoses made with magnifying loupes facilitated the use of large free muscle flaps to cover large tissue defects. After a number of anecdotal reports, the first small series with life table data were published only recently [10-12]. The Rochester Group has increased the number of procedures to 79 after the initial publication [13].

This chapter describes the results of the procedures performed in Helsinki (Finland), Gent (Belgium), and Marseille (France).

The first combined procedure was performed October 2, 1989 in Helsinki, April 9, 1992 in Gent, and June 15, 1999 in Marseille. The current activity of the groups in Helsinki, Gent, and Marseille is described in Table I. The great majority of the patients in Helsinki and Gent are diabetics, their share being 80% and 83%, respectively, in contrast to a much smaller share in Marseille.

There is another indication to use free flaps for advanced leg salvage as well. In addition to covering large tissue defects of the foot, early coverage with free flaps may be used for leg salvage even in case of infected, exposed, or ruptured autogenous vein graft [5,13,14].

The hybrid operation

Not all patients with critical leg ischemia and major tissue loss are candidates for this combined vascular bypass and vascular free graft. Severe coronary or cerebrovascular disease, renal failure requiring long-term dialysis, and high serum concentration of C-reactive protein co-existing with critical ischemia are significant risk factors for early postoperative leg or life loss in infrapopliteal surgery for critical leg ischemia [15]. While 16% to 28% of patients undergoing combined distal bypass with free vascular graft have been reported to have end-stage renal disease [10,11,13], the number is decreasing (Table I). A

Table I	EXPERIENCE OF DISTAL BYPASS COMBINED WITH FREE VASCULAR GRAFT IN THE CENTERS OF HELSINKI, GENT AND MARSEILLE						
Center	Number of patients	Mean age (range)	Male/female	Diabetes %	Free vascular graft		Early failure %	Simultaneous intervention %
Helsinki	75	61 (37-83)	46 / 29	80	- Latissimus dorsi 42 - Rectus abdominus 18 - Radial forearm flap 9 - Omentum 2 - Miscellaneous 4	15	75
Gent	72	62 (29-85)*	46 / 14*	83	- Rectus abdominus 44 * - Latissimus dorsi 8 - Serratus 3 - Fascia-cutaneous flap 4 - Radial forearm flap 1	15	87
Marseille	10	59 (41-76)	9 / 1	30	Serratus 6 Latissimus dorsi 2 Radial forearm flap 1 Omentum 1	10	70

* Indicates diabetic patients only

special problem arises in the postoperative recovery and rehabilitation period after combined arterial reconstruction and free flap transfer in obese and non-compliant patients. Patient selection is therefore of outmost importance.

Selective antegrade lower extremity angiography is performed to evaluate the extent of arterial disease. Endovascular treatment of aorto-iliac stenotic lesions and endovascular treatment of diseased arteries of the lower extremity may sometimes be performed as inflow procedures to enable the anastomosis of free flap pedicle directly to the native vessels. Most often, however, a bypass with infrapopliteal outflow is needed for proper revascularization of the ischemic foot.

Vascular reconstruction and microvascular free flap transfer can be done either simultaneously or on two separate occasions. The simultaneous approach is preferred when the general health allows lengthy operation with large bleeding surfaces, thereby avoiding a second large operation. A simultaneous procedure was chosen in 75%, 87%, and 70% of the cases in Helsinki, Gent, and Marseille, respectively. Simultaneous use of free flap transfer increases the graft flow [16]. Native veins, however, tend to be small in diameter in critically ischemic legs. This, together with shorter operating time and possibility to ensure the patency of the bypass, are factors in favor of the delayed microvascular reconstruction [7].

In cases with fulminant infection or a septic foot, prior debridement or minor amputation is usually performed two to five days before the combined distal bypass and free graft operation. In this hybrid operation a two-team approach should be used. Good teamwork between the vascular and plastic surgeon is mandatory. They may want to perform adequate debridement and primary assessment of the foot viability first. Next, the operation continues from two separate clean fields: the vascular surgeon harvests the vein and performs the bypass while the plastic surgeon raises the flap and performs the microvascular free flap transfer. This allows both teams to start the operation at the same time and obviously shortens the operative time.

The flow to a free microvascular flap depends on the recipient artery as well as on the specific tissue components of the flap (Table II). Muscular flaps resist infection, eliminate dead space, and can easily be tailored to fill in uneven contours. The selection of the muscle depends on the patient, anesthesia, need for tissue coverage, and regional localization of arterial disease. The latissimus dorsi flap (Fig. 2) is preferred in Helsinki over the rectus abdominus flap, as it has a long pedicle that is not affected by atherosclerosis. The vessels to and from the latissimus dorsi flap are well sized, therefore making anastomosing less difficult. Furthermore, there is no donor site morbidity like at the abdomen: when using the rectus abdominus muscle, postoperative pain may hamper respiration, the risk for herniation is increased, and possible kidney transplantation is made more demanding. However, the advantage of the rectus abdominus muscle flap (Fig. 3) is that it can be harvested under regional anesthesia and in supine position. It is the most popular

Table II	DETAILS OF DIFFERENT FREE GRAFTS					
Type	*Outflow (ml/min)*	*Occurence of atherosclerosis at pedicle*	*Complications with harvesting*	*Anesthetic contra-indications*	*On-table position*	*Seize*
Latissimus dorsi	20 - 50	+	+	+++	Lateral decubitus	+++
Rectus abdominus	10 - 20	++	++	++	Dorsal decubitus	++
Gracilis muscle	5 - 15	+++	-	-	Lateral decubitus	+
Serratus muscle	5 - 15	+	-	+++	Lateral decubitus	+
Radial forearm flap	4 - 10	+	++	-/+	Dorsal decubitus	+
Anterior thigh	10 - 20	++	+	-	Dorsal decubitus	++
Omentum	20 - 30	+	++	+++	Dorsal decubitus	++

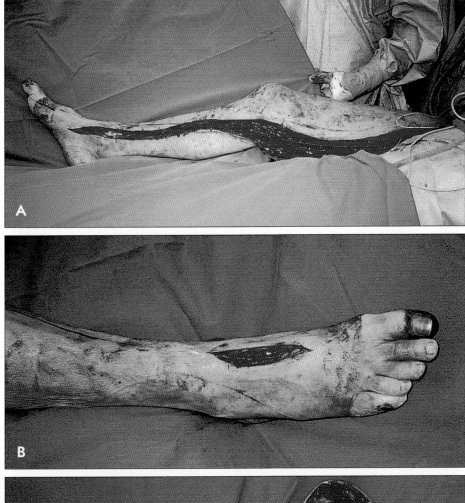

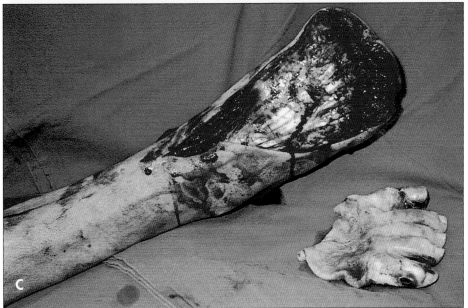

FIG. 2 Distal bypass with latissimus dorsi (LD) graft. A - Femoropedal bypass performed.
B - Distal anastomosis accomplished. C - Non-vital tissue liberally excised. *(To be continued)*

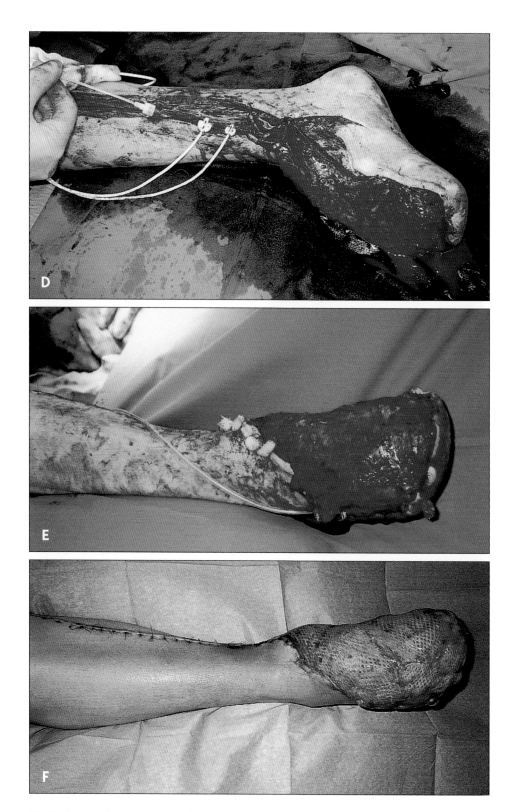

FIG. 2   D - Feeding artery to LD flap anastomosed end-to-side to the vein graft. Note separate flowmetry from the vein graft proximal and distal to the anastomosis and from the feeding artery as well. E - Flap anastomosed and fixed before skin grafting. F - Ten days postoperatively with split thickness skin grafting.

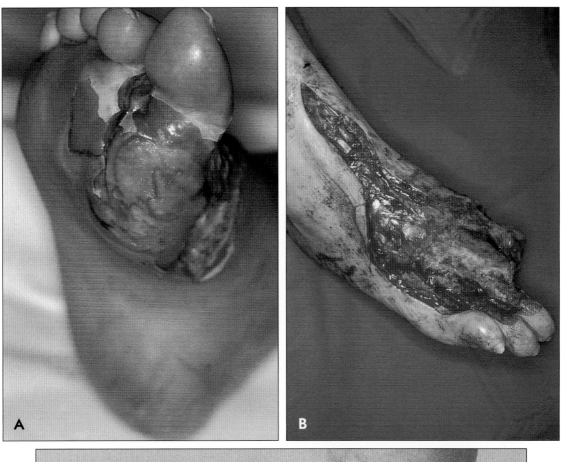

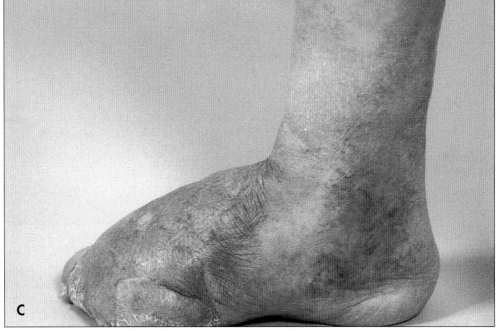

FIG. 3 Rectus abdominus muscle flap. A - Large ischemic ulcer. B - after wound excision. C - Six months after femorodistal bypass and rectus abdominus flap transfer.

graft in Gent as its harvesting is easier and can be performed concomitantly with the revascularization and without special positioning on the operating table. Atherosclerosis of the inferior epigastric artery has not been a clinical problem in the Gent practice. Serratus anterior muscle, especially popular in Marseille (Fig. 4), may also be used, although it does not offer as good coverage as the latissimus dorsi flap. As it is fed by a tributary from the thoracodorsal artery, it can be used as a short segment interposition conduit with own coverage. With this method only autologous arterial material is used at the distal anastomosis.

The muscle flap transfer is completed with split thickness skin graft, meshed if used for immediate coverage. Muscle flaps offer the advantage of filling cavities and covering large tissue loss with tendon and bone exposure. Although free muscle flaps tend to remain bulky, these contour problems subside with muscle atrophy, occurring within a few months [17].

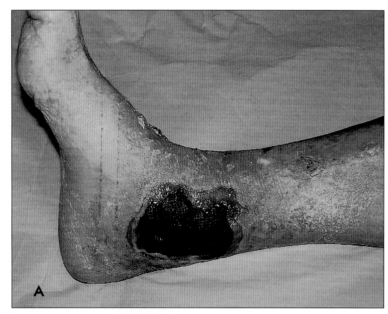

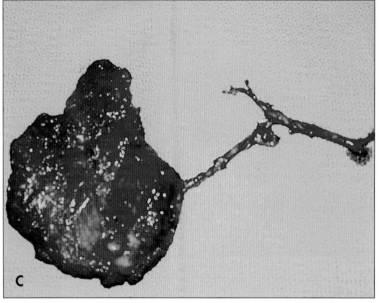

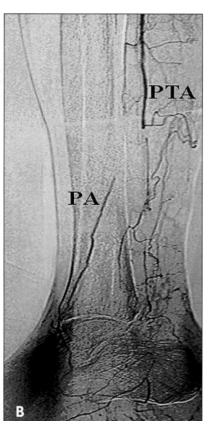

FIG. 4 Serratus anterior muscle flap. A - Widespread necrosis at the internal malleolus. B - Angiogram showing occlusion of anterior tibial artery and peroneal artery. Occlusion of the posterior tibial artery (PTA) at middle third of the leg. Peroneal artery (PA) refilled at inferior third of the leg. C - Operative view of serratus anterior muscle with its feeding artery from thoracodorsal artery.

Fasciocutaneous flaps, like the radial forearm flap (Fig. 5), have a low flow (Table II). They can provide a superior contour and are preferred in smaller wounds of the foot and ankle. Serletti et al. [18] favor the use of the radial forearm flap when the contour is a potential problem. The scapular fasciocutaneous flap is preferred by Serletti et al. [18] for the management of large wounds on the weight-bearing plantar surface because of the thicker skin of this flap. Our experience, however, is that split thickness skin grafting directly on the transferred muscle allows the most tolerable surface for weight bearing. Omentum offers the best length, takes whatever shape is needed, and can be used to cover long lesions extending over the whole leg (Fig. 6).

After completion of the end-to-side anastomosis between the vein graft and the recipient artery, the anastomosis between the feeding artery of the flap and the inflow vessel is preferably performed in an end-to-side fashion, whenever possible with continuous 8-0 polypropylene sutures using ordinary vascular technique and with the aid of 4.5-fold

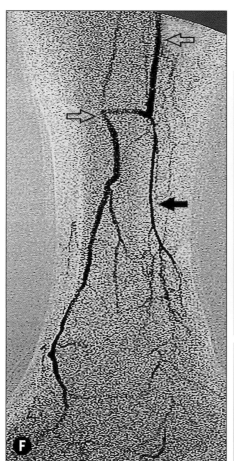

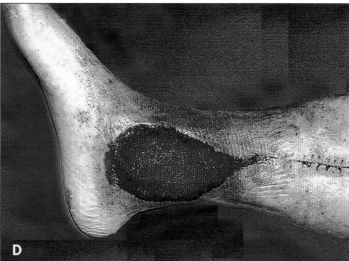

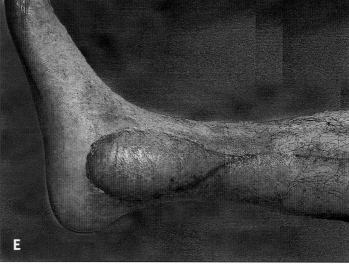

FIG. 4 D - flap covering tissue loss before the skin graft. E - result at 10 months. F - Angiogram performed at 10 months showing patency of interposed thoracodorsal artery (open arrows) between posterior tibial artery and peroneal artery and patency of the artery feeding the muscle (black arrow).

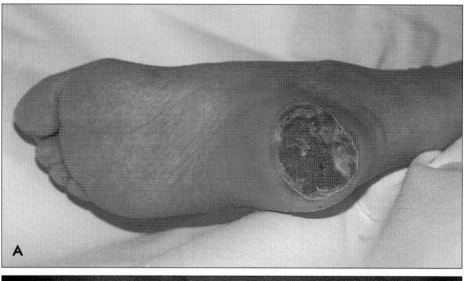

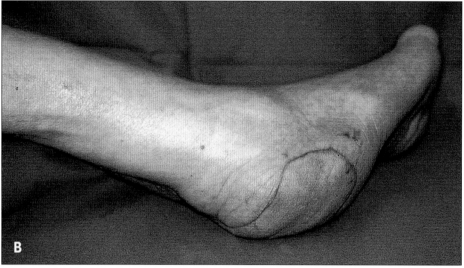

FIG. 5 Distal bypass with radial forearm flap. A - Necrotic lesion involving the underlying calcaneus. B - Femorotibial bypass performed and heel reconstructed with the radial forearm flap after wound excision.

magnifying loupes. This is the technique most often used in Helsinki (Fig. 7A). An alternative, often used in Gent, is to perform a side-to-side anastomosis between the vein graft and the recipient artery and use the distal part of the vein graft as a feeding artery to the flap with an end-to-end anastomosis (Fig. 7B). The Marseille modification [19] with the serratus anterior muscle includes the use of the thoracodorsal artery as the distal part of the conduit, thus providing a distal arterial end-to-side anastomosis (Fig. 7C).

If there is no outflow vessel available for the graft, it still may be used as a conduit between the open inflow artery, for instance the popliteal artery, and the flap artery. Next, the anastomosis is performed in an end-to-end fashion and a free flap with high flow is to be selected (Table II) as otherwise the graft is prone to be occluded. As shown by Shestak et al. [9], Serletti et al. [18], and our own experience [20], this indirect revascularization of the leg by infra-inguinal bypass to a free muscle flap in patients with unreconstructable arteries may also be

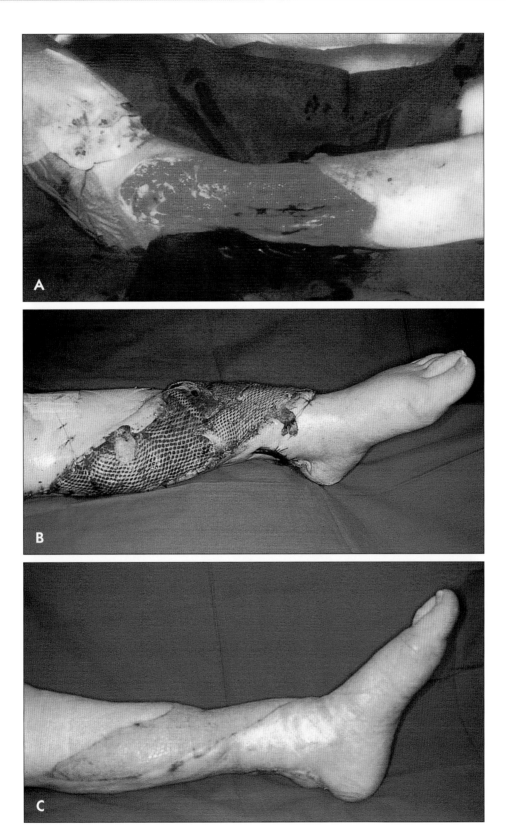

FIG. 6 Distal bypass with omentum graft. A - Large circumferential defect. B - Omental flap with split thickness skin graft. C - Result at six months.

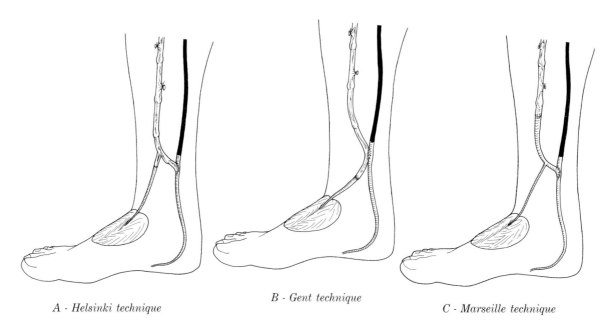

A - Helsinki technique   *B - Gent technique*   *C - Marseille technique*

FIG. 7   Different ways of anastomosing the vein bypass to the recipient artery and the feeding artery of the flap (see text).

successful. This extremely aggressive procedure is seldom indicated and every effort should be made to find an outflow artery for the distal bypass [21]. However, in such cases a neovascular network between the flap and the neighboring tissue may develop, and signs and symptoms of ischemia may subside [8,9,18,20,22]. The venous anastomosis is performed in an end-to-end fashion to one of the concomitant deep veins with interrupted sutures to avoid narrowing of the anastomosis.

Postoperative treatment and surveillance

Antibiotics are given for three to four weeks according to culture results, wound healing, and kidney function. In case of deep infection of the foot or if osteomyelitis is present, a long 6- to 12-month or even lifelong therapy may be needed. A continuous epidural anesthetic block is used during the first postoperative days. Bed rest with slight limb elevation is indicated for about seven days. At times, the heel should be floating to prevent heel ulceration or destruction of the flap, which occasionally can be achieved by suspension with Kirschner wires or external fixation. Ambulation is started very gradually, with exercises in a standing position

for 10 minutes at a time to start, but weight bearing is not allowed until after four to six weeks, when the flap covers the plantar surface of the foot.

Graft patency after bypass grafting and free flap transfer is preferably assessed by duplex scanning rather than by direct pulse palpation and doppler ankle-brachial index measurement only. The viability of the free flap is clinically assessed every one to two hours during the first postoperative day and thereafter every three to four hours with decreasing frequency. Arterial inflow to the free flap is open if the flap oozes a drop of fresh arterial blood when punctured repeatedly with a needle. Alternative methods are microdialysis technique and transcutaneous oxygen tension measurement, the latter requiring intact skin for measurements. If the venous outflow is obstructed, the flap swells, bleeds, and turns cyanotic. Immediate re-intervention is mandatory in any case of early occlusion, the problem most often situating at the site of the venous anastomosis.

All free flaps become sympathectomized when they are removed from their original site. The initial swelling of muscle flaps due to this phenomenon may be frightening for the patient. Vein graft surveillance is performed with duplex scanning, whereas angiography is performed whenever signs and symptoms of graft stenosis or ischemia of the distal part of leg or free flap are observed.

Results

Initial failure rate of the bypass, the free flap, or both varied between 8% and 15% (Table I). Limb salvage at three and five years' follow-up were 88% and 63%, respectively. In two thirds of the patients, complete mobility could be achieved (Table III). These operations must be done in centers with sufficient recourses, experience, and good quality control. Patient selection is essential. Uremic patients and patients with poor general condition or lack of motivation and cooperation are poor candidates for the operation [12,23]. Although patients with diabetes and end-stage renal disease have a very poor outcome, encouraging results in end-stage renal disease patients have been reported [24]. Both Helsinki and Gent continue to treat even uremic patients, however, very selectively. Renal transplant patients are more often appropriate candidates for free flap operation [10].

Combining long bypass grafting and free flap transfer, for instance with latissimus dorsi, is a long and tedious procedure. Operative stress and a long postoperative course before eventual recovery expose patients to a number of complications. Diabetic patients are prone to wound edge problems, requiring repeated revisions. No data are available comparing the outcome after below-knee amputation and combined long grafting and free flap transfer. Early reports always tend to give an overly optimistic view of the outcome. Therefore, proper quality of life studies are needed. The preliminary interview data from Helsinki showed that if patients could have chosen they would have undergone the same tedious and heavy process of combined distal bypass and free vascular grafting. In their retrospective view, two of 28 patients had preferred major amputation.

Conclusion

Combining microvascular muscle flap transfer with vascular reconstruction for salvage of legs with extensive ischemic tissue loss offers acceptable results and deserves an attempt in selected patients.

| **Table III** | RESULTS OF VASCULAR RECONSTRUCTIONS WITH FREE VASCULAR GRAFT FOR LIMB SALVAGE |

1st author Year [ref]	Number of patients/ Diabetes/ Renal failure	Most frequently used grafts %	Anastomotic site of freding graft artery	Mean follow-up Years	Early failure	Return to autonomy %	Limb salvage %	Survival (3 years) %	Survival and limb salvage % (3 years)
Tukiainen 2000 [10]	29/80%/ 28%	LD 67 RA 23	VG 90 NV 10	1.5	4	82	82	97	80
Vermassen 2000 [11]	45/100%/ 16%	RA 79 LD 11	VG 74 NV 26	2.2	5	82	88	88	77
Moran 2002 [13]	75/76 %/ 27%	RA 44 RF 30 LD 19	VG 55 NV 45	NA	6	69	75	67 *	NA

* Limb salvage at 5 years

LD: latissimus dorsi
NV: native vessel
RA: rectus abdominus
RF: radial forearm flap
VG: venous graft
NA: not available

REFERENCES

1 Luther M. Treatment of chronic critical leg ischemia. A cost benefit analysis. *Ann Chir Gynaecol Suppl 1997*; 213: 1-142.

2 Eskelinen E, Lepäntalo M, Hietala EM, et al. Lower limb amputations in southern Finland in 2000 and trends up to 2001. *Eur J Vasc Endovasc Surg* 2004 (in press).

3 Luther M, Kantonen I, Lepäntalo M, et al. Arterial intervention and reduction in amputation for chronic critical leg ischaemia. *Br J Surg* 2000; 87: 454-458.

4 Eskelinen E, Luther M, Eskelinen A, Lepäntalo M. Infrapopliteal bypass reduces amputation incidence in elderly patients: a population-based study. *Eur J Vasc Endovasc Surg* 2003; 26: 65-68.

5 Lepäntalo M, Tukiainen E. Advanced leg salvage. In: *Perspectives in vascular surgery and endovascular therapy.* New York, Westminster Publications, Inc 2002; (vol 15): pp 27-41.

6 Gooden MA, Gentile AT, Mills JL, et al. Free tissue transfer to extend the limits of limb salvage for lower extremity tissue loss. *Am J Surg* 1997; 174: 644-649.

7 Cronenwett JL, McDaniel MD, Zwolak RM, et al. Limb salvage despite extensive tissue loss. Free tissue transfer combined with distal revascularization. *Arch Surg* 1989; 124: 609-615.

8 Mimoun M, Hilligot P, Baux S. The nutrient flap: a new concept of the role of the flap and application to the salvage of arteriosclerotic lower limbs. *Plast Reconstr Surg* 1989; 84: 458-467.

9 Shestak KC, Hendricks DL, Webster MW. Indirect revascularization of the lower extremity by means of microvascular free-muscle flap. A preliminary report. *J Vasc Surg* 1990; 12: 581-585.

10 Tukiainen E, Biancari F, Lepäntalo M. Lower limb revascularization and free flap transfer for major ischemic tissue loss. *World J Surg* 2000; 24: 1531-1536.

11 Vermassen FE, van Landuyt K. Combined vascular reconstruction and free flap transfer in diabetic arterial disease. *Diabetes Metab Res Rev* 2000; 16 (suppl 1): S33-S36.

12 Illig KA, Moran S, Serletti J, et al. Combined free tissue transfer and infrainguinal bypass graft: an alternative to major amputation in selected patients. *J Vasc Surg* 2001; 33: 17-23.

13 Moran SL, Illig KA, Green RM, Serletti JM. Free-tissue transfer in patients with peripheral vascular disease: a 10-year experience. *Plast Reconstr Surg* 2002; 109: 990-1006.

14 Tukiainen E, Biancari F, Lepäntalo M. Deep infection of infrapopliteal autogenous vein grafts: immediate use of muscle flaps in leg salvage. *J Vasc Surg* 1998; 28: 611-616.

15 Biancari F, Kantonen I, Alback A, et al. Limits of infrapopliteal bypass surgery for critical leg ischemia: when not to reconstruct. *World J Surg* 2000; 24: 727-733.

16 Lorenzetti F, Tukiainen E, Alback A, et al. Blood flow in pedal bypass combined with a free muscle flap. *Eur J Vasc Endovasc Surg* 2001; 22: 161-164.

17 Salmi A, Ahovuo J, Tukiainen E, et al. Use of ultrasonography to evaluate muscle thickness and blood flow in free flaps. *Microsurgery* 1995; 16: 601-605.

18 Serletti JM, Deuber MA, Guidera PM, et al. Atherosclerosis of the lower extremity and free-tissue reconstruction for limb salvage. *Plast Reconstr Surg* 1995; 96: 1136-1144.

19 Malikov S, Casanova D, Champsaur P, et al. The bypass-flap: an innovating technique of distal revascularization. Anatomical study and clinical application. *Ann Vasc Surg* 2004 (in press).

20 Matzke S, Tukiainen EJ, Lepäntalo MJ. Survival of a microvascular muscle flap despite the late occlusion of the inflow artery in a neuroischaemic diabetic foot. *Scand J Plast Reconstr Hand Surg* 1997; 31: 71-75.

21 McDaniel MD, Zwolak RM, Scheinder JR, et al. Indirect revascularization of the lower extremity by means of microvascular free-muscle flap. A preliminary report. *J Vasc Surg* 1991; 12: 829-830.

22 van Landuyt K, Monstrey S, Blondeel P, et al. Revascularization by ingrowth of a free flap: fact or fiction. *Microsurgery* 1996; 17: 417-422.

23 Karp NS, Kasabian AK, Siebert JW, et al. Microvascular free-flap salvage of the diabetic foot: a 5-year experience. *Plast Reconstr Surg* 1994; 94: 834-840.

24 Gentile AT, Berman SS, Reinke KR, et al. A regional pedal ischemia scoring system for decision analysis in patients with heel ulceration. *Am J Surg* 1998; 176: 109-114.

22

ASSISTED THROMBECTOMY FOR ACUTE LOWER LIMB ISCHEMIA

NICOLAS VALÉRIO, JAN BLANKENSTEIJN

Acute ischemia of the lower limbs is the result of a sudden occlusion of an arterial segment, which may occur in normal arteries due to embolization or, more often, thrombosis of pathological arteries in the course of the atheromatous process.

The usual treatment comprises two steps: removal of the thrombus (thrombo-embolectomy) and causal treatment, which is usually performed during the same procedure when it concerns a thrombosis of pathological arteries. The considerable mortality associated with conventional surgical treatment of acute ischemia is due to the fragility of the group in which it occurs: elderly patients with numerous comorbidities. This has led to the development of less invasive therapies like endoluminal and thrombolytic techniques.

The growth of endovascular techniques and their adoption by vascular surgeons have changed the operating theaters into theaters equipped with digital and mobile interventional imaging devices. Now, digital imaging techniques, angioplasty, and thrombolysis are part of the arsenal of the modern vascular surgeon, who must be familiar with the possibilities offered by these new techniques in the treatment of acute ischemia.

In this chapter we will describe the mechanical and pharmacological possibilities available for endovascular application, which can also be combined with thrombo-embolectomy, as well as the contribution of pre-operative fluoroscopy, in the treatment of acute ischemia. Knowledge of these techniques and their use is essential to the vascular surgeon who is mostly involved in the emergency treatment of these patients when an interventional radiologist is absent.

Thrombo-embolectomy

The classic surgical technique, as described fourty years ago by Fogarty, most commonly consists of surgical access to the common femoral artery. A balloon catheter is introduced into the arterial lumen through an arteriotomy in order to remove the thrombus. This simple technique has the advantage that the obstacle can be removed quickly. The drawback is its blind character, which sometimes makes it traumatic and often incomplete.

Fluoroscopy and the development of balloon catheters based on the endovascular technology nowadays enable us to perform a complete thrombo-embolectomy under fluoroscopic control [1]. A standard J-guidewire or hydrophilic guidewire (0.014 to 0.035) is used for selective catheterization, under fluoroscopic control, of the leg arteries. Under fluoroscopic control, the guidewire is passed distally to the occluded segment using standard guidewire techniques. If necessary, supporting catheters can be used. Next, a double lumen thrombectomy catheter (Fig. 1) is passed over the guidewire and, under fluoroscopic control, the thrombectomy balloon is inflated with diluted contrast and withdrawn. After removal of the bulk of the distal thrombus, a 4F to 7F sheath can be advanced into the distal artery and secured with a silastic vessel-loop for backflow control and easier access.

Completion angiography

After thrombectomy, subjective appreciation of the inflow and the reflux is not sufficient as a guarantee for a good result. Digital angiography on the operating table is necessary to check the complete patency of the arterial segment treated. This angiogram, made with or without subtraction, shows whether the thrombectomy has been complete and can depict the lesion causing the thrombosis that induced the acute ischemia. This completion angiogram should verify the inflow and outflow. In the majority of cases, a manual retrograde injection through an introducer placed in the common femoral artery suffices to visualize the iliac arteries up to the aortic bifurcation. When this is sufficient to obtain a good quality image, one should move a catheter up to the distal aorta and inject using an automatic injector. Distally, the angiogram should show the crural arteries down to the foot to ensure adequate revascularization.

Residual thrombus

When the completion angiogram shows a residual thrombus at a distance from the arterial segment where the arteriotomy was performed, several options can be applied. Thrombo-aspiration is attractive when it concerns a recent and small thrombus. This is performed using a catheter with a large diameter (6F to 8F), which is positioned at the thrombus over a classic (e.g., hydrophilic) guidewire (Fig. 2). Subsequently, the wire is retracted and an empty syringe is attached to the catheter in order to aspire the thrombus. This thrombus is trapped in the tip of the catheter, which is then retracted. This maneuver is repeated several times to make sure the complete thrombus is removed, which may

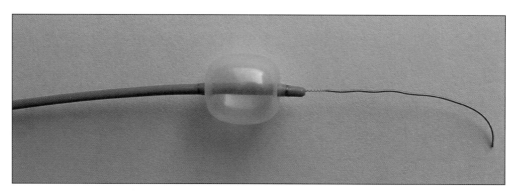

FIG. 1 Double-lumen thrombectomy catheter over a guidewire.

fragment during the thrombo-aspiration [2]. (Fig. 3) Thrombolysis may be applied in combination with thrombectomy when a thrombus exists that extends distally into the calf and foot [3]. A hydrophilic J-guidewire is used to advance a multiperforated catheter (Fig. 4) to make contact with the thrombus. This catheter should be positioned in such a way that the proximal openings are close to the most proximal part of the clot and the distal ones close to the distal part of the clot. Administration

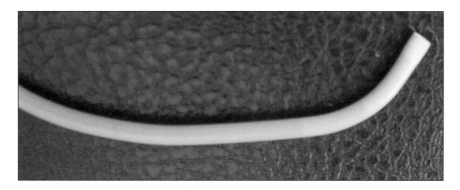

FIG. 2   Thrombo-aspiration catheter.

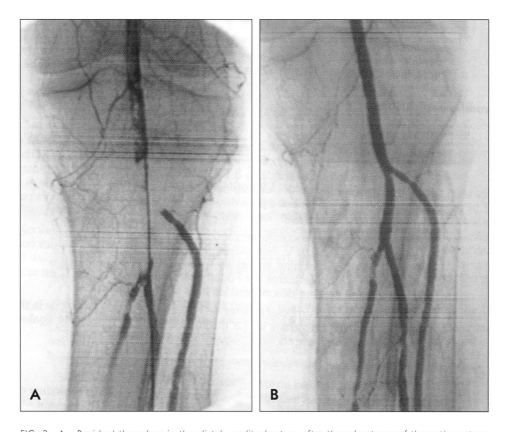

FIG. 3   A - Residual thrombus in the distal popliteal artery after thrombectomy of the native artery.
B - Result after thrombo-aspiration.

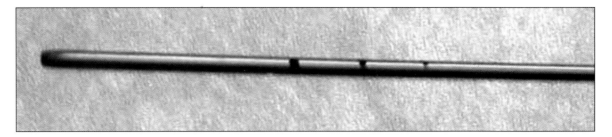

FIG. 4 Straight multiperforated catheter for thrombolysis.

of the thrombolytic agent may be performed continuously, as a bolus, or pulse-sprayed, i.e., a highly concentrated bolus injected under high pressure to hasten the effect of thrombolysis [4]. Of the three commonly used thrombolytic agents (urokinase, streptokinase, and recombinant tissue-type plasminogen activator; rt-PA), we use rt-PA, which we administer as an in-situ bolus in a dosage of 5 mg and which can be repeated three or four times.

More details about thrombolytic agents, the dosages given, and the methods can be found in the literature review by Comerota and Schmieder [5]. When an old, adherent thrombus is present, thrombectomy may be performed by using a Volmar ring or special Fogarty catheters. These helical catheters without a balloon are called Fogarty catheters for thrombectomy of prosthesis or adherent clots (Fig. 5). These two techniques, particularly attractive for thrombectomies of prosthetic bypasses, may also be used with care in healthy native arteries. Fluoroscopy and road mapping can be used to check the mechanical thrombectomy. These traumatizing techniques may induce iatrogenic lesions,

which frequently require angioplasty with or without a stent.

Several percutaneous thrombectomy options have been developed in recent years. These may be applied in addition to surgical thrombectomy. The mechanical procedures are based on the dissolution, fragmentation, and aspiration of clots. In general, two types of recirculation mechanisms exist: recirculation by means of rotation, in which turbulence is generated by the high rotation velocity, and hydraulic recirculation, in which the high injection speed induces a Venturi effect that catches, resolves, and evacuates the clots. The primary function of other devices is to fragment and aspire the thrombus. These devices are associated with a considerable risk of embolization and arterial damage [6].

Causal treatment

After removal of the thrombus the recanalization of the artery may be insufficient because of remaining atherosclerotic lesions. These lesions are mostly

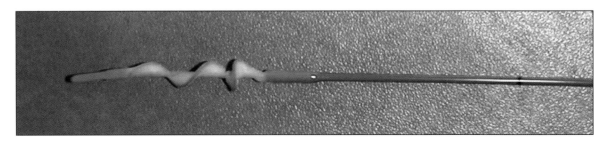

FIG. 5 Fogarty catheter for thrombectomy of a prosthesis.

the cause of the extensive thrombosis that has led to the acute ischemia. It is therefore necessary to treat the lesions as found by completion angiography. These lesions should be treated whenever possible during the same procedure by means of less aggressive endovascular procedures or by endarterectomy. Bypass reconstructions are an alternative in case of extended lesions or failure of the previous techniques.

DISTAL LESION

In the majority of cases the cause of the acute ischemia is located in the femoropopliteal tract. In case of a short, severe stenosis, balloon angioplasty with or without a stent may effectively treat the lesion. Very extended lesions require a bypass reconstruction. Lesions causing acute ischemia are usually multifocal and may reach down to the crural arteries. Balloon angioplasty of a lesion in the crural arteries improves the outflow and diminishes peripheral resistance and, thus, the postoperative risk of re-thrombosis (Fig. 6).

PROXIMAL LESION

A proximal cause should be searched for systematically during the completion angiography, especially when no local or distal cause can be found. These lesions, mostly at the iliac level, may generally be treated by means of angioplasty with or without a stent (Fig. 7). In the rare cases in which no flow is obtained after thrombectomy, an alternative to an extra-anatomical bypass (femorofemoral or axillofemoral) is to perform a retrograde angiogram via a puncture of the contralateral femoral artery. Thus, a pigtail angiographic catheter can be placed in the distal aorta in order to perform an angiogram via an injector of the occluded iliac tract. This contralateral endovascular access may enable a recanalization of the occluded iliac tract from the other side.

ENDARTERECTOMY

In case the lesion cannot be passed by means of guidewires or catheters, endarterectomy may be an alternative before performing a bypass procedure. This may be an open procedure for limited lesions at the femoral bifurcation, but also a remote procedure for proximal (iliac arteries) lesions or distal lesions (superficial femoral and popliteal artery lesions). In this case, the endarterectomy is commenced from the arteriotomy via a ringed device introduced between the atheromatous sequester and the arterial wall. The ring with a matching diameter creates a cleavage plain between wall and atheroma down to just beyond the lesion to be treated.

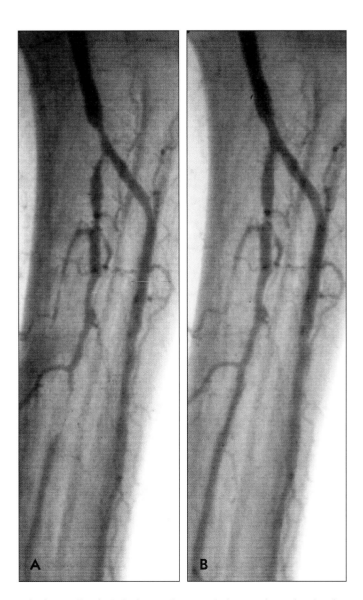

FIG. 6 A - Fig. 6. A. Peri-operative completion arteriography showing severe lesions of the crural arteries distal to a thrombectomy of a femoropopliteal bypass. B - Completion angiography after dilatation.

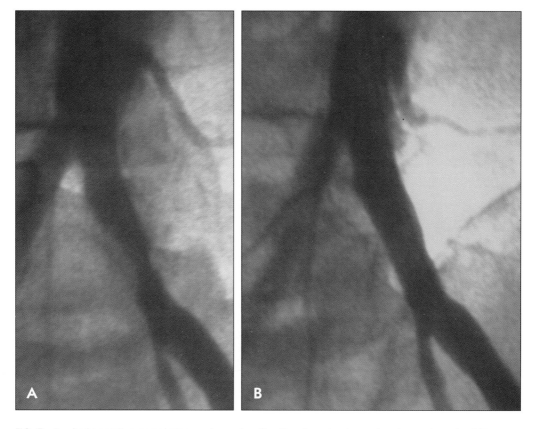

FIG. 7 A - Peri-operative completion angiography after iliac thrombectomy showing a stenosis of the common iliac artery. B - Completion angiography after stenting.

Certain rings contain a system that can dissect the distal end of the plaque under fluoroscopic control [7]. The plaque is then removed completely via the arteriotomy. The novel aspect of this technique (see chapter 20) as compared with procedures performed in the 1970s, is the angiographic control of the distal limit of the endarterectomy. Once the endarterectomy is completed and the plaque removed, a smooth J-guidewire is introduced just beyond the distal limit of the endarterectomy. This is easily estimated by the length of the removed plaque. During this maneuver, one should ensure that the guidewire does not enter the endarterectomy plain, but descends easily into the arterial lumen. Angiographic control is performed after declamping, with the guidewire insitu. In case of an irregularity at the level of the end of the desobstruction, an introducer is placed and a stent is positioned there to fix the distal intimal layer (Fig. 8).

Discussion

Despite early and suitable treatment for acute ischemia, the mortality after surgical treatment has not decreased significantly during the last thirty years [8]. This is in contrast with the progress made in conventional vascular surgery with still improving results. Moreover, the progress in anesthesiology has led to a better peri-operative treatment of these patients, whose medical condition is often compromised. The severe pathology in a precarious area per se is not sufficient to explain the lack of improvement of the results. Obviously another explanation is the fact that these patients are frequently treated in general surgery units and do not benefit from the latest technologies, particularly of fluoroscopy in the operating theater. Furthermore, surgeons who treat them do not always master the pharmacological and endovascular techniques, which can be successfully combined with thrombo-embolectomy.

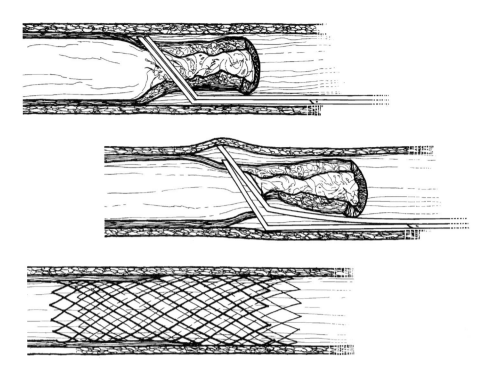

FIG. 8   Scheme showing the principle of distant endarterectomy with fixation of the distal endothelium with a stent.

The reduction in mortality of acute ischemia is due to a reduction in the treatment delay and a reduced invasiveness of the, particularly surgical, therapy. Fluoroscopy points out the lesions to be treated and, thus, reduces the surgical invasiveness by diminishing the need for major reconstructive surgical procedures. Endovascular techniques allow a quick and high-quality revascularization in the case of limited lesions. Single thrombolysis has the drawback of a long latency time, which may be incompatible with limb salvage. Applied in combination with thrombectomy, it has a major influence on the restoration of the outflow toward the calf and foot.

Conclusion

Nowadays, the modern treatment of acute ischemia no longer consists of the choice between thrombolysis and surgical treatment. Fluoroscopically controlled thrombectomy in combination with one or more endovascular or fibrinolytic techniques offers an effective and durable treatment for acute ischemia. Knowledge and control of the total arsenal of these new techniques allows us to choose the best revascularization strategy in order to improve the treatment of these patients and to diminish the mortality of this pathology.

REFERENCES

1 Parsons RE, Martin ML, Veith FJ, et al. Fluoroscopically assisted thromboembolectomy: an improved method for treating acute arterial occlusions. *Ann Vasc Surg* 1996; 10: 201-210.

2 Wagner HJ, Starck EE, Reuter P. Long-term results of percutaneous aspiration embolectomy. *Cardiovasc Intervent Radiol* 1994; 17: 241-246.

3 Gonzalez-Fajardo JA, Perez-Burkhardt JL, Mateo AM. Intraoperative fibrinolytic therapy for salvage of limbs with arterial ischemia: an adjunct to thromboembolectomy. *Ann Vasc Surg* 1995; 9: 179-186.

4 Valji K, Roberts AC, Davis GB, et al. Pulsed-spray thrombolysis of arterial and bypass graft occlusions. *AJR Am J Roentgenol* 1991; 156: 617-621.

5 Comerota AJ, Schmieder FA. Intraoperative lytic therapy: agents and methods of administration. *Sem Vasc Surg* 2001; 14: 132-142.

6 Ouriel K. Endovascular techniques in the treatment of acute limb ischemia: thrombolytic agents, trials, and percutaneous mechanical thrombectomy techniques. *Sem Vasc Surg* 2003; 16: 270-279.

7 Moll FL, Ho GH, Joosten PPh, et al. Endovascular remote endarterectomy in femoropopliteal long segmental occlusive disease. A new surgical technique illustrated and preliminary results using a ring strip cutter device. *J Cardiovasc Surg* 1996; 37: 39-40.

8 Dormandy J, Heeck L, Vig S. Acute limb ischemia. *Sem Vasc Surg* 1999; 12: 148-153.

23

VENOUS THROMBECTOMY
COMBINED WITH ILIOCAVAL STENTING

ROLF GÜNTHER, JOACHIM WILDBERGER
PATRICK HAAGE, THOMAS SCHMITZ-RODE, KARL SCHÜRMANN

Management of venous disease is usually conservative. Even minimally invasive techniques like percutaneous interventions are rarely applied, except in failing hemodialysis fistulas, where balloon dilatation and stenting are frequently used for the management of central and peripheral venous stenoses and occlusions. In thrombosis of deep leg and iliac veins as well as the inferior vena cava (IVC), catheter thrombolysis offers a therapeutic option. The combined approach of percutaneous thrombectomy and iliocaval stenting may be applied successfully in isolated cases of acute thrombosis due to underlying venous stenoses. In chronic venous iliac vein occlusion, the combination of balloon angioplasty and stent implantation without thrombectomy may be considered.

Stent implantation and percutaneous management of thrombotic occlusions are accepted modalities of treatment, mainly in arterial rather than in venous disease. Concomitant acute deep venous thrombosis of the iliac veins may be treated by thrombolysis, surgery, or direct venous interventions. In this chapter the available techniques, indications, and results are presented; we emphasize that the majority of the data available are based on experimental rather than on clinical results.

Options for thrombus removal

During the last ten years, several non-surgical techniques have been developed to treat thrombotic occlusions, including thrombolysis, thrombus frag-mentation, aspiration, and extraction [1]. The table summarizes the experimental and clinical techniques. Catheter-directed thrombolysis has been applied extensively for lower extremity deep venous thrombosis. Mewissen et al. [2] analyzed the results

Table	PERCUTANEOUS THROMBECTOMY MODALITIES

✓ Catheter-directed lysis

✓ Ultrasonic energy-assisted lysis

✓ Oscillating wire enhanced lysis

✓ Mechanical catheter thrombus fragmentation

✓ Rotational recirculation fragmentation

✓ Catheter-based manual thrombus aspiration

✓ Hydrodynamic fragmentation and aspiration

✓ Dormia basket thrombectomy

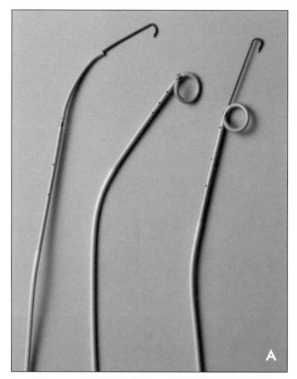

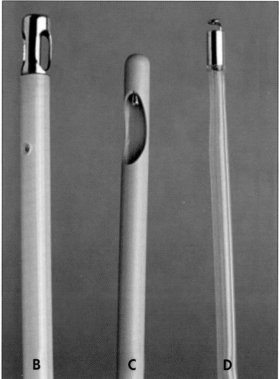

FIG. 1 Devices for fragmentation and removal of thrombus. A - Schmitz-Rode rotating pig-tail catheter (5F). B - Amplatz rotational recirculation catheter (7F). C - D - Rheolytic catheters, Hydrolyser 7F and Possis 5F.

in a national multicenter registry comprising 312 urokinase infusions in 303 limbs (287 patients) affected by symptomatic lower extremity deep venous thrombosis, and concluded that catheter-directed thrombolysis is safe and effective. Thrombolysis and fragmentation can also be achieved by application of ultrasonic energy to a titanium wire [3] or ultrasound-assisted pharmacological lysis. Segmental occlusions can be treated by oscillating sine-shaped wire-enhanced lysis with subsequent aspiration. Figure 1 shows percutaneous mechanical devices for thrombus fragmentation and removal, including the Schmitz-Rode rotateable pigtail catheter, Amplatz recirculation catheter, and rheolytic catheters. These mechanical devices have been applied in experimental and clinical studies [4-7]. Uflacker [7] performed a feasibility study of the Amplatz thrombectomy device in a variety of vascular territories with acute or subacute thrombosis. Technical success was achieved in 11 of 13 patients, and he concluded that this device is useful for recanalization of acute and subacute clotted native vessels and grafts. It should be noted, however, that large prospective studies are not available to confirm these results.

Hydrodynamic fragmentation and thrombus aspiration based on the Venturi effect have been developed and several catheters introduced, including the Hydrolyser, Oasis, and Possis [8-10]. Finally, thrombectomy can be achieved with a Dormia basket (Fig. 2C).

As a general rule, thrombotic material should be removed as early as possible. It has been shown that the leukocyte adhesion molecule P-selectin activates the leukocytes that emigrate in the venous wall resulting in an inflammation, which may be reversible in the early phase [11]. It is not the intention of this chapter to describe the above-mentioned techniques, mainly experimental, in detail but rather to focus on clinically applicable thrombectomy modalities as described in the literature and our personal experience in a limited number of patients.

Caval protection during thrombectomy

Percutaneous thrombectomy can be performed with or without a caval protection device against pulmonary embolism using a transjugular approach, particularly if mechanical thrombectomy and fragmentation are intended. During pharmacological thrombolysis such a protection seems to be unnecessary except in the presence of free-floating iliocaval thrombi.

Venous stenoses may function as a natural barrier against migration of large thrombi and do not necessitate additional caval protection against pulmonary embolization. Under these circumstances thrombectomy does not seem risky since proximal thrombus embolization may be sufficiently prevented by the stenosis proximal to the thrombosed segment. Also, a transfemorally placed Fogarty balloon in the ipsilateral vein can prevent thrombus migration during hydrodynamic thrombectomy in the iliac veins.

During pharmacological lysis of free-floating femoral and iliocaval thrombi, caval filters may be used for temporary protection against pulmonary embolism; however, they are not very suitable for protection during mechanical thrombus manipulation because the interspaces of the filter legs are usually too large to effectively filtrate the resulting multiple thrombotic particles.

Two different devices have been used clinically for that purpose: an expandable caval sheath with a shaft inside diameter (ID) 12F, outside diameter (OD) 15F, expanded sheath length 70 millimeters,

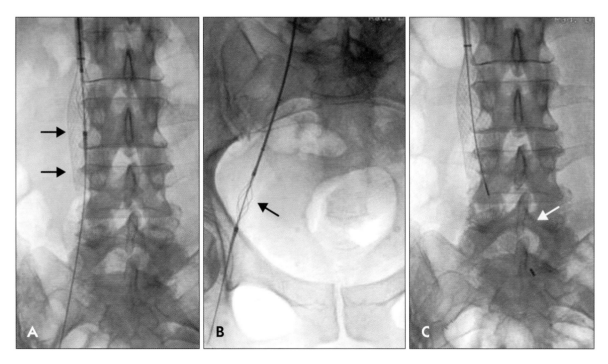

FIG. 2 Caval protection during thrombectomy of a free-floating iliocaval thrombus. A - Expandable sheath *(arrow)*. B - *Arrow-Treretora* device in the right iliac vein *(arrow)* for thrombus fragmentation. C - Thirty millimeter Dormia basket in the left iliac vein *(arrow)* for thrombus extraction. Because of renal insufficiency, no contrast medium was applied during the procedure.

30 millimeters in diameter (Fig. 2) [12], and a large balloon (shaft ID 12F, OD 18F, balloon size 25 millimeters) [13], which can be introduced into the IVC during thrombus removal and fragmentation.

Percutaneous thrombectomy

Thrombectomy in the IVC is usually performed with a Dormia basket, expandable up to 30 millimeters in diameter. All material is removed through the large bore 12F expandable sheath, introduced via a transjugular approach (Fig. 2). The basket extraction technique can also be used for the iliac veins with simultaneous caval protection. Mechanical fragmentation in the femoral veins, however, should not be applied because of the potential damage to the valves.

Mechanical fragmentation of thrombi in the iliac veins can also be performed with an 8F *Arrow-Treretora* motor-driven rotation basket (speed approxi-mately 3000 revolutions per minute) used over a 0.035 inch guidewire [4] (Figs. 2,3). Because of the maximum diameter of the expanded basket of 15 millimeters, the system is too small for the IVC in humans. The same limitation is true for the re-circulation devices *(Amplatz Clot Buster)* and rhe-olytic catheters. Thus, the efficacy of these devices depends on the ratio of the vessel and the catheter diameter.

Apart from the basket extraction technique, thrombectomy can be performed with 5F to 7F rhe-olytic catheters [10]. During the procedure, careful attention must be given to the amount of aspirated blood in order to avoid significant blood loss. Anti-coagulant agent (5000 IU heparin) is administered during the procedure and the need for additional thrombolysis is rare.

Sometimes the results of thrombus removal are disappointing because of the ineffectiveness of a small-caliber device in a relatively large vein, the lack of steerability, or the already organized throm-

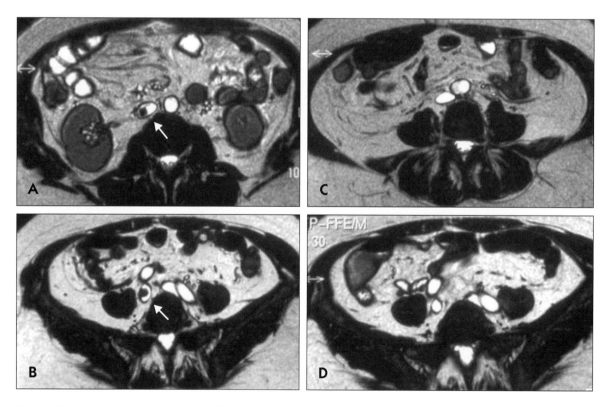

FIG. 3 Magnetic resonance image (True-FISP) before (A,B) and after (C,D) successful thrombectomy of a free-floating thrombus *(arrow)*.

bus. Fresh thrombus is easier to remove than old, organized, and wall-adherent material. There seems to be a time limitation of about ten days after which the success rate of percutaneous thrombus removal drops significantly. After three weeks thrombi are wall-adherent and partly organized so that percutaneous thrombectomy fails.

Stenting

Stents are intravascular devices that serve as a scaffold to maintain lumen patency. In addition, the stent wire mesh leads to compression of thrombotic material and fixation to the vessel wall.

Venous stenting was introduced for stenoses and occlusions of peripheral and central veins draining hemodialysis fistulae [14]. In these patients central venous obstruction often leads to arm edema due to a high volume flow created by the shunt in place. Severe edema in non-shunt leading veins remains rare when sufficient collateralization are present, but may result in constant swelling of the extremity and chronic venous insufficiency.

A large variety of stents are available, ranging from balloon-expandable to self-expandable stents, bare and covered stents, made of nitinol, stainless steel, or different alloys. There are three important criteria for the selection of venous stents: stents should adapt themselves smoothly to the venous wall, they should not migrate, and they should be large enough in diameter (e.g., up to 20 millimeters and more for the IVC) to comply with the size of the veins. Stents suitable for that purpose are self-expandable Wallstents® [9] (Figs. 4,5) or Gianturco® stents [15]. In case of severe stenosis

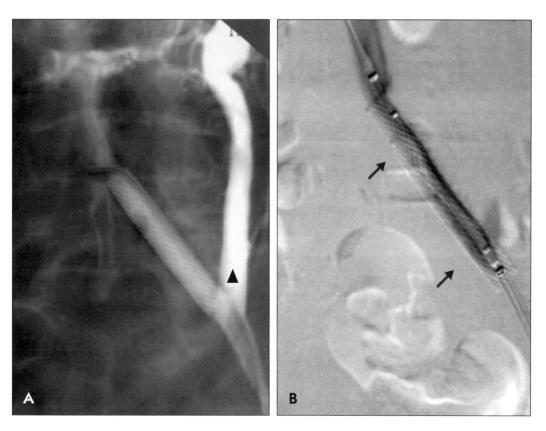

FIG. 4 Pelvic vein spur leading to venous flow obstruction of the left lower extremity. A - Venography during implantation of the first stent (self-expandable *Wallstent*) shows large collateral pathway via the left ascending lumbar vein *(arrowhead)*. B - After placement of a second overlapping stent *(arrows)* free flow has been restored.

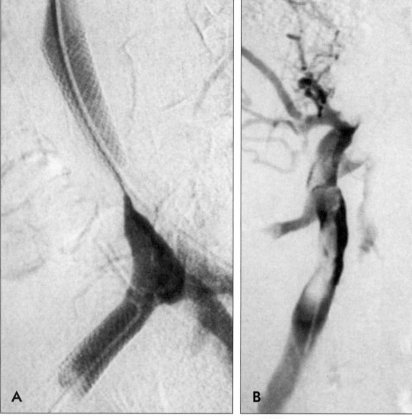

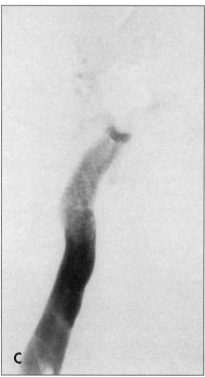

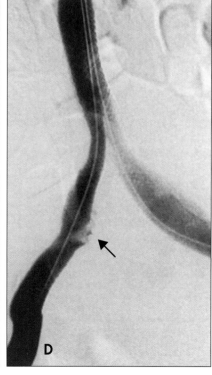

FIG. 5 A 64-year-old patient with retroperitoneal fibrosis treated with caval and right iliac vein stenting because of bilateral leg edema [9].

A - Four weeks later, recurrent edema occurred due to severe stenosis of the IVC beneath the stent and high-grade stenoses of both common iliac veins close the caval junction as shown by iliac venography (percutaneous transfemoral catheter in the right iliac vein and transjugular catheter in the left iliac vein).

B - Two days later, right-sided venography shows fresh thrombus in the external iliac vein and occlusion of the common iliac vein.

C - After hydrodynamic thrombectomy, the external iliac vein is free from thrombus but occlusion of the common iliac vein persists.

D - After bilateral stenting, crossing of the internal iliac vein on the right side, patency of both iliac veins is restored. Small residual thrombus is seen in the orifice of the right internal iliac vein *(arrow)*.

where the expansion force of self-expandable stents is not sufficient, an additional balloon-expandable stent (e.g., Palmaz-Stent) can be inserted within the self-expandable stent for stabilization. Covered stents are not required for venous stenting. Long-term anticoagulation is indicated in iliac veins, whereas in IVC stents short-term anticoagulation suffices in our experience.

Side effects of stenting are related to stent thrombosis and intimal hyperplasia. Stent thrombosis is usually an early complication, whereas intimal hyperplasia may develop within six months as a mid-term side effect.

Indications

General indications for percutaneous thrombectomy in the venous system are mainly acute superior caval thrombosis, subclavian vein thrombosis, thrombosis of hemodialysis fistulas and grafts, and acute iliocaval thrombosis.

Iliofemoral vein thrombosis is an indication for thrombolysis rather than percutaneous thrombectomy, whereas in iliocaval thrombosis the above techniques of percutaneous thrombectomy can be applied, particularly if there are contra-indications to systemic or local lysis.

General indications for venous stenting in the iliocaval system include symptomatic stenoses and occlusions in pelvic vein spur, retroperitoneal fibrosis, stenosis following surgery, irradiation or thrombosis, peri-iliocaval tumors, and Budd-Chiari syndrome (associated with caval stenosis).

Venous thrombectomy associated with stenting in iliocaval thrombosis can be considered as a hybrid procedure, combining both thrombolysis and/or percutaneous thrombectomy with additional iliocaval stenting. This hybrid approach is indicated if thrombosis is a secondary phenomenon caused by an underlying iliac or caval vein stenosis, as listed above (Fig. 5). Thrombosis can be acute or chronic. In both instances balloon angioplasty (percutaneous transluminal angioplasty [PTA]) is performed prior to stenting. Since lumen increase obtained by PTA is unlikely to be maintained and recurrent stenosis occurs, early stenting is helpful to stabilize the venous segment treated. Apart from percutaneous thrombectomy, alternative forms of treatment to be considered prior to stenting are systemic thrombolysis and surgical thrombectomy. Also surgical thrombectomy can be combined with additional stent implantation [16].

Results

Catheter-directed thrombolysis has been used successfully for the treatment of iliofemoral thrombosis [2], although there is yet no sufficient evidence for the clinical efficacy of this intervention on a larger basis. Isolated cases have been reported where mechanical fragmentation [7,9] or hydrodynamic/rheolytic devices [10] without additional stenting were applied.

Mechanical thrombectomy may damage the endothelium and cause valve injury, as observed in animal experiments [17,18]. Since valve integrity is of major concern, mechanical thrombectomy using rotating devices should be avoided in the femoral vein, in contrast to the iliocaval veins.

Regarding the combination of percutaneous thrombectomy and stent placement, there are few clinical reports addressing acute thrombosis and demonstrating the feasibility of this approach [9,15] (Fig. 5); however, there are no larger series. The combination of balloon angioplasty and stenting without thrombectomy has also been described by some authors in chronic iliac venous occlusion [19, 20].

Potential complications of percutaneous thrombectomy and stent implantation include recurrent thrombosis due to endothelial injury during mechanical thrombectomy and stent thrombogenicity. The risk of pulmonary embolism is rare when adequate technical precautions are taken during manipulation of fresh thrombosis as described above. Stented venous segments are also prone to neointimal growth and may develop restenosis.

Mickley et al. [16] reported on their results of surgical thrombectomy combined with an inguinal arteriovenous fistula in 76 patients and subsequent stenting. A total of 26 stents were implanted for 20 stenoses (8 spurs, all post-thrombotic and post-operative stenoses). In 25 of 26 patients the venous lumen was completely restored. Three of four restenoses were successfully treated by another intervention. There was one late failure at 60 months. The cumulative primary and secondary patency rates were 72% and 88%, respectively.

Conclusion

Percutaneous thrombectomy may be applied in acute iliocaval thrombosis. If thrombosis is caused by an underlying venous stenosis, thrombectomy can be combined with balloon angioplasty and stent implantation. Thus, this hybrid percutaneous approach offers a minimally invasive alternative to surgery in the treatment of those lesions.

REFERENCES

1 Sharafuddin MJ, Hicks ME. Current status of percutaneous mechanical thrombectomy. Part II. Devices and mechanisms of action. *J Vasc Interv Radiol* 1998; 9: 15-31.

2 Mewissen MW, Seabrook GR, Meissner MH, et al. Catheter-directed thrombolysis for lower extremity deep venous thrombosis: report of a national multicenter registry. *Radiology* 1999; 211: 39-49.

3 Polak JF, Chen F, Marciante R, et al. Thrombolysis by application of ultrasonic energy to a titanium wire: estimation of particle size. *J Vasc Interv Radiol* 2002; 13: S76.

4 Haage P, Tacke J, Bovelander J, et al. Prototype percutaneous thrombolytic device: preclinical testing in subacute inferior vena caval thrombosis in a pig model. *Radiology* 2001; 220: 135-141.

5 Gandini R, Maspes F, Sodani G, et al. Percutaneous ilio-caval thrombectomy with the Amplatz device: preliminary results. *Eur Radiol* 1999; 9: 951-958.

6 Gu X, Sharafuddin MJ, Titus JL, et al. Acute and delayed outcomes of mechanical thrombectomy with use of the steerable Amplatz thrombectomy device in a model of subacute inferior vena cava thrombosis. *J Vasc Interv Radiol* 1997; 8: 947-956.

7 Uflacker R. Mechanical thrombectomy in acute and subacute thrombosis with use of the Amplatz device: arterial and venous applications. *J Vasc Interv Radiol* 1997; 8: 923-932.

8 Tacke J, Vorwerk D, Bucker A, et al. Experimental treatment of early chronic iliac vein thrombosis with a modified hydrodynamic thrombectomy catheter: preliminary animal experience. *J Vasc Interv Radiol* 1999; 10: 57-63.

9 Vorwerk D, Günther RW, Wendt G, et al. Iliocaval stenosis and iliac venous thrombosis in retroperitoneal fibrosis: percutaneous treatment by use of hydrodynamic thrombectomy and stenting. *Cardiovasc Intervent Radiol* 1996; 19: 40-42.

10 Reekers JA, Blank LE. Iliocaval thrombosis: percutaneous treatment with hydrodynamic thrombectomy. *Eur Radiol* 2000; 10: 326-328.

11 Downing LJ, Wakefield TW, Strieter RM, et al. Anti-P-selectin antibody decreases inflammation and thrombus formation in venous thrombosis. *J Vasc Surg* 1997; 25: 815-828.

12 Schmitz-Rode T, Vorwerk D, Schurmann K, Günther RW. Experimental impeller fragmentation of iliocaval thrombosis under tulip filter protection: preliminary results. *Cardiovasc Intervent Radiol* 1996; 19: 260-264.

13 Wildberger JE, Schmitz-Rode T, Reffelmann T, et al. Percutaneous transjugular thrombectomy in iliocaval thrombosis. Initial experience with a newly developed 12F balloon sheath. *Rofo Fortschr Geb Rontgenstr Neuen Bildgeb Verfahr* 2000; 172: 651-655.

14 Haage P, Vorwerk D, Piroth W, et al. Treatment of hemodialysis-related central venous stenosis or occlusion: results of primary Wallstent placement and follow-up in 50 patients. *Radiology* 1999; 212: 175-180.

15 Yamauchi T, Furui S, Katoh R, et al. Acute thrombosis of the inferior vena cava: treatment with saline-jet aspiration thrombectomy catheter. *AJR Am J Roentgenol* 1993; 161: 405-407.

16 Mickley V, Schwagierek R, Schutz A, et al. Stent implantation after thrombectomy of pelvic veins. Indications, results. *Zentralbl Chir* 1999; 124: 12-17.

17 van Ommen V, van der Veen FH, Daemen MJ, et al. In vivo evaluation of the Hydrolyser hydrodynamic thrombectomy catheter. *J Vasc Interv Radiol* 1994; 5: 823-826.

18 Sharafuddin MJ, Gu X, Han YM, et al. Injury potential to venous valves for the Amplatz thrombectomy device. *J Vasc Interv Radiol* 1999; 10: 64-69.

19 Raju S, McAllister S, Neglen P. Recanalization of totally occluded iliac and adjacent venous segments. *J Vasc Surg* 2002; 36: 903-911.

20 Neglen P, Raju S. Balloon dilation and stenting of chronic iliac vein obstruction: technical aspects and early clinical outcome. *J Endovasc Ther* 2000; 7: 79-91.

24

EMBOLIZATION COMBINED WITH OPEN SURGERY TO TREAT COMPLEX CONGENITAL VASCULAR MALFORMATIONS

CHANTAL VAN DER HORST

Vascular anomalies can be subdivided in hemangiomas and vascular malformations. The prevalence of hemangiomas in the general newborn population is 10%. Only a small amount (7%) of children with problematic hemangiomas due to ulceration or complications related to localization are seen by specialists. Vascular malformations like capillary malformations are seen in 3 per 1000 newborns. Venous, arterio-venous or lymphatic malformations are even more rare.

Vascular malformations can cause significant morbidity in children and in adults. Most patients with a problematic vascular malformation or hemangioma are sent to centers where they are seen in a combined outpatient clinic in which physicians of different subspecialties like vascular surgery, radiology, dermatology and plastic surgery combine their skills to provide these patients with a adequate treatment plan.

This is also the case in our center for vascular anomalies. When additional knowledge is required an orthopedic surgeon or pediatrician with special knowledge of vascular anomalies is added to the team. Since similar teams are mainly organized in tertiary referral centers, knowledge about these anomalies is not wide spread among general physicians.

Most patients referred to our center have already been treated before without improvement and without sufficient information as to what to expect from the treatment.

Before focusing on these treatments in which embolization and open surgery are combined, it is appropriate to describe the process of achieving the correct diagnosis since misdiagnoses lead to disappointing results.

Diagnosis

Although already in 1982 Mulliken and Glowacki published their classification on hemangiomas and vascular malformations based on natural history, cellular turnover and histology, still a lot of confusion exists about the nomenclature of these anomalies (Table) [1].

HEMANGIOMAS

Hemangiomas are in 75% of the cases absent at birth and in 25% visible as a white spot or reddish patch with visible small vessels. After birth a hemangioma shows a tendency of fast growth (proliferative phase) approximately until the age of one year. After the proliferative phase a hemangioma enters a stationary phase (no growth) lasting one to several years and a phase of involution (regression) varying from very fast to prolonged regression, sometimes lasting until adolescence. In 5% of the patients a hemangioma does not regress completely. Tele-angiectasias, fibrofatty tissue and skin discoloration can stay after involution. In the proliferative phase ulcerations, bleeding, obstruction of the visual axis or airway and "cosmetic" problems are the reasons for clinical presentation (Fig. 1).

Table	TRANSLATION OF OLD TERMINOLOGY TO NEW TERMINOLOGY (CLASSIFICATION)
Old terminology	*New terminology*
	Hemangioma
Strawberry	Strawberry hemangioma
Capillary	Capillary hemangioma
Capillary cavernous	Capillary cavernous hemangioma
	Malformation
Port-wine	Port-wine malformation
Cavernous	Venous malformation
Venous	Venous malformation
Hemangio-lymphangioma	Venous-lymphatic malformation
Lymphangioma	Lymphatic malformation
Arteriovenous	Arteriovenous malformation

VASCULAR MALFORMATIONS

Vascular malformations are always present at birth (although not always recognized) and enlarge in proportion with the growing child. These malformations never regress spontaneously and remain present during the patient's life. Especially during adolescence or during/after pregnancy, under influence of hormones, or after trauma, patients present themselves with complaints of their malformation. Vascular malformations are divided in capillary, venous, lymphatic arteriovenous or mixed malformations on the basis of their histologic composition.

Confusion on diagnosis is also created by pathology reports. Only in the case of a hemangioma in the proliferative phase a proper discernment could be made, in the past, with respect to vascular malformations. In the stationary and involutionary phase all hemangiomas were mentioned cavernous hemangiomas, sharing this kind of description with venous malformations. Immunohistochemical studies from North et al. [2] have recently demonstrated a fundamental similarity between the vasculature of infantile hemangiomas and the placenta. Infantile hemangiomas in all stages of evolution express tissue-specific markers like glucose transporter proteine isoform 1 (Glut-1), Lewis-antigen, Fc gamma receptor ll and merosine which are not expressed in normal skin or in vascular malformations. In case of doubt on the diagnosis pathology reports can currently distinguish between hemangiomas and vascular malformations [2].

Capillary malformations (CM) are composed of distended capillaries in skin and mucosal membranes. Endothelial lining of the capillaries are normal. CM offer a psychological burden to patients, especially when affecting the face. When distended capillaries are not only present in the skin but also in subcutaneous tissue, muscle and mucosa, the patient presents with hypertrophy of the affected part of the face. Treatment can be performed with a pulsed-dye laser [3]. Sometimes a capillary malformation on the face occurs with glaucoma and epilepsia, together forming the Sturge-Weber syndrome (Fig. 2). Capillary malformation on the extremities combined with overgrowth and venous abnormalities is called Klippel-Trenaunay syndrome. Evidence for a genetic cause is growing [4].

Lymphatic malformations aggravate during infections (upper airway) and are prone to infection. The lymphatic malformation can subsequently swell enormously and patients are severely ill (Fig. 3). The most common locations of lymphangiomas are

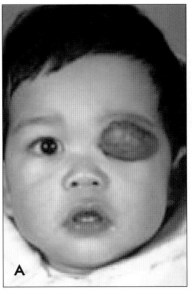

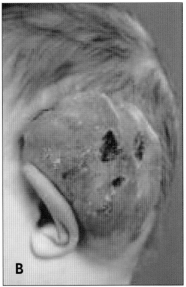

FIG. 1 A - Hemangioma causing amblyopia because of localization before eye axis. B - Ulcerated and bleeding hemangioma.

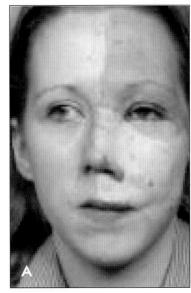

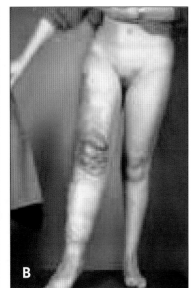

FIG. 2 Capillary malformations in Sturge Weber syndrome (A), and in Klippel-Trenaunay syndrome (B).

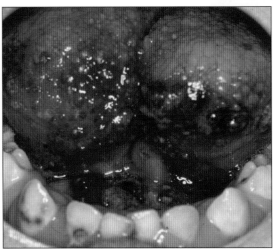

FIG. 3 Lymphatic malformation of a tongue.

neck (75%) and axilla, sometimes with extensions in mediastinum, retroperitoneum and pelvis. When present in the neck a lymphatic malformation is often called hygroma colli cysticum, referring to the presence of big cysts. A lymphatic malformation in bone can lead to overgrowth of the bone. Compression during physical examination is not possible. Patients with a lymphatic malformation usually do not present themselves with pain, unless infected. Resection is advised in cases of macro-cystic disease, whereas microcystic lymphatic malformations are treated by embolization (alcohol 98%, OK-234, glue or Ethiblock) [5].

Pain, however, is the main reason for patients with venous malformations to seek medical attention. This pain is mainly due to trombo-embolic processes taking place in venous malformations, leading to calcifications which can be palpated as little balls (fleboliths) in the subcutaneous tissues. These round balls can be seen on plain X-ray and are pathognomonic for venous malformations. Clinical presentation with venous malformations can also be induced by cosmetic reasons or sudden swelling (intramuscular tumor). When present in the skin, blue discoloration can be seen. Depending on localization and extent of the affected area, swelling can lead to impressive effects, for example breathing problems when a venous malformation is localized in the neck area.

Physical examination provides additional information on venous malformations since they can be emptied when the affected extremity is elevated or compressed and filled with leg dependency or when compression is released. On the contrary, an arteriovenous malformation cannot be compressed. In these cases pulsations can be detected by palpation or doppler signal.

ADDITIONAL ASSESSMENT

Additional investigations to acquire a proper diagnosis can be performed by magnetic resonance imaging (MRI) and sonography. Duplex scanning is the easiest and first choice method of assessment, allowing depiction of the vascular mass and its extension. Doppler analysis is highly effective in confirming the presence of hyperperfusion (high-flow), which is typical for arteriovenous malformations. Venous malformations are characterized by low-flow patterns. Apart from diagnostic arguments, diagnosing a high-flow malformation is important with regard to therapy and prognosis because hyperperfusion is the main cause of symptoms, complications

and treatment difficulties of arteriovenous malformations. MRI is the gold standard in the evaluation of vascular malformations, being able to give information on anatomical extension of the malformation and on flow characteristics [6-8]. High-flow voids seen on MRI are indicative of an arteriovenous malformation, low-flow of a venous, lymphatic or capillary malformation. A flow void in a mainly venous malformation may be a phlebolite.

Only when dealing with a high flow malformation an angiography is performed. MR-images after gadolinium enhancement help to differentiate between lymphatic and venous malformations. Lymphatic malformations do not exhibit central enhancement with gadolinium. Besides this, fluid-levels can be present only in lymphatic malformations.

High-flow vascular malformations are formed by arteriovenous fistulas, arteriovenous malformations (AVM) and by hemangiomas in the proliferating phase. All these entities share the same symptoms on physical examination: warm and pulsating on palpation. Sometimes a thrill is palpable. Hemangiomas are discerned from arteriovenous malformations and fistula by their history: no swelling present at birth and fast growth directly after birth. Arteriovenous fistulas are mainly seen after trauma like a history of a stab wound. Also hair transplants can lead to arteriovenous fistulas. AVMs consist of multiple direct connections between arteries and veins, without capillary connections. They may be present in childhood and progress during puberty or pregnancy. Also use of oral contraceptives can cause exacerbation of the AVM. AVMs are rare compared to other vascular malformations. Presenting symptoms can be severe bleeding, ulceration, pain, congestive heart failure or cosmetic problems. Congestive heart failure is only seen as a complication of extensive, often abdominal AVM.

Therapeutic options for AVMs are embolization, operative resection or operative resection and reconstruction with a free flap.

Embolization

Embolization with different materials like glue, ethanol, coils and/or particles is the treatment of choice either alone or in combination with operation. Embolization is performed via arterial catheterisation in case of arteriovenous malformations. Venous or lymphatic access via direct puncture or guided by ultrasound is performed in case of venous or lymphatic malformations. Embolization has to be performed supraselectively because when proximal vessels are embolized, recruitment of other feeding vessels to the AVM can occur or collateral vessels formed, which subsequently leads to revascularization of the AVM. A hybrid procedure combining embolization and surgery is indicated if the symptoms and/or the occurrence of complications justify resection of the vascular malformation. These procedures should follow the same principles as in oncology surgery in which the malformation is radically excised. Embolization is performed prior to surgery in order to decrease intra-operative blood loss. The delay between embolization and surgery should be limited to one or two weeks in order to prevent new arterial pedicels to grow. Complications are seen in 20% of the cases, especially after embolization with ethanol. The latter is the most effective material to embolize, however, it can lead to extensive skin necrosis.

Embolization can be performed without anesthesia only if particles or glue are used. General anesthesia is necessary when using alcohol because of extreme pain and cardiotoxity. Alcohol can only be used in experienced hands because of the chance of necrosis (Fig. 4,5).

Surgery

Operative resections are indicated if patients have severe complaints (bleeding and/or pain). Before operating, embolization with particles can be performed to limit blood loss. Surgery is only considered when resection can be complete. Leaving tissue which is affected by AVM may cause repeated complaints of the AVM. Sometimes, amputation is the only option left and can be a relief for patients suffering from recurrent bleeding.

OPERATIVE RESECTION AND RECONSTRUCTION WITH A FREE FLAP

AVMs can be very troublesome during periods of bleeding and pain. We have to realize, however, that AVMs represent a benign lesion. An example of a dilemma is resection of a hemifacial AVM. The possible postoperative hemifacial paralysis is only justified when the AVM is severely bleeding. Likewise, resection of an AVM residing in several muscle groups in a leg is only acceptable when pain in this

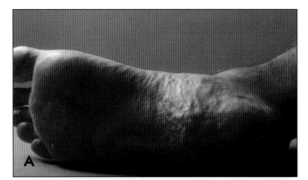

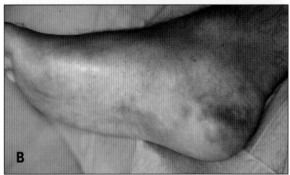

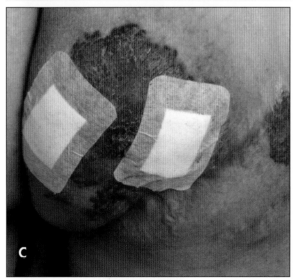

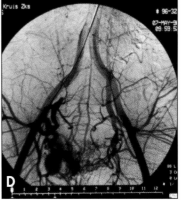

FIG. 4 A - AVM of the sole of the foot. B - After transarterial embolization, circulation in medial heel was marginal. Sensation was disturbed during six months. Pain of the AVM is cured for four years now. C - AVM re buttock pre-embolization. D - Angiography before embolization.

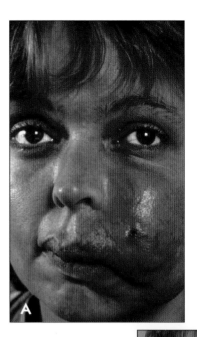

FIGURE 5
Arteriovenous malformation of the left side of the face.

A - Just after severe bleeding which stopped after two hours of compression.

region is permanent and severely invalidating. In Fig. 6 an AVM is shown in the thenar and thumb of a 27 years old man who did not dare to leave his house anymore because of repeated arterial bleeding. Multiple sessions with embolizations did not lead to control of bleeding. He wanted to avoid amputation of the first ray of his hand to any means. Resection was performed of the AVM of his thenar. His thumb was sceletonized up to the bone and digital nerves. Only unaffected skin and soft tissue on the tip of the thumb were left and a radial forearm flap was used to cover the bare area of the thumb. In the years after the tip started to bleed again. He refused amputation.

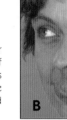
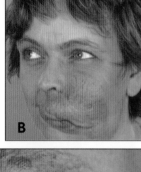

B - Eight years later after several sessions of transarterial and venous side embolization acute arterial bleeding started again intra-orally.

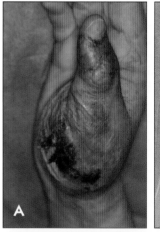
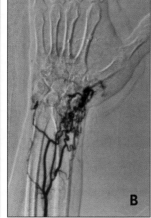

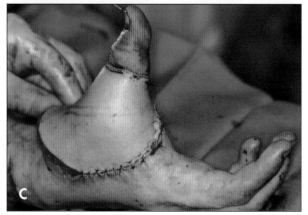

C - After 98% alcohol embolization on the venous side of the AVM, necrosis occurred.

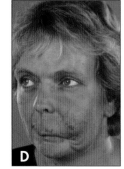

D - One year after heeling of the necrosis. No recurrence of bleeding, no pulsations palpable.

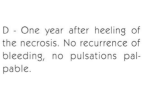

FIG. 6 A - Severe bleeding of thumb AVM. B - After pre-operative embolization. C - After resection and reconstruction with radial forearm flap.

Conclusion

Vascular anomalies constitute a major challenge for the patient and the physician. Proper diagnosis is crucial before treatment modalities are considered. Hemangiomas and vascular malformations require a multidisciplinary approach, allowing the most optimal hybrid treatment to handle these relatively rare disorders.

REFERENCES

1 Mulliken JB, Glowacki J. Hemangiomas and vascular malformations in infants and children: a classification based on endothelial characteristics. *Plast Reconstr Surg* 1982; 69: 412-422.

2 North PE, Waner M, Mizeracki A, et al. A unique microvascular phenotype shared by juvenile hemangiomas and human placenta. *Arch Dermatol* 2001; 137: 559-570.

3 van der Horst CM, Koster PH, de Borgie CA, et al. Effect of timing of treatment of port-wine stains with the flash-lamp-pumped pulsed-dye laser. *N Engl J Med* 1998; 338: 1028-1033.

4 Breugem CC, Alders M, Salieb-Beugelaar GB, et al. A locus for hereditary capillary malformations mapped on chromosome 5q. *Hum Genet* 2002; 110: 343-347.

5 Giguere CM, Bauman NM, Smith RJ. New treatment options for lymphangioma in infants and children. *Ann Otol Rhinol Laryngol* 2002; 111: 1066-1075.

6 Breugem CC, Maas M, Breugem SJ, et al. Vascular malformations of the lower extremity with osseous involvement. *J Bone Joint Surg Br* 2003; 85: 399-405.

7 Breugem CC, Maas M, Reekers JA, van der Horst CM. Use of magnetic resonance imaging for the evaluation of vascular malformations of the lower extremity. *Plast Reconstr Surg* 2001; 108: 870-877.

8 Hein KD, Mulliken JB, Kozakewich HP, et al. Venous malformations of skeletal muscle. *Plast Reconstr Surg* 2002; 110: 1625-1035.

9 Lee BB, Bergan JJ. Advanced management of congenital vascular malformations: a multidisciplinary approach. *Cardiovasc Surg* 2002; 10: 523-533.

25

HYBRID PROCEDURES IN VASCULAR ACCESS FOR HEMODIALYSIS

VOLKER MICKLEY

Thrombosis is a common complication in arteriovenous shunts for hemodialysis. In most cases, one or more stenoses can be identified as the cause(s). Correction of these stenoses is an integral part of any declotting procedure, in which surgical bypass or patch or balloon angioplasty with and without stent implantation are therapeutic options.

In the literature, autogenous arteriovenous access studies comparing the relative values of surgical and interventional declotting procedures and comparing the different options to treat a stenosis are lacking. From recently published surgical and interventional series, however, it can be deducted that the preferred treatment of the most frequent type of stenosis (located closely to the arteriovenous anastomosis) consists of performing a more central new anastomosis. Thus, there seem to be limited options for hybrid procedures in thrombosed arteriovenous fistulae (AVF).

Hemodialysis artificial access grafts are implanted when an autogenous arteriovenous access cannot or can no longer be created due to hypoplasia or absence of superficial arm veins. Therefore, in case a graft fails, any procedure that salvages the venous system should be preferred over an operation, which could potentially cause further damage. Therefore, correction of a local stenosis with patch or balloon angioplasty is preferred to surgical bypass whenever possible. For hemodialysis patients with a thrombosed access graft, the endovascular surgeon is potentially the ideal partner because following catheter thrombectomy and on-table angiography, he is free to choose the best interventional or surgical treatment option, depending on the site and the extent of the obstruction.

Arteriovenous access thrombosis

The native AVF has been shown to provide the most reliable and durable method of access for hemodialysis. Complication rates are lower than those associated with arteriovenous grafts (AVGs) and central venous catheters (CVCs). Furthermore, AVF patient survival is significantly longer, even when corrected for comorbidity [1,2]. However, when hypoplastic or absent peripheral veins or severely diseased peripheral arteries hinder the construction of an autogenous access, a synthetic graft or even a catheter will be required to start or maintain renal replacement therapy.

The most frequent acute complication of arteriovenous access for hemodialysis is thrombosis. Of course, access thrombosis can be bridged with a CVC for hemodialysis until the planned intervention the next day or even some days later. However, one must not forget that implantation of a CVC is burdened with a high rate of acute and late complications [3]. The well-known disadvantages and potential dangers of CVC for hemodialysis should encourage immediate declotting of a thrombosed access with subsequent correction of any underlying stenosis, in a such way that the access can be used again for the next planned hemodialysis session.

The different surgical and interventional alternatives for the treatment of stenosed and thrombosed AVF and AVGs have been dealt with extensively in earlier EVC textbooks [4,5]. Therefore, this chapter only addresses their combination as hybrid procedures in acute thrombosis, based on the author's experience and the admittedly scarce literature on this subject.

Hybrid procedures in thrombosed vascular access grafts

PART I
PROSPECTIVE RANDOMIZED STUDY COMPARING CONVENTIONAL AND ENDOVASCULAR REPAIR OF VENOUS ANASTOMOTIC STENOSES

Thirty-six patients presenting with acute occlusion of their forearm looped expanded polytetra-fluoroethylene (ePTFE) AVG were enrolled in a prospective study if, after Fogarty catheter thrombectomy, on-table angiography demonstrated obstruction at the graft-to-vein anastomosis as the only reason for graft thrombosis.

The graft was opened through a traverse skin incision over the distal part of the venous limb of the loop at the greatest possible distance from the venous anastomosis. After thrombectomy, the arterial graft limb and the feeding artery were opacified first to rule out residual clot and inflow stenosis. The injection was performed through a short, large-bore cannula (not via an introducer sheath) in order not to miss midgraft stenoses. Following this, the same was done for the venous graft limb and the venous outflow.

If on-table angiography demonstrated a stenosis at the graft-to-vein anastomosis longer than 5 centimeters or a complete occlusion of the outflow vein, graft extension to a more proximal vein was performed (13 patients) using a 6 or a 7 millimeter standard wall ePTFE graft. The remaining patients were randomly allocated to either patch angioplasty (12 patients) or dilatation of their venous anastomotic stenoses (11 patients). For the patches, thin-walled ePTFE was used. Angioplasty was performed with high-pressure balloons. In most patients a balloon with a diameter one millimeter larger than the graft diameter was chosen in order to completely re-open or even slightly over-dilate the stenosis. A Wallstent® was implanted in 2 of 11 patients because of elastic recoil of their stenosis (Figs. 1 through 5).

All patients could be followed-up with a mean of 12 months. Primary patency was defined to end with the first re-thrombosis of the access, irrespective of its cause. After declotting the newly thrombosed access, angioplasty was the treatment of choice if the venous anastomosis was stenosed again. Secondary patency of the corrected venous anastomoses ended if bypass surgery was required again. Results were calculated according to the life-table method (Table I).

Graft extension seemed to have a better primary patency rate at six months, but the differences between the treatment modalities were no longer significant at one year. To gain the secondary patency rates given in Table I, approximately four re-interventions per patient and per year were necessary, without significant differences between the groups.

PART II
PROSPECTIVE STUDY ON THE RESULTS OF PRIMARY INTRA-OPERATIVE STENT IMPLANTATION FOR VENOUS ANASTOMOTIC STENOSES OF AVGs

Because of the disappointing results of balloon dilatation, a second study was performed in 40 consecutive patients with a thrombosed forearm or upper arm access graft in whom, after surgical thrombectomy and angioplasty, a Wallstent® was implanted into the stenosis. The surgical and endovascular techniques have been detailed in Part I. The definitions of primary and secondary patency were the same as in the first study. Overall primary patency rates were better for angioplasty with stent implantation than for angioplasty alone, but a subgroup analysis according to the site of the venous anastomosis showed that stents deployed in joint regions (elbow, axilla) did not help to extend patency, whereas stents implanted into a venous graft anastomosis located in the upper arm performed fairly well (Figs. 6 and 7).

Discussion

AVF THROMBOSIS

Since the publication by Dapunt et al. in 1987 [6], no study has been published comparing the treatment results of interventional and surgical treatment of AVF stenosis and thrombosis. Unfortunately, surgical treatment was not standardized in this study. In some of the patients only thrombectomy was performed, and an eventually underlying stenosis remained untreated. Consequently, patency rates after surgery were significantly worse than after angioplasty.

Publications on hybrid procedures in thrombosed AVF are completely lacking. Provided that modern

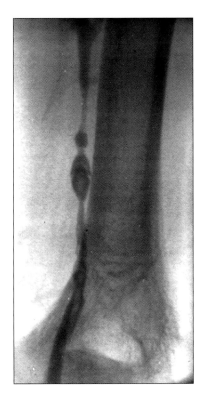

FIG. 1 *String of beads* -like stenoses of the venous anastomosis and of the draining brachial vein of a forearm looped 6 millimeter AVG detected during surgical thrombectomy.

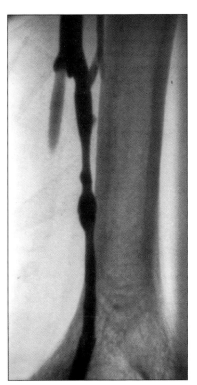

FIG. 2 Significant residual stenoses due to elastic recoil of the dilated vein segment despite prolonged dilatation with a 7 millimeter high-pressure balloon.

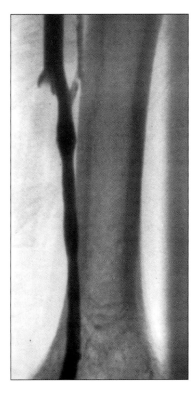

FIG. 3 Satisfying result after implantation of a *Wallstent*® (8 mm x 8 cm) into the stenotic area.

Table I

PATENCY RATES OF DIFFERENT THERAPEUTIC MODALITIES FOR THE TREATMENT OF A VENOUS ANASTOMOTIC OBSTRUCTION DETECTED DURING SURGICAL THROMBECTOMY OF A THROMBOSED ARTERIOVENOUS GRAFT

| Method | Number of patients | Primary patency rates - % | | | | | Secondary patency rates - % | | | | |
		0*	6	12	18	24	0*	6	12	18	24
Graft extension	13	100	42	11	-	-	100	66	30	-	-
Patch angioplasty	12	100	8	8	-	-	100	45	27	-	-
Balloon angioplasty	11	100	19	4	-	-	100	100	76	-	-
Balloon angioplasty with stent implantation	40	100	60	21	11	7	100	95	64	44	36

* Procedural success

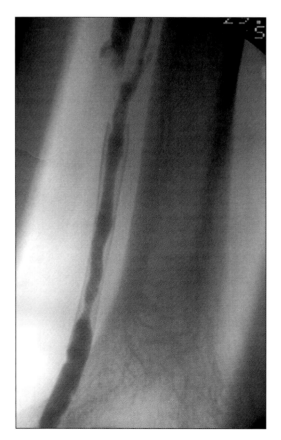

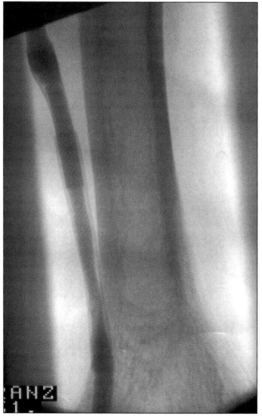

FIG. 4 Excessive intimal hyperplasia within the stented vein segment and short occlusion of the main draining vein detected during graft thrombectomy 16 months after stent implantation.

FIG. 5 Mild residual stenosis after in-stent dilatation and re-opening of the main draining vein with implantation of another overlapping *Wallstent*®.

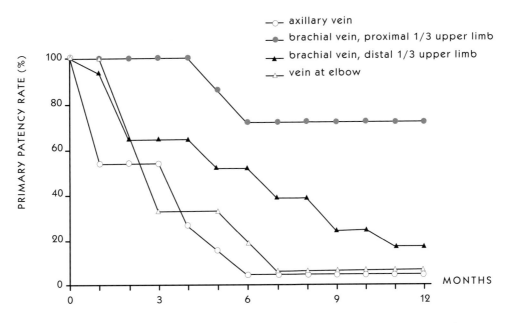

FIG. 6 Primary patency rates of venous anastomotic stents implanted during surgical thrombectomy of AVG depending on the location of the anastomosis.

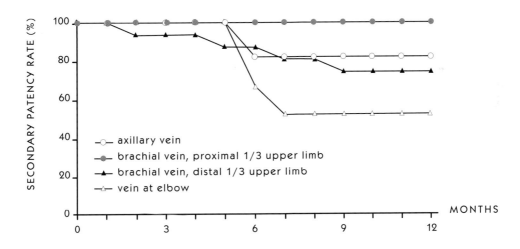

FIG. 7 Secondary patency rates of venous anastomotic stents implanted during surgical thrombectomy of AVG depending on the location of the anastomosis.

interventional declotting techniques are as effective in a hemodialysis fistula as is surgical thrombectomy, the potential results of combined surgical and interventional procedures can be deducted from the recent radiological literature (Table II) [7-14].

About 80% of stenoses leading to occlusion of AVF are found at the arteriovenous anastomosis or close to it. Surgical dissection and mobilization of the vein on one hand and the extremely turbulent flow within a functioning arteriovenous connection

| Table II | | PRIMARY AND SECONDARY PATENCY RATES FOLLOWING INTERVENTIONAL AND SURGICAL THERAPY OF ARTERIOVENOUS FISTULAE-STENOSES ACCORDING TO THE LITERATURE | | | | | | | | | | | | |

1st author [ref.]	*Year of publication*	*Number of patients*	*Primary patency rates - %* MONTHS					*Secondary patency rates - %* MONTHS				
			0❶	6	12	18	24	0❶	6	12	18	24
Interventional radiology												
Lay et al. [7]	1998	36	90	77	64		39	90	85	81		65
Zaleski et al. [8]	1999	17	82	71	64			82	82	82		
Haage et al. [9]	2000	54	89	52	27			89	65	51		22
Rocek et al. [10]	2000	10	90	60				90	80			
Turmel-Rodrigues et al. [11]	2000	54❷	93	70	49		45	93	84	81		76
		17❸	76	18	9			76	68	50		28
Manninen et al. [12]	2001	53	92	58	44		40	92		85		79
Clark et al. [13]	2001	65	94		26			94		82		
Liang et al. [14]	2002	42	93	81	70	63		93	84	80	80	
Surgery												
Oakes et al. [15]	1998	19❹	100	100	81	67		100	100	89	89	
Mickley et al. [16]	2003	30	100	96	80	67	67	100	100	95	87	87

❶ Procedural success
❷ Forearm fistulae
❸ Upper arm fistulae
❹ Separately analyzed subgroup of "hemodynamically stable patients with mature fistulae amendable to more proximal arteriovenous anastomoses"

on the other hand have been incriminated to be the causes. In most cases these fibrotic stenoses afford high-pressure balloons and prolonged dilatation times. Long-term results of percutaneous transluminal angioplasty (PTA), however, are so disappointing that even dedicated interventionalists recommend surgical revision [12]. Therefore, in thrombosed AVF there is little room, if any, for hybrid procedures. Distal ligation of the stenotic vein segment and creation of a new proximal anastomosis of the cephalic vein to the radial artery is the easiest and most durable way of reconstruction [15,16].

AVG THROMBOSIS

The great majority of grafts occlude due to progressive stenosis of their venous anastomosis. Despite the fact that the first case reports on angioplasty of a venous anastomotic stenosis during surgery for graft occlusion were published in the late 1980 [17,18], and a large number of purely radiological series have been published, and although there are even some prospective randomized studies comparing surgery and interventional radiology for this indication [19], results of hybrid procedures are rarely reported.

In a retrospective analysis, Anain et al. [20] compared the results of surgical thrombectomy and balloon dilatation with those of urokinase thrombolysis and PTA in thrombosed hemodialysis grafts. At three months, primary patency in the surgical group was 33%, compared to only 11% in the radiological group. Ko et al. [21] reported on a consecutive series of 13 surgical patients with a primary graft patency at three and six months of 62% and 38%, respectively, following Fogarty catheter thrombectomy and balloon dilatation. Our own results of the conventional and the endovascular approach are quite comparable with these publications and equally disappointing. They simply bear witness to the fact that a patient with an access graft has a permanent access problem.

Once a hemodialysis access graft is thrombosed, neither color-coded duplex ultrasound nor arteriography or phlebography help to detect the causative stenosis. In consequence, after declotting, on-table angiography of the AVG including both anastomoses together with the feeding artery and the draining vein is mandatory to define and immediately treat the cause of thrombosis. On-table diagnostic angiography is the first step to a hybrid procedure. Introducing a guidewire and a balloon catheter seems to be most straightforward in this setting. With the significant lack of literature-based evidence in mind, however, we have to ask ourselves whether there are arguments beyond technical convenience for the endovascular treatment of venous anastomotic stenoses.

Per definition, AVG patients are patients with absent peripheral veins. Treatment of AVG stenosis must therefore not only aim at preservation of the graft at the puncture site but also at preservation of the patient's already reduced venous capital. In contrast to conventional surgery, hybrid procedures possibly can help to prevent graft extension to a more proximal (venous) anastomotic site. This advantage makes them an intriguing alternative for the treatment of the majority of AVG stenoses, although surgical thrombectomy and graft revision has been shown to be more effective in most trials comparing open graft revision with interventional radiology [19]. Dilatation of a venous anastomotic stenosis often needs a high-pressure balloon but otherwise is easy, safe, and quick. In thrombosed prosthetic vascular access, hybrid procedures allow to combine the simple and inexpensive technique of Fogarty catheter thrombectomy with the most vein preserving treatment option for the underlying stenosis. A growing number of patients present with more than one stenosis at the time of access thrombosis [22]. After complete on-table angiography of the feeding artery and the venous outflow, only the endovascular approach allows the treatment of all stenoses with minimal invasiveness and limited consumption of time.

Primary stent implantation for venous anastomotic stenosis is not recommended because there are no data in the literature proving the superiority of this expensive tool to dilatation alone. Stent implantation is indicated in elastic recoil of the stenosis, which is a frequent problem in venous stenoses [23], and in the rare case of dissection or rupture unresponsive to prolonged balloon inflation.

Complete occlusions of the draining vein, that cannot be re-opened with a guidewire or a coronary probe, afford graft extension to a more proximal vein segment. Graft extension should also be considered for bypassing a stenosis located in a joint region and for a more "definite" treatment of early or repeat restenoses after PTA.

Conclusion

Due to a significant lack of pertinent publications, the role of hybrid procedures in vascular access for hemodialysis still remains to be defined. Whereas endovascular therapy seems to be of limited value in stenosed autogenous fistulae, patients with graft access might profit from the application of vein-saving procedures. Dedicated endovascular surgeons would be the ideal partners for hemodialysis patients with a stenosed or occluded arteriovenous access graft. Endovascular surgeons are free to choose or combine conventional surgical and endovascular procedures according to the nature and location of the access problem, and hopefully they are motivated enough to further report their results.

REFERENCES

1 Dhingra RK, Young EW, Hulbert-Shearon TE, et al. Type of vascular access and mortality in U.S. hemodialysis patients. *Kidney Int* 2001; 60: 1443-1451.
2 Pastan S, Soucie JM, McClellan WM. Vascular access and increased risk of death among hemodialysis patients. *Kidney Int* 2002; 62: 620-626.
3 Mickley V. Central venous catheters: many questions, few answers. *Nephrol Dial Transplant* 2002; 17: 1368-1373.
4 Tordoir JH, van de Sande F, Leunissen KM. Complications of vascular access for hemodialysis. In: Branchereau A, Jacobs M (eds). *Complications in vascular and endovascular surgery* (Part I). Armonk, Futura Publishing Inc. 2001: pp 225-237.

5 Mickley V. Acute complications of arteriovenous fistula for hemodialysis. In: Branchereau A, Jacobs M (eds). *Vascular Emergencies*. Elmsford, Blackwell Publishing Inc., Futura Division 2003: pp 217-229.

6 Dapunt O, Feurstein M, Rendl KH, Prenner K. Transluminal angioplasty versus conventional operation in the treatment of haemodialysis fistula stenosis: results from a 5-year study. *Br J Surg* 1987; 74: 1004-1005.

7 Lay JP, Ashleigh RJ, Tranconi L, et al. Result of angioplasty of Brescia-Cimino haemodialysis fistulae: medium-term follow-up. *Clin Radiol* 1998; 53: 608-611.

8 Zaleski GX, Funaki B, Kenney S, et al. Angioplasty and bolus urokinase infusion for the restoration of function in thrombosed Brescia-Cimino dialysis fistulas. *J Vasc Intervent Radiol* 1999; 10: 129-136.

9 Haage P, Vorwerk D, Wildberger JE, et al. Percutaneous treatment of thrombosed primary arteriovenous hemodialysis access fistulae. *Kidney Int* 2000; 57: 1169-1175.

10 Rocek M, Peregrin JH, Lasovickova J, et al. Mechanical thrombolysis of thrombosed hemodialysis native fistulas with use of the Arrow-Trerotola percutaneous thrombolytic device: our preliminary experience. *J Vasc Intervent Radiol* 2000; 11: 1153-1158.

11 Turmel-Rodrigues L, Pengloan J, Rodrigue H, et al. Treatment of failed native arteriovenous fistulae for hemodialysis by interventional radiology. *Kidney Int* 2000; 57: 1124-1140.

12 Manninen HI, Kaukanen ET, Ikaheimo R, et al. Brachial arterial access: endovascular treatment of failing Brescia-Cimino hemodialysis fistulas. Initial success and long-term results. *Radiology* 2001; 218: 711-718.

13 Clark TW, Hirsch DA, Jindal KJ, et al. Outcome and prognostic factors of restenosis after percutaneous treatment of native hemodialysis fistulas. *J Vasc Intervent Radiol* 2002; 13: 51-59.

14 Liang HL, Pan HB, Chung HM, et al. Restoration of thrombosed Brescia-Cimino dialysis fistulas by using percutaneous transluminal angioplasty. *Radiology* 2002; 223: 339-344.

15 Oakes DD, Sherck JP, Cobb LF. Surgical salvage of failed radiocephalic arteriovenous fistulae: techniques and results in 29 patients. *Kidney Int* 1998; 53: 480-487.

16 Mickley V, Cazzonelli M, Bossinger A. The stenosed Brescia-Cimino fistula: operation or intervention? *Zentralbl Chir* 2003; 128: 757-761.

17 Smith TP, Hunter DW, Darcy MD, et al. Thrombosed synthetic hemodialysis access fistulas: the success of combined thrombectomy and angioplasty (technical note). *AJR Am J Roengenol* 1986; 147: 161-163.

18 Kistler D, Bohndorf, Gunther RW. Combined surgical-radiological procedure in occlusion of a hemodialysis shunt. *Chirurg* 1990; 61: 84-86.

19 Green LD, Lee DS, Kucey DS. A metaanalysis comparing surgical thrombectomy, mechanical thrombectomy, and pharmacomechanical thrombolysis for thrombosed dialysis grafts. *J Vasc Surg* 2002; 36: 939-945.

20 Anain P, Shenoy S, O'Brien-Irr M, et al. Balloon angioplasty for arteriovenous graft stenosis. *J Endovasc Ther* 2001; 8: 167-172.

21 Ko PJ, Liu YH, Hsieh HC, et al. Initial experience during balloon angioplasty assisted surgical thrombectomy for thrombosed hemodialysis grafts. *Chang Gung Med J* 2003; 26: 178-183.

22 Guerra A, Raynaud A, Beyssen B, et al. Arterial percutaneous angioplasty in upper limbs with vascular access devices for haemodialysis. *Nephrol Dial Transplant* 2002; 17: 843-851.

23 Kolakowski S Jr., Dougherty MJ, Calligaro KD. Salvaging prosthetic dialysis fistulas with stents: forearm versus upper arm grafts. *J Vasc Surg* 2003; 38: 719-723.

Conception et réalisation
ODIM, z.a. La Carretière
04130 VOLX

Achevé d'imprimer sur ses presses
en février 2004
N° d'imprimeur : 04.065
Dépôt légal : 1er trimestre 2004

Imprimé en FRANCE